ATLAS OF
BREAST SURGERY

ATLAS OF
BREAST SURGERY

SAMUEL A. WELLS, JR., M.D.

Bixby Professor and Chairman, Department of Surgery,
Washington University School of Medicine,
St. Louis, Missouri

V. LEROY YOUNG, M.D.

Professor of Surgery, Division of Plastic and Reconstructive Surgery,
Washington University School of Medicine,
St. Louis, Missouri

DOROTHY A. ANDRIOLE, M.D.

Assistant Professor, Department of Surgery,
Washington University School of Medicine,
St. Louis, Missouri

297 Illustrations by
Leon Schlossberg

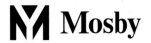

St. Louis Baltimore Boston Chicago London Madrid Philadelphia Sydney Toronto

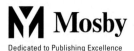

Dedicated to Publishing Excellence

Publisher: George Stamathis
Editor: Susie Baxter
Developmental Editor: Anne Gunter
Project Manager: Patricia Tannian
Production Editor: Barbara Jeanne Wilson
Senior Book Designer: Gail Morey Hudson
Manufacturing Supervisor: Betty Richmond
Cover art: Leon Schlossberg

Printed in the United States of America
Composition by Graphic World, Inc.
Printing/binding by Maple Vail Book Mfg. Group

Mosby–Year Book, Inc.
11830 Westline Industrial Drive
St. Louis, Missouri 63146

Library of Congress Cataloging in Publication Data

Wells, Samuel A.
   Atlas of breast surgery / Samuel A. Wells, Jr., V. Leroy Young,
Dorothy A. Andriole
      p.   cm.
   ISBN 0-8151-9216-9
   1. Breast—Surgery—Atlases. 2. Breast—Cancer—Surgery—Atlases.
3. Breast—Biopsy—Atlases.   I. Young, V. Leroy. II. Andriole,
Dorothy A. III. Title.
   [DNLM: 1. Breast Diseases—surgery—atlases. 2. Mammoplasty—
atlases. WP 17 W456a 1993]
RD539.8.W45 1993
618.1′9059—dc20
DNLM/DLC
for Library of Congress   93-28315
                                                                            CIP

ISBN 0-8151-9216-9

93 94 95 96 97 / 9 8 7 6 5 4 3 2 1

Preface

Breast diseases are so prevalent that physicians in almost every specialty of medicine will be confronted at some time by a patient seeking medical advice for a disorder of the mammary gland. The *Atlas of Breast Surgery* is written primarily for clinicians concerned with the operative management of patients with benign or malignant diseases of the breast. The text begins with a review of the general anatomy of the breast and related structures. The remainder and largest portion of the book describes and illustrates the operative procedures most commonly used in therapeutic, reconstructive, and cosmetic breast surgery. In each chapter a discussion of the indications and contraindications of a given operative procedure is followed by a consideration of the potential complications of the procedure, the preoperative preparation of the patient, the operative technique, and the postoperative care. The detailed steps of each operation are outlined sequentially as the operation is to be performed. Frequently, more than one operative technique may be used to treat a given breast condition, and there may be controversy regarding the single best procedure. In such cases we have emphasized the procedures that have been used extensively with good results. We realize that future technologic advances, as well as an improved understanding of the biology of breast diseases, will eventually modify the indications for many of the procedures described in this atlas. The majority of the operations, however, will almost certainly be used for years to come. We hope the reader finds this book useful in understanding the central role of the surgeon in managing patients with breast diseases.

Samuel A. Wells, Jr.
V. Leroy Young
Dorothy A. Andriole

Contents

Contents

ATLAS OF
BREAST SURGERY

I

ANATOMY

A detailed description of the anatomy of the breast and chest wall is presented in this section. A thorough understanding of the pertinent anatomy facilitates performance of the wide spectrum of surgical procedures that will be described. As well as the overview provided here, additional detailed anatomic illustrations and descriptions of the muscles used for reconstruction by myocutaneous flap transposition (Chapter 20: "Latissimus Dorsi Flap"; Chapter 21: "Breast Reconstruction Using the Pedicled TRAM Flap") or free flap transfer (Chapter 22: "Microvascular Free Flap Reconstruction" in Part V: "Reconstructive Procedures") are included.

1

Anatomy

Introduction

The breast is a modified compound alveolar secretory gland derived from apocrine epithelium. The mammary gland proper consists of approximately 20 irregular lobes radiating from the central nipple area. Each of the lobes has an excretory duct that opens into the lactiferous sinus situated beneath the nipple. In addition, fibrous and adipose tissues, as well as lymphatic channels, are interspersed among the lobes of the mammary gland. Nerves and blood vessels are present throughout the breast parenchyma. The axilla contains lymph node groups that frequently become involved when pathologic processes develop in the breast.

ANATOMIC ILLUSTRATIONS

Breast Topography (Figure 1-1)

When making an incision in the skin overlying the breast, it is important to follow the lines in the skin that demarcate the direction of natural tension. These skin tension lines, known as Langer's lines, are depicted in the left breast in Figure 1-1, and the suggested sites of several skin incisions are shown in the right breast. When a breast biopsy is performed, the incision should be placed so that the incised skin and the underlying breast parenchyma can be incorporated easily within the resected tissue block, should partial or total mastectomy become necessary. Depending on the location of a breast lesion, a linear incision may provide the optimal therapeutic result, even though a circumareolar incision is preferable cosmetically. Generally, a radial incision directly perpendicular to Langer's lines is avoided because it may give a poor cosmetic result and distort the contour of the breast.

A periareolar incision usually heals well, with an excellent cosmetic result. This incision can be safely extended halfway around the nipple-areolar complex, and adequate exposure can be obtained for biopsy of masses several centimeters from the nipple. However, one should be cautious when using this incision for biopsy of a mass that is not immediately beneath the nipple-areolar complex because the wound may be seeded with tumor cells if the lesion is malignant.

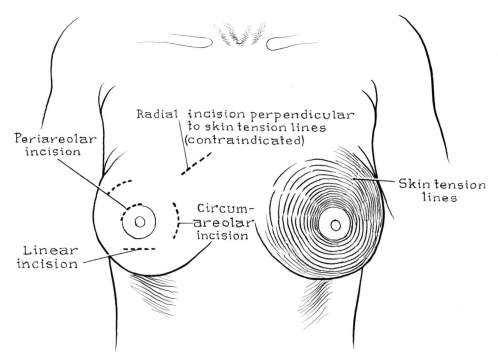

Fig 1-1.   Breast topography.

Gross Anatomy of the Breast and Related Structures (Figure 1-2)

This figure depicts the macroscopic appearance of the right breast (stippled area) as it appears with the skin and subcutaneous tissues dissected away from the upper torso. The left breast (also stippled) is shown with the pectoralis major muscle removed to emphasize the relationship of the breast to the underlying pectoralis minor muscle and to the axillary structures.

Although there is individual variation in the size of the breast, the following anatomic guidelines defining the extent of the breast on the anterior chest wall are relatively constant. The breast parenchyma extends superiorly to the clavicle and inferiorly to the sixth costal cartilage. This may not be evident grossly; however, it is readily demonstrable histologically. This constancy is significant in determining the extent of dissection in surgical procedures intended to remove the total breast. The breast extends medially as far as the midsternal line at the level of the fourth rib and laterally to the midaxillary line, where the axillary tail of Spence is formed. This structure is the superolateral extent of breast parenchyma in the axillary region. The intercostobrachial nerve courses through the axilla in close proximity to this breast tissue. The breast overlies the pectoralis major muscle and fascia medially and superolaterally, and it overlies the serratus anterior, external oblique, and rectus abdominis muscles laterally and inferiorly.

On the right chest the axillary tail of Spence is partially covered by the pectoralis major, which forms the anterior axillary fold. The cephalic vein lies superior to the pectoralis major and inferior to the deltoid muscle in the deltopectoral groove. This groove is variably evident, depending on how well these muscles are developed in an individual patient. The cephalic vein and

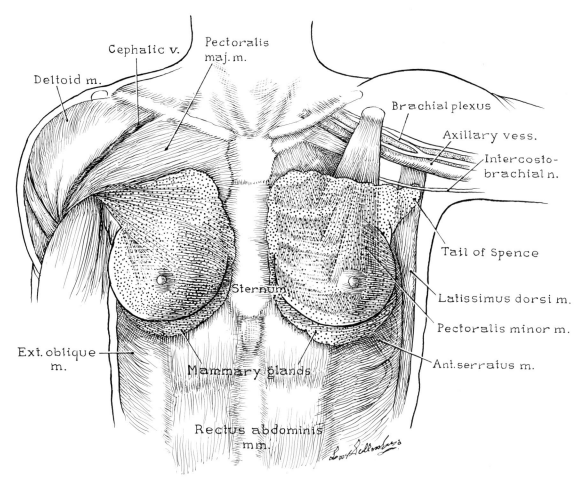

Fig 1-2. Gross anatomy of the breast and related structures.

the deltopectoral groove are important landmarks for the superior limit of the pectoralis major muscle.

Chest Wall Musculature (Figure 1-3)

The pectoralis major arises from the anterior surface of the medial (sternal) aspect of the clavicle, the anterior surface of the sternum inferiorly to the level of the sixth or seventh rib, the cartilages of the 12 ribs, and the aponeurosis of the external oblique muscle (Figure 1-3, A). Over the sternum, tendinous fibers decussate with fibers from the opposite side. A separate abdominal slip may also attach to the anterior surface of the rectus abdominis muscle fascia. The pectoralis major converges from its broad origin to form a 5-cm-wide tendon that inserts into the crest of the greater tubercle of the humerus, just lateral to the point of insertion of the latissimus dorsi muscle. The lateral border of the muscle in the axillary region forms the anterior axillary fold. The pectoralis major has a dual blood supply from the thoracoacromial artery (not shown here) and the internal mammary artery. The muscle functions in adduction and medial rotation of the humerus, and it also contributes to deep forced respiratory efforts. Removal of the entire muscle results in an unsightly chest wall defect; however,

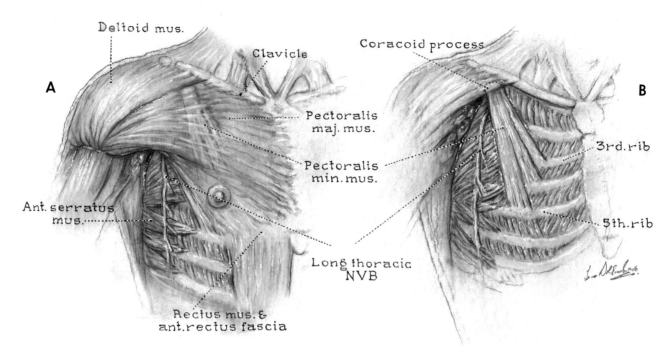

Deltoid mus.

Clavicle

Coracoid process

A

B

Pectoralis
maj. mus.

Pectoralis
min. mus.

3rd. rib

Ant. serratus
mus.

5th. rib

Long thoracic
NVB

Rectus mus. &
ant. rectus fascia

Fig 1-3. Chest wall musculature.

there is only a minimal or moderate functional deficit. The nipple-areolar complex is illustrated to show its positional relationship to the pectoralis major.

In Figure 1-3, *B,* the pectoralis major muscle has been removed to show the pectoralis minor, a relatively small, triangular muscle that originates anteriorly from the third to the fifth ribs. It inserts by a flat tendon on the medial border and upper surface of the coracoid process of the scapula. The pectoralis minor is innervated predominantly by the medial pectoral (anterior thoracic) nerve. It contributes to scapular motion and rotation; however, its removal is not associated with any significant cosmetic or functional deficit.

The serratus anterior muscle is a broad, flat muscle, originating from the anterior surfaces of the uppermost eight ribs and from the intercostal muscle fascia. It inserts onto the deep surface of the scapula on its medial border. The serratus anterior receives its innervation from the long thoracic nerve. This nerve courses vertically along the superficial surface of the serratus anterior in the region of the axilla. The serratus anterior functions to draw the scapula forward, particularly in reaching or pulling efforts. This muscle, along with the trapezius muscle, functions in raising the arms above the head. Inadvertent damage to the long thoracic nerve during the course of a mastectomy or an axillary dissection may cause paralysis of the serratus anterior and result in a winged scapula, which is associated with severe cosmetic and functional deficits.

The long rectus abdominis muscle spans the anterior surface of the abdomen. It is enclosed anteriorly and posteriorly by the rectus sheath, an aponeurosis of the oblique and transversus abdominis muscles. The rectus abdominis originates from tendons attached to the crest of the pubic bone and to the symphysis pubis (not shown). It inserts on the fifth to seventh costal cartilages and the xiphoid process of the sternum. The rectus abdominis is segmentally innervated by ventral rami of the lower six thoracic nerves. It functions as part of the abdominal wall musculature to provide a firm, protective covering for the contents of the peritoneal cavity. The anatomy of the rectus abdominis pertaining to breast reconstruction is further discussed in Chapter 21.

Posterior and Lateral Chest Wall Musculature (Figure 1-4)

The latissimus dorsi is a large, flat, triangular muscle, originating posteriorly from the six lower thoracic spines (by means of the lumbodorsal fascia to which it is attached) and from the lumbosacral spines and the posterior aspect of the iliac crest. The fibers of the latissimus dorsi converge anteriorly and superiorly to form a long tendon that inserts on the anterior surface of the upper aspect of the humerus. This insertion is located posterior to the brachial plexus, the axillary vessels, and the intercostobrachial nerve (see Figure 1-2). The lateral border of the latissimus dorsi forms the posterior axillary fold as it crosses the axillary space. The latissimus dorsi is innervated by the thoracodorsal nerve. Its blood supply is from the thoracodorsal artery, which originates from the subscapular artery. The infraspinatus, teres minor, and teres major muscles lie medial to the latissimus dorsi muscle. The trapezius overlies the latissimus dorsi superiorly and medially. Each of these muscles lies posterior to the scapula. The latissimus dorsi functions to adduct, extend, and medially rotate the humerus. Denervation or removal of the muscle is not associated with a significant functional deficit. The latissimus dorsi may be used as a myocutaneous flap, in breast reconstruction, or for coverage of a chest wall defect. Denervation or removal of the muscle eliminates a useful source of autogenous tissue. Therefore most surgeons preserve the thoracodorsal vessels and nerve during the course of an axillary dissection, unless they must be sacrificed to remove bulky nodal disease. The anatomy of the latissimus dorsi pertaining to breast reconstruction is discussed in Chapter 20.

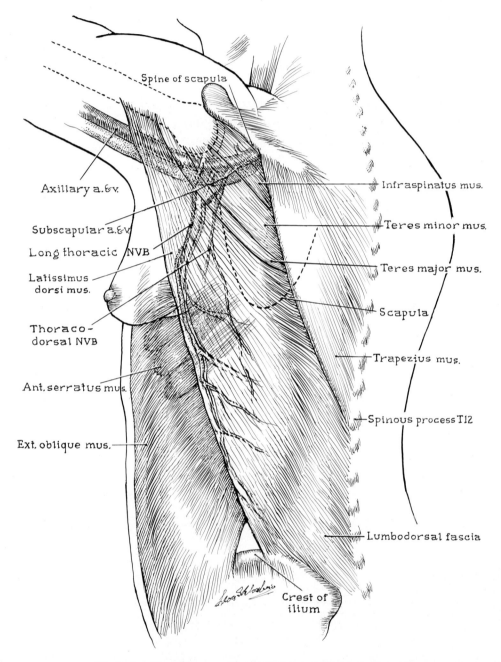

Spine of scapula

Axillary a.&v.

Subscapular a.&v.

Long thoracic NVB

Latissimus dorsi mus.

Thoraco-dorsal NVB

Ant. serratus mus.

Ext. oblique mus.

Infraspinatus mus.

Teres minor mus.

Teres major mus.

Scapula

Trapezius mus.

Spinous process T12

Lumbodorsal fascia

Crest of ilium

Fig 1-4. Posterior and lateral chest wall musculature.

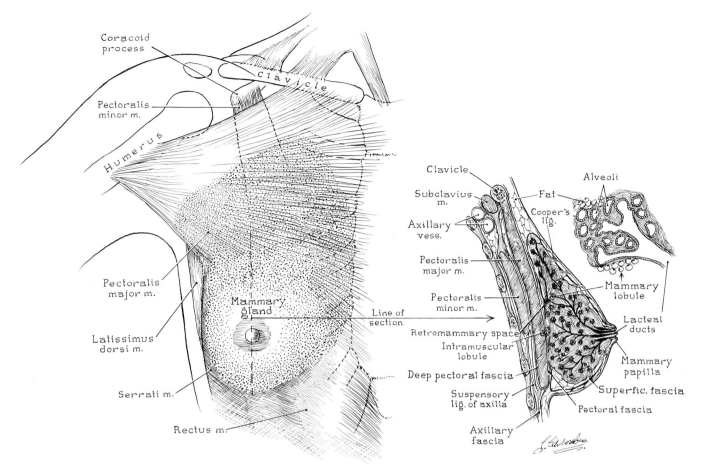

Fig 1-5. **Frontal view and sagittal section of the breast.**

Frontal View and Sagittal Section of the Breast (Figure 1-5)

The left side of this illustration depicts the relationship of the breast (stippled area) to the underlying chest wall muscles. The right side of the illustration depicts a sagittal section of the breast and chest wall as it appears at the midline of the nipple. Also shown (in the inset) is the microscopic appearance of breast parenchyma. The breast is suspended in the subcutaneous tissue on the anterior chest wall primarily overlying the pectoralis major fascia. On the sagittal section are shown clusters of mammary lobules, connected by interposed fibrous tissue and blood vessels to form lobes. Each mammary lobe is composed microscopically of a collection of lobules surrounding alveoli embedded in fat. All lobules in a single lobe drain into a single common lacteal duct. There are about 15 to 20 lacteal ducts in the breast, which all converge in the areolar to form the mammary papilla, a conical projection containing the orifices of the ducts that open to the nipple. The superficial fascia is a thin, wispy layer of fascia in the subcutaneous tissue between the breast parenchyma and the skin. Cooper's ligaments, derived from this fascial layer and the parenchyma beneath it, suspend the breast from the skin.

The pectoral fascia defines a plane between the breast parenchyma superficially and the underlying pectoralis major muscle. The region between the breast parenchyma and the pectoral fascia is composed of a thin layer of loose, connective tissue known as the retromammary space. Occasionally a small intramuscular lobule of mammary tissue extends across the retromammary space, through the pectoral fascia, and into the pectoralis major muscle.

The relationship of the clavicle, the axillary vessels and supporting muscles in the retromammary area, and the chest wall is shown in this figure. The clavicle lies superficial to the axillary vessels. The pectoralis major lies inferior to the clavicle. The pectoralis minor lies entirely deep to the pectoralis major and in the same plane as the superiorly located subclavius muscle. Laterally the two layers of the pectoral fascia fuse to form the axillary fascia, which extends across the axillary space.

Axillary Musculature, Arterial Supply, and Innervation of the Breast and Axilla (Figure 1-6)

The macroscopic extent of the breast (stippled) is shown. The pectoralis major is not illustrated. A segment of the pectoralis minor muscle has been removed to show the deep axillary musculature and the arterial supply to the breast and to the axilla.

The axillary space, located in the region lateral to the serratus anterior muscle on the chest wall, is defined by an anterior border, a posterior border, a medial border, and an apex. Anteriorly, the axillary space extends to the pectoralis major muscle. The lateral border of this muscle forms the anterior axillary fold. Posteriorly, it is bound by the subscapularis, teres major, and latissimus dorsi muscles. The posterior axillary fold is formed by the lateral border of the latissimus dorsi muscle. The medial border is the serratus anterior muscle on the chest wall. The superior extent of the axillary space is defined by the axillary vessels and by the apex of the axilla.

The teres major muscle is a thick, flat muscle that originates from the dorsal surface of the inferior border of the scapula and inserts, by way of a flat tendon, on the medial aspect of the intertubercular sulcus of the humerus. The teres major is innervated by the subscapular nerve and functions in adduction, extension, and medial rotation of the arm. The subscapularis, a large, triangular muscle, originates from the scapula on the medial aspect of the subscapular fossa. It inserts, by a tendon, on the lesser tubercle of the humerus and the anterior aspect of the shoulder joint capsule. The subscapularis is innervated by the upper and lower subscapular nerves and functions to medially rotate the arm. It also contributes to adduction, abduction, flexion, and extension of the arm. Multiple branches of the subclavian artery supply the breast and related structures.

The internal mammary artery branches from the inferior surface of the first part of the subclavian artery and courses directly and inferiorly behind the cartilages of the uppermost six ribs, approximately 1 cm lateral to the border of the sternum. The internal mammary artery supplies the breast through anterior intercostal branches, particularly the fourth and fifth, and through the perforating arteries. Anterior intercostal branches arise from the internal mammary artery in each of the upper six intercostal spaces. These intercostal branches run posteriorly along the inferior surfaces of the ribs

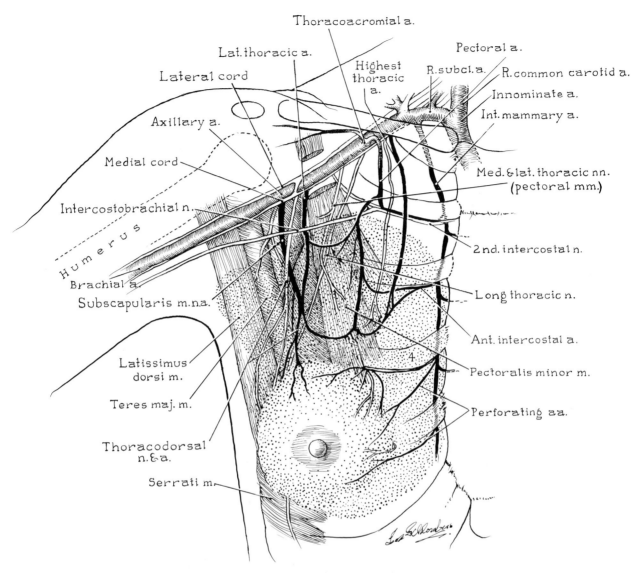

Fig 1-6. Axillary musculature, arterial supply, and innervation of the breast and axilla.

and send branches through the intercostal muscles to the pectoral muscles, the breast, and the overlying skin. The internal mammary artery also gives off perforating arteries that emerge through the upper six intercostal spaces through the pectoralis major muscle, supplying it and the overlying skin. The perforating arteries also course anteromedially on the chest to supply the breast.

The subclavian artery travels laterally deep to the clavicle. Distal to the clavicle, the subclavian artery becomes the axillary artery. The axillary artery extends to the lateral border of the teres major muscle, where it becomes the brachial artery. The axillary artery is divided into three parts. The first part of the artery is proximal to the pectoralis minor muscle and is enclosed in the axillary sheath along with the axillary vein and brachial plexus. The second part of the artery is posterior to the pectoralis minor, and the third part of the artery is lateral to the pectoralis minor. The highest thoracic artery usually arises directly from the first part of the axillary artery. Occasionally it branches from the thoracoacromial artery and courses down the chest wall, medial to the pectoralis major and minor muscles. The thoracoacromial artery branches from the first, or occasionally the second, part of the axillary artery. It divides into the pectoral artery and into other unnamed branches that supply the shoulder region. The pectoral artery passes between the pectoralis major and minor muscles and branches into them. The lateral thoracic artery, a more distal branch of the axillary artery, courses along the lateral border of the pectoralis minor. It supplies the serratus anterior, the pectoral, and the subscapularis muscles. The lateral thoracic artery also gives off lateral mammary branches that provide the predominant blood supply to the breast. The subscapularis artery is a large branch of the third part of the axillary artery. It sends branches to supply the shoulder joint and its musculature. Beyond these branches, the subscapularis artery becomes the thoracodorsal artery, which accompanies the thoracodorsal nerve, to supply the latissimus dorsi muscle. The thoracodorsal artery also sends branches to the serratus anterior. Therefore the breast parenchyma receives its blood supply from multiple sources, including the intercostal arteries, the highest thoracic artery, the pectoral artery, and the lateral thoracic artery. These vessels anastomose extensively to provide a network blood supply to the breast.

The anterior chest wall and axilla are innervated by the lower four cervical nerves and by the uppermost thoracic nerve. The long thoracic nerve travels posteriorly behind the brachial plexus and axillary artery. It then courses downward along the surface of the serratus anterior, which it innervates. The medial and lateral thoracic nerves originate from the brachial plexus and course inferiorly to provide motor innervation to the pectoralis major and minor muscles. The thoracodorsal nerve also originates from the brachial plexus and courses posteroinferiorly to provide motor innervation to the latissimus dorsi. The intercostobrachial nerve is the lateral cutaneous branch of the second intercostal nerve. This nerve crosses the axilla as it emerges from the chest wall to innervate the skin on the medial aspect of the upper arm and in the axilla.

Branches of the upper six thoracic nerves supply the cutaneous surface of the anterior and lateral chest wall, including the breast, by way of the anterior and lateral cutaneous branches. The posterior, lateral, and medial cords of the brachial plexus are closely associated with the axillary artery in the shoulder region and then with the brachial artery in the arm.

Arterial Supply and Innervation of the Breast (Figure 1-7)

A more detailed illustration of the multiple origins of arterial blood supply to the breast parenchyma is shown in Figure 1-7, *A*. The internal mammary artery, the highest thoracic artery, the lateral thoracic artery, and the intercostal arteries provide branches that directly supply the breast and anastomose extensively within it.

The innervation to the breast parenchyma in its lower aspect is shown in Figure 1-7, *B*. Multiple nerves arise directly from the medial and lateral intercostal nerves and travel through the breast. Innervation to the nipple is supplied by the lateral and medial branches of the fourth intercostal nerve.

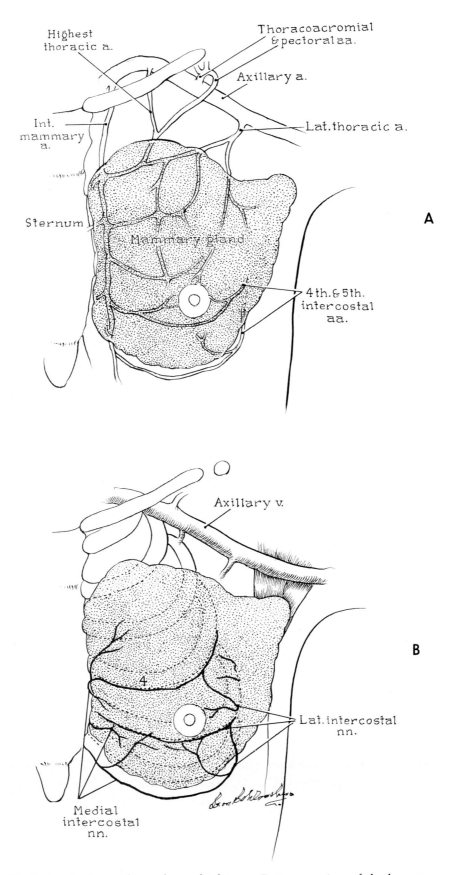

Fig 1-7.   **A,** Arterial supply to the breast. **B,** Innervation of the breast.

Venous and Lymphatic Drainage of the Breast and Axilla (Figure 1-8)

The pectoralis major and minor muscles are shown divided and partially excised where they overlie the axillary vessels and lymph nodes.

Generally the venous drainage of the breast and axillary region parallels the arterial supply. The axillary vein, which begins at the lower border of the teres major muscle, is the continuation of the basilic vein from the arm. The axillary vein lies medial to and partially anterior to the axillary artery. At the outer border of the clavicle, the axillary vein becomes the subclavian vein. The axillary vein receives multiple, variable tributaries from the chest wall, the breast, and the pectoral muscles. Named branches include the subscapular vein and the lateral thoracic vein, which travel with their corresponding arteries. The cephalic vein, which drains the arm, joins the axillary vein just below the clavicle. Tributaries from the breast drain into the axillary vein and the subclavian vein. The internal mammary vein travels with the corresponding artery and drains into the subclavian vein. The intercostal veins receive tributaries from the breast as they course posteriorly around the chest wall and drain into the superior vena cava by way of the vertebral and azygos veins (not shown).

The breast and axillary regions contain a network of lymphatic channels that anastomose extensively throughout the skin, subcutaneous tissue, and parenchyma of the breast. Also, a dense collection of lymphatic channels exists in the subareolar region of the breast, extending peripherally to form a circumareolar plexus of lymphatic channels. Multiple routes of lymphatic drainage from the breast are indicated by the arrows and dotted lines in the figures. The three main routes for lymphatic drainage from the breast to the regional lymph nodes are the axillary, the interpectoral, and the internal mammary.

The axillary route, which is described anatomically as five separate groups of lymph nodes, is the major route for lymphatic drainage from the breast. The external mammary nodes are close to the breast on its lateral aspect and receive drainage from the lateral half of the breast parenchyma. The subscapular nodes lie along the course of the subscapular and thoracodorsal vessels. These nodes are more posteriorly and superiorly placed than the external mammary nodes. The central nodes lie close to the axillary vein. The subclavicular nodes are located at the apex of the axilla and receive drainage from all the other groups of axillary lymph nodes. The subclavicular nodes then may drain into the central venous system or into the supraclavicular lymph node group, which is situated at the junction of the subclavian and internal jugular veins. Metastases to the supraclavicular lymph node group signify incurable disease in the patient with a breast malignancy.

Surgically, lymph nodes in the axillary region are described by levels. Level I defines lymph nodes located laterally to the pectoralis minor. Level II lymph nodes are behind the pectoralis minor. Level III lymph nodes are medial to the pectoralis minor. Axillary nodes obtained during the course of an Auchincloss modified radical mastectomy or an axillary dissection alone usually include those at level I and level II. In addition to these nodes, lymph nodes in level III are removed in the radical mastectomy procedure and in the Patey modified radical mastectomy.

The second main route for lymphatic drainage from the breast is the interpectoral route. These interpectoral lymph nodes (Rotter's nodes) receive

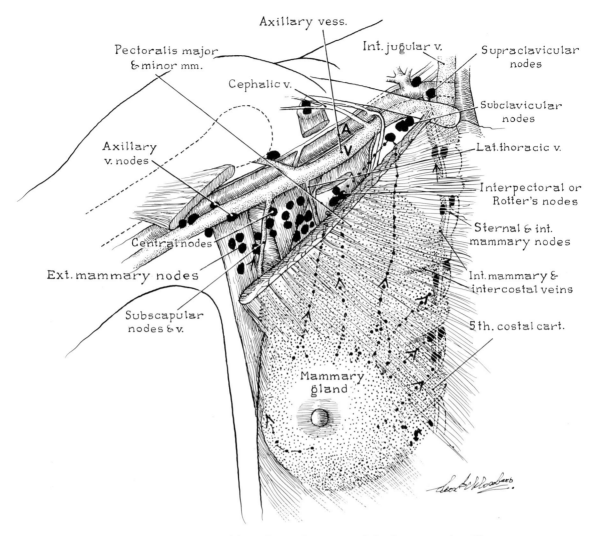

Fig 1-8. **Venous and lymphatic drainage of the breast and axilla.**

lymphatic drainage from the posterior aspect of the breast by way of channels that originate in the retromammary region and perforate the pectoralis major muscle. These interpectoral nodes then drain directly into the subclavicular lymph nodes. The subclavicular nodes also receive some lymphatic channels that course from the breast beneath the pectoral muscles.

The final route for lymphatic drainage from the breast is the internal mammary route. Lymph nodes situated along the course of the internal mammary vessels receive lymphatic drainage from the breast (predominantly the medial half of the breast). These lymphatic channels follow the course of the perforating vessels through the pectoralis major. The internal mammary nodes are most numerous in the upper four intercostal spaces. They ultimately drain into the central venous system on the right side by way of the right lymphatic duct and on the left side by way of the thoracic duct.

II

BIOPSY
PROCEDURES

A wide range of relatively simple biopsy procedures are available to aid in diagnosing a breast mass. The procedures must be performed in a manner that will not compromise a subsequent operation if the mass is malignant.

Fine needle aspiration cytology, core needle biopsy, incisional biopsy, and excisional biopsy can establish the tissue diagnosis of a palpable mass. Nonpalpable breast masses are often detected by mammography or ultrasound, and the techniques of fine needle aspiration cytology and excisional biopsy are especially useful in evaluating these lesions.

In addition to a histologic or cytologic examination, other studies, particularly the qualitative and quantitative determination of sex steroid receptors and DNA phase analysis, are performed if sufficient tissue is obtained. These tests yield important prognostic and therapeutic information.

Generally the likelihood of establishing the correct histologic diagnosis with a given procedure increases in direct proportion to the magnitude of its invasiveness. Fine needle aspiration, the least invasive procedure, yields a cytologic, rather than a histologic, diagnosis. Depending on the size of the mass, an approximate 20% false negative rate is possible for the diagnosis of breast carcinoma. The false positive rate is <1%. Therefore a negative result is inconclusive, and a diagnosis of carcinoma on the basis of fine needle aspiration may be provisional, rather than definitive. Immunohistochemical staining can sometimes yield qualitative estrogen and progesterone receptor information on a fine needle aspiration cytology specimen; however, quantitative hormone receptor studies and DNA phase analysis cannot be determined.

The tissue obtained by core needle biopsy is sufficient for a definitive histologic diagnosis. Although the false positive rate is nil, the false negative rate is approximately 5%. Therefore a benign histologic diagnosis in a patient with a palpable breast mass is inconclusive, particularly if on clinical examination the mass is suspected to be carcinoma. Qualitative hormone receptor studies and DNA phase analysis may be performed on a core needle biopsy specimen if the amount of tissue obtained is sufficient. However, there is usually insufficient tissue for quantitation of hormone receptors.

An incisional or excisional biopsy procedure yields sufficient tissue for histologic and biochemical studies. An excisional biopsy may be diagnostic and therapeutic when the mass is completely removed. Finally, needle localization biopsy is an open biopsy technique used for the diagnosis of a nonpalpable, mammographically detected mass.

For all open biopsy techniques the placement of the incision and the subsequent dissection must be carefully planned. Incision placement and dissection have great importance relative to the resection procedure that must be performed if the mass is malignant and relative to the performance of a reconstructive procedure. The inappropriate placement of an incision or inadvertent widespread tissue contamination during the biopsy procedure markedly limits the choice of subsequent therapeutic and reconstructive procedures.

2

Fine Needle Aspiration Cytology

Introduction

A breast mass can be evaluated by fine needle aspiration (FNA) with cytologic examination of the aspirated material. In many cases cytologic evaluation can readily define masses as malignant. However, at present a definitive role for FNA in the diagnosis of breast carcinoma is not universally established because the accuracy of the cytologic diagnosis is variable and depends largely on the skill and experience of the cytologist. However, a provisional positive diagnosis of carcinoma established by FNA is useful in directing patient discussions and in planning the best definitive surgical approach.

Because of the significant false negative rate with the procedure, a benign diagnosis on an FNA cytology specimen (or a nondiagnostic acellular aspirate) does not exclude the presence of a carcinoma and should not reassure the surgeon that a clinically suspicious mass is benign. Frequently, the patient with a solid breast mass and a negative fine needle aspiration subsequently undergoes a core needle biopsy or an open biopsy procedure for diagnosis.

Indications

Fine needle aspiration is used to obtain a cellular specimen from a solid mass. With the widespread use of mammography, nonpalpable breast lesions are frequently identified and ultrasound-directed FNA may be used to establish a diagnosis. The role of stereotaxically directed FNA in the cytologic diagnosis of a solid mass detectable only on mammography is under investigation.

Contraindications

There are no absolute contraindications to FNA cytology; however, it must be performed with caution in patients with masses deep in the breast, with masses near the chest wall, or in patients with bleeding disorders.

Complications

Theoretically, inadvertently advancing the needle deep to the breast parenchyma could cause perforation of the pleural cavity or significant chest wall bleeding. Generally, however, the only morbidity associated with fine needle aspiration is ecchymosis at the site of aspiration.

Preoperative Preparation

Fine needle aspiration is readily performed in the office setting. The cytologic specimen should be appropriately processed as soon as it is obtained. If indicated, it is often preferable to perform mammography before undertaking FNA because FNA could distort the radiographic appearance of the breast and make mammographic interpretation more difficult.

OPERATIVE PROCEDURE
Fine Needle Aspiration of a Solid Breast Mass
Patient Positioning and Aspiration (Figure 2-1)

The patient is generally placed in the supine position for FNA. Occasionally, for aspiration of a mass in the lateral breast or in the axilla, a lateral position may be more appropriate. A hand-held device that accommodates a 20-ml syringe attached to a 23-gauge needle or a syringe and a 23-gauge needle is used. The breast mass is immobilized. A small wheal may be raised by injecting local anesthetic in the skin overlying the palpable mass. The overlying skin is then cleansed, and the needle, attached to the syringe, is inserted through the skin (Figure 2-1, *A*) at an oblique angle and into the palpable mass. The needle should not be advanced directly perpendicular to the chest wall, particularly if the mass is deep in the breast. When the needle has been advanced into the palpable breast mass, the plunger is retracted to produce negative pressure in the syringe, and then the plunger is slowly released. This is repeated several times while the position of the needle is moved around (Figure 2-1, *B*) so that samples from several different areas of the mass will be included in the aspirate.

When FNA is completed, negative pressure in the syringe is released and the needle is slowly withdrawn from the breast. The contents of the needle are then expressed onto a glass slide. This may be facilitated by first removing the needle and aspirating air directly into the syringe. The plunger is then advanced to expel the contents of the needle barrel onto the slide. A second slide is used to thinly coat the material on the first slide, which is then immersed in 95% methyl alcohol fixative. A cytologic diagnosis may be obtained within 24 hours at most centers.

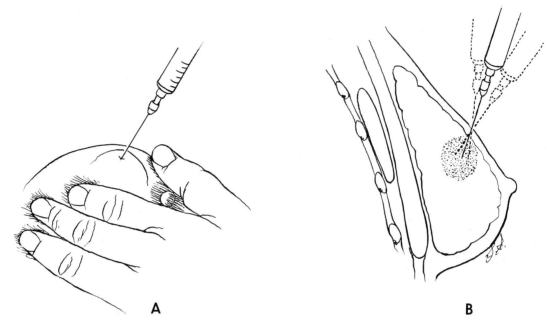

Fig 2-1.   Patient positioning and aspiration.

Postoperative Care

Some ecchymosis at the aspiration site may develop; if so, it generally resolves in a few days. No limitations on activity are necessary after FNA. The further management of the patient with a solid breast mass varies, depending on the FNA cytologic results and on the results of other diagnostic tests.

3

Core Needle Biopsy

Introduction

A histologic diagnosis of carcinoma may be established by examination of tissue obtained percutaneously with a core needle apparatus. The procedure can be performed readily in the outpatient setting with minimal patient discomfort. With recently developed immunoperoxidase staining techniques, the qualitative determinations of estrogen receptor can be performed on tissue samples. However, open biopsy is usually necessary to obtain sufficient tissue for quantitative hormone receptor studies.

Indications

The core needle biopsy is used to establish a histologic diagnosis in the patient with a clinically suspect palpable breast mass. A diagnosis of carcinoma on tissue obtained at core needle biopsy obviates the need for an open biopsy. Although the procedure is generally performed in the office setting, it may be used intraoperatively for the patient undergoing a one-stage procedure, with core biopsy, frozen section confirmation of carcinoma, and immediate definitive surgery (mastectomy or breast conservation surgery and axillary dissection). In this setting the tissue is sent unfixed to the pathologist for immediate frozen section. In some centers ultrasound guidance is used for core needle biopsy of nonpalpable masses. The use of stereotaxically directed core needle biopsy is under investigation.

Contraindications

Core needle biopsy of a breast mass deep in the breast or in the axillary tail must be performed with caution because of the close proximity of the pleural cavity and neurovascular structures. In addition, particular care must be taken in performing core needle biopsy in a woman with either a breast implant or a bleeding disorder.

Complications

Complications occur infrequently and include ecchymosis, hematoma formation, and wound infection. Significant bleeding or pneumothorax is a rare complication that could occur with inadvertent advancement of the needle through the breast into the underlying chest wall musculature or the chest cavity.

Preoperative Preparation

Core needle biopsy is readily performed in the office setting. The tissue obtained may be sent to the pathologist for immediate frozen section or placed in fixative solution for permanent sectioning. If mammography is indicated, it is often preferable to perform the test before undertaking any diagnostic procedures, including FNA, which could distort the radiographic appearance of the breast and make accurate mammographic interpretation more difficult.

OPERATIVE PROCEDURE
Core Needle Biopsy
Patient Positioning; Core Needle Apparatus Insertion (Figure 3-1)

With the patient in the supine position, the palpable mass is gently but firmly immobilized, usually by an assistant. The skin is cleansed, and a wheal is raised with a local anesthetic at the planned site of needle insertion. A small incision can be made with a scalpel in the anesthetized skin, as shown in Figure 3-1, *A,* to facilitate advancement of the cannula and obturator

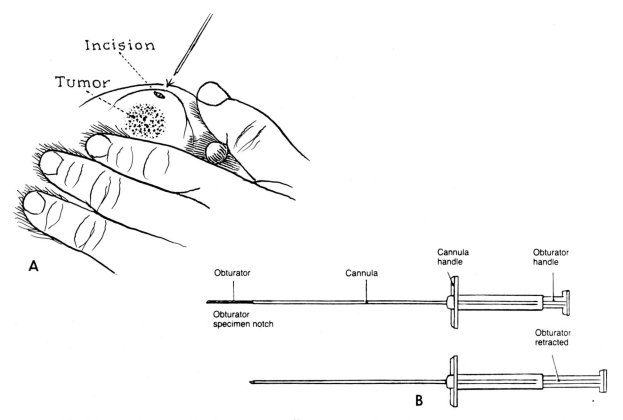

Fig 3-1. Patient positioning; core needle apparatus insertion.

needle (Figure 3-1, *B*). The apparatus is advanced through the skin at an oblique angle to the chest wall. Care should be taken not to advance the core needle apparatus perpendicular to the chest wall because this increases the possibility of pneumothorax or intercostal artery laceration, as well as the risk of spreading the tumor cells to the normal tissues deep to the mass.

Tissue Sampling (Figure 3-2)

The core needle apparatus is advanced through the skin to the palpable mass with the cannula handle fully extended so that the cannula completely covers the specimen notch on the obturator needle as shown in the sagittal section in Figure 3-2, *A*.

As the core needle apparatus is positioned adjacent to the mass, the obturator is advanced through the cannula so that the needle with the specimen notch is lodged in the palpable mass (Figure 3-2, *B*.) The cannula handle is then advanced over the obturator handle, while the obturator needle is held stationary, so that the breast tissue lying in the specimen notch is cut from the surrounding tissue by the sharp edge of the obturator, (Figure 3-2, *C*). The core needle apparatus is withdrawn from the breast in this position, with the specimen notch fully covered by the cannula. The specimen is removed and sent for frozen section. After the specimen is removed, the biopsy procedure can be repeated through the same entry site, if necessary.

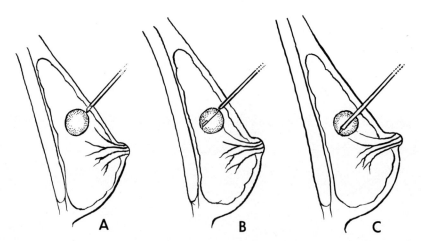

Fig 3-2. Tissue sampling.

Postoperative Care

The biopsy site is covered with a dry sterile dressing. Specific activity restrictions are not necessary following core needle biopsy. Additional diagnostic procedures and follow-up examinations are determined on the basis of the biopsy results.

4

Incisional Biopsy

Introduction

An incisional biopsy is an open procedure involving removal of a wedge of tissue from a palpable breast mass. The major portion of the mass remains intact in the breast after the procedure.

Indications

Incisional breast biopsy is indicated for the evaluation of a large breast mass, suspected to be malignant, when a definitive diagnosis cannot be established by fine needle aspiration or core needle biopsy. When a tissue diagnosis has already been established by core needle biopsy, incisional biopsy is sometimes performed to obtain additional tissue for quantitative hormone receptor analysis before induction chemotherapy for a locally advanced breast carcinoma. Incisional biopsy is also occasionally performed to establish a tissue diagnosis of fibroadenoma before excision of a large, benign-appearing mass in a young woman.

Contraindications

There are no absolute contraindications to incisional breast biopsy. However, the procedure should not be performed unnecessarily if a core needle biopsy can provide sufficient diagnostic information to direct definitive therapy or if a mass is small enough that an excisional biopsy can readily be performed.

Complications

A significant, although infrequent, complication is wound infection. This can delay a definite surgical procedure for carcinoma and may increase the likelihood of a subsequent wound infection following definitive surgery. When an incisional biopsy is obtained from a large carcinoma with overlying skin changes, wound healing may be delayed because of the extensive tissue infiltration with malignant cells.

Preoperative Preparation

Diagnostic mammography should be performed on the patient before incisional biopsy is performed. The biopsy procedure can be done on an outpatient basis, using either local or general anesthesia, depending on the location of the mass and the preferences of the surgeon and the patient.

OPERATIVE PROCEDURE

Location of Mass and Planned Skin Incision (Figure 4-1)

The patient is placed in a supine position with the arm abducted on an armboard. The precise location of the mass is confirmed by palpation. The margins of the mass can be marked on the skin if the mass is difficult to localize because distortion of the breast parenchyma may occur following infiltration with a local anesthetic agent. After the breast has been cleansed and draped in a sterile manner, a small incision is made directly overlying the palpable mass (Figure 4-1, A) to minimize contamination of surrounding, uninvolved breast parenchyma. The incision should be made only long enough to obtain the required tissue. Whenever possible, the incision must be oriented in such a manner that it can be easily incorporated in a subsequent tylectomy or mastectomy incision.

A skin ellipse should be included in the biopsy specimen of any mass with overlying cutaneous changes, such as edema of the skin (Figure 4-1, B). The presence of tumor emboli in the dermal lymphatics is indicative of inflammatory carcinoma and has significant prognostic and therapeutic implications.

Incisional Biopsy, Sagittal Section (Figure 4-2)

The incision is placed directly over the palpable mass, and a wedge-shaped specimen is obtained from the most superficial aspect of the mass. The normal breast tissue is unviolated.

The scalpel, rather than the electrocautery, should be used in obtaining the biopsy specimen to minimize tissue distortion. It is also important to avoid cauterizing the tissue because sex steroid receptors are extremely heat labile. Frozen section is usually performed for histologic diagnosis after the specimen is removed because, occasionally, extensive necrotic tissue is present in a large carcinoma or because tissue that appears malignant may show only reactive changes microscopically. In such cases additional tissue can be excised as necessary. After sufficient tissue has been removed, the wound is irrigated with saline solution, and hemostasis is achieved with electrocautery. With adequate hemostasis a drain is unnecessary, and the incision is closed by reapproximating the skin with nonabsorbable sutures.

Postoperative Care

The dressing is removed 1 or 2 days after the biopsy procedure. No special activity limitations are necessary, and the skin sutures may be removed 1 week after the biopsy if the wound is healing satisfactorily. Further management is directed by results of the biopsy.

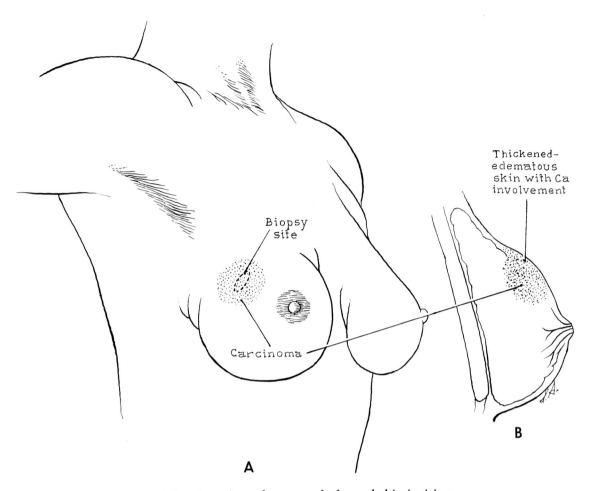

Fig 4-1.   Location of mass and planned skin incision.

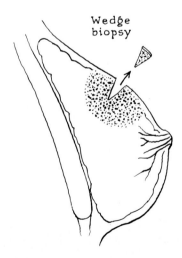

Fig 4-2.   Incisional biopsy, sagittal section.

5

Excisional Biopsy

Introduction

Excisional biopsy involves complete removal of a palpable mass. A variable amount of surrounding, normal-appearing breast parenchyma may also be removed, depending on the size of the mass and on its location. For benign disease the excisional biopsy is therapeutic and diagnostic. For invasive carcinoma, if the microscopic margins of resection are clearly uninvolved by tumor, the excisional biopsy procedure is sufficient for local disease control when followed by radiation therapy. Frequently, however, an excisional biopsy for invasive carcinoma must be followed by a tylectomy to ensure complete removal of the tumor with clear resection margins.

Indications

Excisional biopsy is indicated for evaluation of a relatively small mass (less than 2.5 cm) for which a positive diagnosis of carcinoma has not been established by aspiration cytology or core needle biopsy. Larger, benign-appearing masses, particularly in young women, may also be treated by excisional biopsy.

Contraindications

Excisional biopsy is generally contraindicated for the removal of a large mass that is suggestive of carcinoma because such biopsy may result in extensive tissue contamination and will make a subsequent definitive procedure for local control of disease more difficult to perform adequately. Preferably, incisional biopsy to confirm the suspected diagnosis should be performed if core needle biopsy and aspiration cytology are nondiagnostic. Definitive treatment can then be planned.

Preoperative Evaluation

Incision placement should be planned preoperatively, based on the location of the mass. If malignancy is suspected, the incision is placed directly over the mass in a circumferential or linear orientation. A periareolar incision may be used because of its excellent cosmetic result when a clinically benign mass is excised. This approach should be used only in carefully selected cases. Biopsy of a carcinoma in the periphery of the breast, through a peri-areolar incision, may result in contamination of the breast pocket if the tumor capsule is ruptured. The ability to perform a subsequent satisfactory breast conservation procedure may then be compromised. Occasionally the anatomic location of the mass is such that an inframammary incision is most appropriate for excision.

At present, excisional biopsy to establish a tissue diagnosis is usually the first step of a staged treatment plan for the woman with a small carcinoma of the breast. When carcinoma is suspected, the patient should be appropriately counseled before excisional biopsy regarding therapeutic options and the timing of definitive surgery.

Excisional biopsy may be performed using either local anesthesia or general anesthesia. Choice of anesthesia depends on the location of the mass and on the patient's and the surgeon's preferences. Local anesthesia is most appropriate for very small, superficially located masses. Masses deep in the breast and all larger masses are best excised using either general anesthesia or local anesthesia with intravenous sedation. Younger women and adolescents are particularly reluctant to have breast procedures performed with local anesthesia. General anesthesia is usually appropriate for them.

OPERATIVE PROCEDURE

Location of Mass and Planned Incision (Figure 5-1)

The patient is placed in a supine position, and the location of the mass is confirmed by palpation. After thorough cleansing of the breast and satisfactory anesthetic preparation, the incision is made. Generally, as shown in Figure 5-1, *A*, a circumareolar incision is made directly over the mass. Occasionally, a different incision may be more appropriate; however, the incision should conform to Langer's lines as much as possible.

The dissection will proceed directly through the parenchyma from the skin incision to the palpable mass (Figure 5-1, *B*).

Parenchymal Dissection and Specimen Removal (Figure 5-2)

After the skin incision is made, the skin edges are retracted and the tissue overlying the palpable mass is divided by sharp dissection with the scalpel or scissors. The mass should be handled as little as possible during biopsy to prevent disruption and tumor spillage. A forceps is used to grasp the edge of the tissue surrounding the mass. The mass, with a surrounding rim of normal-appearing breast parenchyma, is then sharply dissected free from the surrounding tissue circumferentially. A thin rim of normal-appearing breast parenchyma should be included with the specimen to be excised when possible (Figure 5-2, *A*). However, when a benign-appearing, well-circumcised mass, typically of fibroadenoma, is excised in a young woman, it is not necessary to include a margin of normal breast tissue. Rather, only the mass is excised.

After excision the specimen should be sent unfixed to the pathologist and the margins of the specimen should be marked with ink, even if the

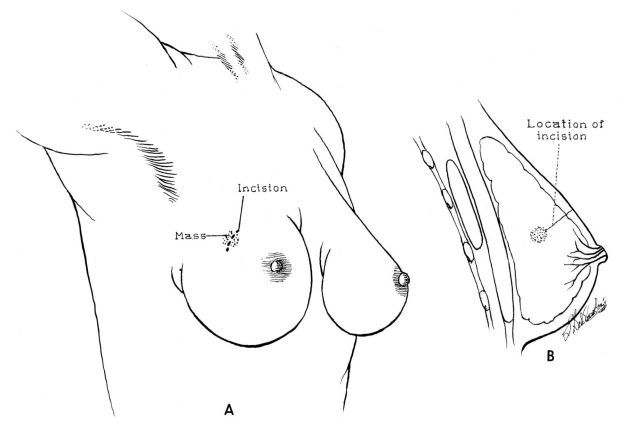

Fig 5-1.   Location of mass and planned incision.

suspicion of malignancy is low. Involvement of the margin with tumor is a major factor in determining the need for additional surgery before radiation therapy in women who are candidates for breast conservation surgery. As shown in Figure 5-2, *B,* an extensive raw surface may exist, particularly following removal of a mass deep in the breast. Meticulous attention to hemostasis is important.

After complete hemostasis has been achieved, the skin is closed with a running subcuticular suture. Deep sutures to reapproximate the breast tissue or drains are generally not necessary. Adhesive strips are applied, and a dry gauze bandage is placed over the incision.

Postoperative Care

Because little normal breast parenchyma is excised during this procedure, a satisfactory cosmetic appearance should result. This may not be apparent immediately following the procedure; however, with time the breast will remold to its former size and shape. Patients should wear an elastic support brassiere for several weeks postoperatively. Most patients can resume routine activities within a week.

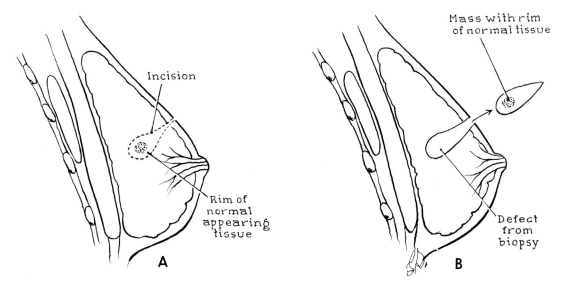

Fig 5-2. Parenchymal dissection and specimen removal.

6

Needle Localization Biopsy

Introduction

As the use of screening mammography has increased, nonpalpable breast abnormalities suggestive of carcinoma are being detected in more asymptomatic women. Over the last decade such women have represented an increasing proportion of patients seen by breast surgeons. Approximately 10% to 20% of asymptomatic patients with suspect abnormalities detected on mammography have breast carcinoma; this percentage may be higher in symptomatic women. Needle localization biopsy is the procedure most often used to obtain a tissue diagnosis in this clinical setting.

Close cooperation among the operating surgeon, the radiologist, and the pathologist is essential to enhance the diagnostic accuracy of this procedure. Because nonpalpable, mammographically visualized abnormalities are typically small, complete removal of the abnormality with a surrounding margin of normal breast parenchyma is the treatment of choice.

Indications

Needle localization biopsy is indicated for the patient with a nonpalpable, mammographically detected abnormality that is suggestive of carcinoma.

Contraindications

Needle localization biopsy is unnecessary in the patient with a palpable breast mass that is suggestive of carcinoma on mammography. It is not necessary to perform a biopsy on lesions that are cystic on ultrasound or that appear benign and unchanged on repeated mammograms over several years.

Complications

Needle or hookwire dislodgement is the most frequent complication of the needle localization procedure. Dislodgement can be avoided by suturing the needle and hookwire to the skin when placement is final. The patient is kept supine or semirecumbent on a stretcher during transport from the radiology department to the operating room suite. A rare complication is the inadvertent advancement of the needle or hookwire through the chest wall, resulting in pneumothorax or hemorrhage. The complication of wire fragment retention in the breast caused by inadvertent transection of the hookwire during the biopsy can be avoided by frequent palpation of the tissue being excised to confirm the relationship of the needle and hookwire to the plane of dissection. Special precautions must be taken in performing needle localization biopsy when a breast implant is in place, or the breast implant may be perforated.

Occasionally the mammographic abnormality is not in the excised tissue specimen. This problem can be avoided by a radiograph of the specimen. If the mammographic lesion is not present therein, additional tissue must be excised until the mammographic abnormality is removed. If the adequacy of the biopsy is in doubt when a final pathology report is obtained, the patient should have mammography repeated. Persistence of a mammographically suspect abnormality necessitates repeating the needle localization biopsy procedure.

Preoperative Evaluation

Evaluation of a patient referred for needle localization biopsy includes physical examination to confirm that the abnormality is not palpable, review of mammograms, and, in selected cases, ultrasound or aspiration cytology. Planned needle placement should be discussed with the radiologist who will perform the needle localization to avoid placment of the needle biopsy site in an area that could compromise future surgical procedures if a malignancy is present. Abnormalities close to the chest wall or in the axillary portion of the breast may be more difficult to localize, and the needle insertion site must be carefully planned. Needle localization biopsy is an outpatient procedure and may be performed under general or local anesthesia, depending on the preferences of the surgeon and the patient and on the anticipated difficulty of the procedure.

OPERATIVE PROCEDURE

Needle Hookwire Apparatus (Figure 6-1)

The first step in the needle localization biopsy procedure is accurate localization of the abnormality. The patient is referred to the radiology department, the mammogram is repeated, and the site of the abnormality is confirmed. After sterile preparation of the breast the skin is anesthetized, and a needle then is placed through the skin into the breast parenchyma adjacent to the abnormality. Most radiologists use a localization apparatus that is composed of a needle and a hookwire or localizer, such as that shown in Figure 6-1. The needle containing the hookwire is inserted through the skin into the breast parenchyma near the abnormality. The hooked wire is straight while it is contained within the needle barrel; however, it develops a bend or barb when the needle is retracted. The hook holds the wire in

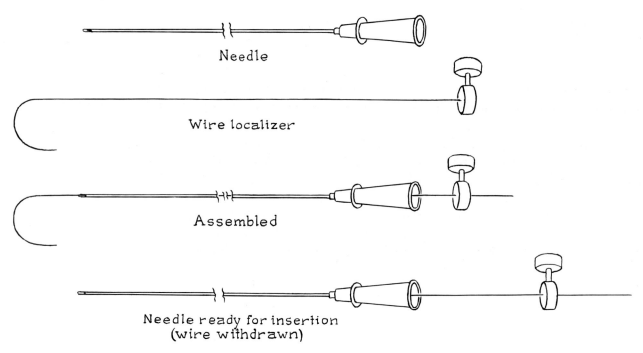

Needle

Wire localizer

Assembled

Needle ready for insertion
(wire withdrawn)

Fig 6-1.   Needle hookwire apparatus.

place near the abnormality. The mammogram is repeated when the needle is in place to confirm its relationship to the lesion in the breast.

Incision Placement (Figure 6-2)

Figure 6-2 shows the appearance of the needle and hookwire apparatus after the hookwire has been satisfactorily placed adjacent to a cluster of microcalcifications (stippled). The wire is secured to the patient's skin with a suture (not shown) to prevent needle or hookwire displacement during transport to the operating suite. The patient must be moved carefully to prevent dislodgement of the apparatus. In the operating room any dressings on the patient's breast are removed. After anesthetic administration the breast is cleansed and draped to include the entire breast in the operative field, taking care to avoid dislodgement of the hook wire apparatus. The skin incision encircling the hookwire insertion site in the skin is shown. When feasible a circumareolar incision is used because this incision produces a minimally disfiguring scar and will not compromise future incisions. Occasionally, when the needle enters the skin at a site distant from the abnormality, the incision may be placed over the region of the abnormality rather than around the hookwire. This will avoid extensive tunneling through the breast during the dissection.

Skin Incision and Tissue Dissection (Figure 6-3)

The elliptical incision incorporating a margin of skin around the hookwire is shown. This incision is extended by sharp dissection with the scissors or a scalpel through the subcutaneous tissue into the breast parenchyma. The planned extent of tissue resected is illustrated in this figure by the dashed

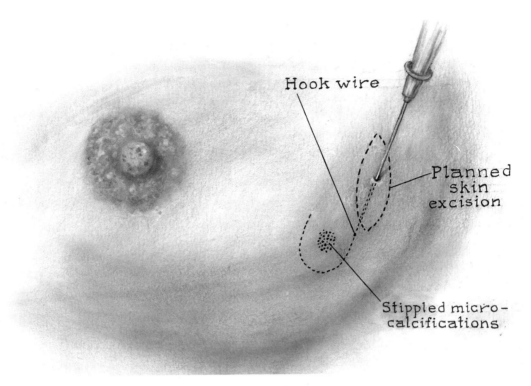

Fig 6-2. Incision placement.

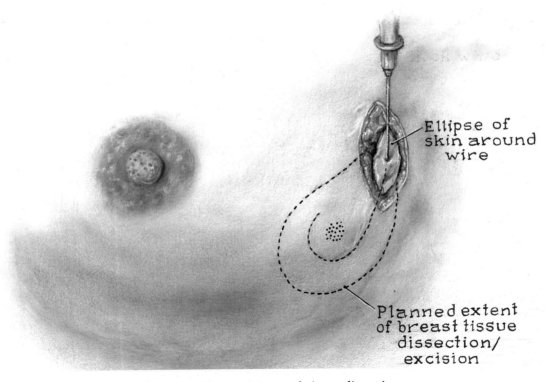

Fig 6-3. Skin incision and tissue dissection.

line. A rim of normal-appearing tissue, completely surrounding the hookwire and the mammographic abnormality, should be obtained to ensure complete removal of the mammographic abnormality.

35

Completion of Dissection; Excised Specimen (Figure 6-4)

As shown in Figure 6-4, *A,* gentle traction may be placed on the ellipse of skin and on the tissue specimen as sharp dissection of the breast parenchyma proceeds. The needle and hookwire apparatus should not be used as a retractor, and manipulation of the apparatus should be avoided. Careful palpation of the tissue specimen and the hookwire at frequent intervals is necessary to confirm that an adequate core of tissue is being excised to include 1 to 2 cm of normal tissue surrounding the hookwire. Sharp dissection rather than electrocautery should be used to minimize destruction of the tissue margins. If necessary, the elliptical skin incision can be lengthened at either end to increase visualization and to obtain a wider core of tissue. When an incision has been made at a site other than around the hookwire, it is extended sharply through the breast parenchyma until the hookwire is identified several centimeters proximal to the abnormality.

Figure 6-4, *B* shows that rake retractors placed on either side of the incision facilitate exposure. Most of the sharp dissection, with the exception of the completion of the dissection at the base of the wedge-shaped tissue block (in the deepest part of wound), should be done under direct vision.

Figure 6-4, *C* shows the appearance of the excised specimen. A margin of 2 cm of normal breast parenchyma surrounding the mammographic abnormality is evident. Only a thin core of breast tissue is excised around the hookwire proximal to this core of tissue. The skin ellipse and hookwire should be left in place for specimen orientation. Radiography of the specimen is performed to confirm that the entire mammographic abnormality is contained in the tissue block. The entire specimen should be inked by the pathologist to define the margins, and a frozen section of any suspicious area should be obtained. If the histologic interpretation suggests or is positive for carcinoma, tissue should be preserved for sex steroid receptor studies. The remainder of the tissue is processed appropriately for permanent sectioning and staining.

Finally, the wound is irrigated, hemostasis is established, and the skin is closed with a running subcuticular suture. Deep sutures are generally avoided because they may distort the breast contour. Drainage of the wound is unnecessary.

Postoperative Care

When the patient is awake and alert, she may be discharged from the outpatient surgical suite. The continuous use of an elastic sports brassiere for 7 to 10 days minimizes ecchymosis and discomfort. Patients generally resume all normal activities within a week. Pain is usually minimal and controlled with oral analgesics. Further follow-up is planned based on the results of the final pathology report.

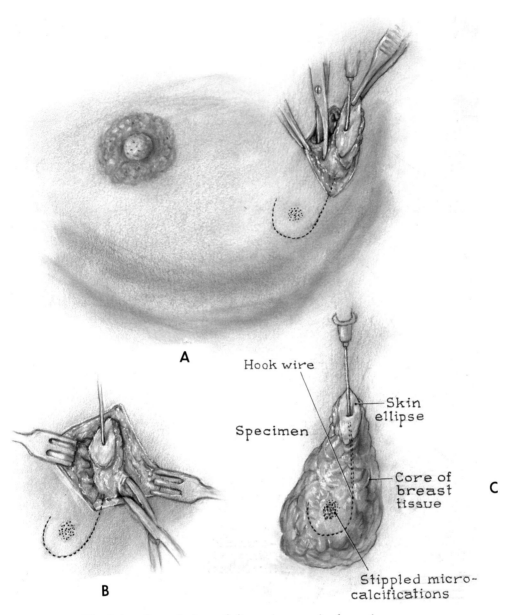

A

B

C

Hook wire

Specimen

Skin ellipse

Core of breast tissue

Stippled micro-calcifications

Fig 6-4.   Completion of dissection; excised specimen.

III

Procedures for the Treatment of Benign Breast Disease

Most breast diseases are benign, and, although the diagnoses and treatments for these disorders are relatively simple, careful patient selection and careful planning are necessary to achieve satisfactory therapeutic and cosmetic results. The operations for benign breast disease vary widely in complexity and in frequency of use. For example, gross cystic disease, one of the most common causes of a palpable breast mass, generally is treated readily by needle aspiration alone. However, occasionally an excisional biopsy is required, as described in Part II, "Biopsy Procedures." Little controversy exists about the appropriate management of gross cystic disease, and most physicians agree on the indications for surgical intervention. In contrast, a patient with either a strong family history of breast cancer and extensive benign breast disease or a biopsy demonstrating cellular atypia may undergo either a subcutaneous mastectomy as described in this section or a total mastectomy (Part IV, "Procedures for the Treatment of Breast Carcinoma") for breast cancer prophylaxis. The role of surgery in breast cancer prophylaxis at present is not well established. There is widespread controversy both regarding the indications for surgical intervention and the appropriate procedures. Therefore the guidelines for use of a specific procedure in the treatment of a benign disease are general recommendations only, and for the individual patient, treatment may differ significantly.

7
Cyst Aspiration

Introduction

Gross cystic disease is the most common cause of a benign breast mass in premenopausal women between the ages of 30 and 55 years. It is unusual in women less than 25 years of age or in postmenopausal women, unless they are taking oral estrogens. Complete aspiration of a cystic breast mass is usually curative because the cyst rarely recurs. Ultrasound-directed aspiration may be successful if previous aspiration attempts have failed to eliminate a cystic mass. The presence of green or clear aspirated fluid associated with complete disappearance of the palpable mass is consistent with the diagnosis of a benign breast cyst. However, the inability to obtain fluid, the recurrence of a palpable mass after fluid aspiration, the continued presence of a mass after aspiration, or the presence of a bloody aspirate is an indication for further evaluation and possible biopsy.

Indications

Cyst aspiration is indicated in patients who have either a simple cyst or a complex cyst. Occasionally women have multiple, bilateral cystic masses, each of which may be treated similarly with aspiration.

Contraindications

There are no absolute contraindications to cyst aspiration, although the procedure must be performed with caution in women with breast implants or bleeding disorders. Ultrasound guidance may make cyst aspiration safer in these situations.

Complications

Bleeding or hematoma formation at the aspiration site is rare. Failure to fully eliminate a palpable cystic mass following aspiration occasionally occurs when the cyst is thick walled. However, if repeated aspiration fails to eliminate the mass, further evaluation is required.

Preoperative Evaluation

The diagnosis of gross cystic disease may be made on the basis of physical examination alone. Also gross cysts are generally identifiable by mammographic or ultrasound examination. However, it is not necessary to perform these examinations routinely before attempting aspiration of a palpable mass. Aspiration can be both diagnostic and therapeutic when the palpable breast mass yields nonbloody fluid and when no palpable abnormality remains after the procedure is completed.

OPERATIVE PROCEDURE

Patient Positioning (Figure 7-1)

A 21-gauge needle attached to a syringe is used for aspiration. A hand-held pistol device, if available, facilitates aspiration without assistance. The skin overlying the palpable mass may be locally infiltrated with 1% lidocaine to raise a small wheal before cyst aspiration. The overlying skin is cleansed, and the breast tissue encompassing the cyst is stabilized by compressing the breast on the chest wall. Cyst aspiration is usually performed with the patient in a supine position. Occasionally a laterally located cyst is more easily aspirated when the patient is lying on her side.

Sagittal Sections of Breast During and After Cyst Aspiration (Figure 7-2)

The needle, attached to the syringe, is inserted through the skin overlying the cyst, and negative pressure is applied to completely aspirate all fluid (Figure 7-2, A). The needle may be redirected within the breast as necessary, with gentle pressure on the mass to aid in complete removal of all free fluid. When aspiration is completed, the negative pressure is gently released, and the needle is withdrawn.

After the needle is removed, the breast is palpated to confirm that the mass is no longer present. A few milliliters of fluid may be aspirated, although large cysts may yield up to 50 milliliters. The fluid is not routinely sent for cytologic evaluation because the incidence of malignancy is extremely low in these cases. However, if the fluid is bloody, rather than clear or greenish tinged, cytologic examination should be performed. As shown in Figure 7-2, B, the breast retains its normal appearance and contour after aspiration because the cyst has collapsed.

Postoperative Care

For the majority of women with gross cystic disease, cyst aspiration completely eliminates the palpable mass. The patient is reexamined 4 to 6 weeks following aspiration to ensure that the mass has not recurred. Cyst recurrence, following aspiration, requires further evaluation.

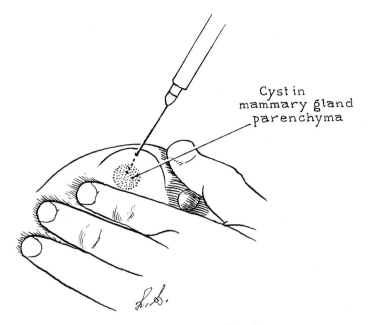

Fig 7-1. Patient positioning.

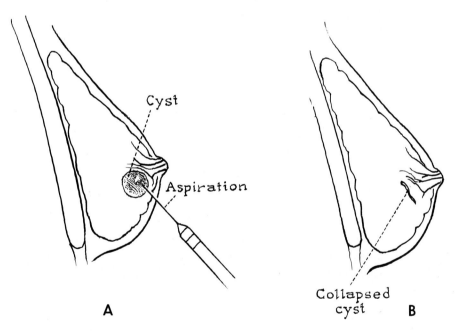

Fig 7-2. Sagittal sections of breast during and after cyst aspiration.

8

Excision of an Intraductal Papilloma

Introduction

An intraductal papilloma is a benign breast tumor resulting from the local proliferation of ductal epithelial cells. The papilloma is usually pedunculated and visible to the unassisted eye on inspection of the opened breast duct at surgery. The growth is typically solitary and develops in a single duct near the areola as shown on the sagittal section in Figure 8-1. Multiple intraductal papillomas are uncommon and usually develop in a cluster of ducts in the periphery of the breast. An intraductal papilloma rarely develops within the nipple.

Although solitary intraductal papillomas may develop in women of any age, most occur in the fourth or fifth decade of life. Spontaneous nipple discharge, often bloody, is the most common presenting symptom. In about 40% of patients the papilloma is palpable, usually in the breast close to the areola. If no mass is palpable, the papilloma can usually be located by gently palpating the breast in a clockwise direction around the nipple-areolar complex. Drainage from the nipple, when a breast segment is palpated, localizes the duct that contains the papilloma. Excision of the involved duct with a surrounding wedge of breast tissue is curative. The patient with multiple intraductal papillomas frequently presents for treatment with a solitary mass and typically does not have nipple discharge. The diagnosis is established pathologically only after the mass has been excised.

Indications

The presence of drainage from the nipple should be thoroughly evaluated and the cause defined. If an intraductal papilloma is definitively diagnosed or if its presence is suspected, it should be excised.

Contraindications

Solitary ductal excision through a periareolar incision is contraindicated in the presence of clinical or radiographic findings suggestive of malignancy. When a malignancy is suspected, a biopsy (as previously described in Part II) should be performed. Solitary ductal excision should not be performed

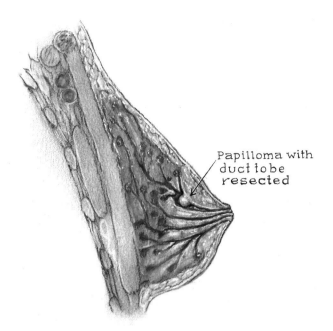

Papilloma with duct to be resected

Fig 8-1. Sagittal section of the breast with intraductal papilloma.

in the patient with bilateral or nonspontaneous discharge. Since the underlying cause is unlikely to be an intraductal papilloma, a more extensive study, including an endocrine evaluation, may be indicated. Ductal excision is not done if the surgeon is unable to localize the duct of origin of the discharge at the time of surgery.

Complications

Incomplete ductal excision, usually attributable to an error in identification of the involved duct at the time of surgery, may result in recurrence of the symptoms. Careful patient evaluation and confirmation of the involved duct intraoperatively reduce the possibility of incomplete excision of the papilloma or of inadvertent excision of an uninvolved duct.

Preoperative Evaluation

Mammography is generally indicated in the preoperative evaluation of patients with spontaneous nipple discharge (especially bloody discharge) because of the possible association of a breast malignancy. This is particularly important in older patients, for whom the frequency of malignancy in the presence of a bloody nipple discharge may be 10% to 15%. In the absence of a palpable mass, a ductogram (a radiograph obtained after contrast material is injected by needle into a breast duct) may be useful to delineate the involved duct.

Cytology of the patient's discharge fluid is typically nondiagnostic and is therefore of limited utility. The patient should be advised to avoid manipulation of the breast for a few days before surgery so that nipple discharge can be readily elicited before the skin incision is made. This procedure may be performed on an outpatient basis under general or local anesthesia.

OPERATIVE PROCEDURE

Periareolar Incision (Figure 8-2)

The inset in Figure 8-2 demonstrates the location of a small, solitary papilloma in the upper, outer quadrant of the left breast, near the nipple-areolar complex. Before making a skin incision, the surgeon must confirm the location of the duct to be excised. This is established either by the palpation of a mass or by the elicitation of nipple discharge following sequential clockwise pressure in the periareolar area. If ductography has been successfully performed, the involved duct will be easily identified. The radiographs should be available in the operating room during the procedure for review by the surgeon.

After the involved duct has been localized, the skin is cleansed and the entire breast is draped in the operative field. With satisfactory anesthesia a periareolar incision is made. As shown by the dotted line, the incision can be extended around half the circumference of the areola. The papilloma (shown) is a small, dark, friable mass adherent to the wall of the involved duct and partially obstructing the lumen. The periareolar incision is extended through the subcutaneous tissue. The duct containing the papilloma is usually filled with dark fluid and is easily identified. Extension of the incision around both sides of the involved duct produces the most satisfactory exposure. An areolar flap is then elevated by sharp dissection.

Dissection of Involved Duct (Figure 8-3)

By sharp dissection the involved duct is isolated circumferentially from the surrounding breast tissue at the areola. The duct is then transected close to the undersurface of the areola, and a clamp is applied to the end of the duct extending into the breast parenchyma. After the involved duct has been divided, the overlying skin and subcutaneous tissue are undermined to further expose the ductal system.

Completion of Ductal Excision (Figure 8-4)

As shown on the sagittal section in Figure 8-4, *A*, the intraductal papilloma is evident in the middle of the involved duct, which is being sharply excised with a margin of surrounding breast parenchyma. Gentle traction on the cut end of the duct facilitates its identification because the ductal system branches deep in the breast. Elevation of the incision edges with skin hooks (Figure 8-4, *B*), permits most of the dissection to be performed under direct vision. A wedge-shaped core of tissue, with its broad base deep in the breast and its apex at the cut end of the duct, is developed to ensure inclusion of the ductal papilloma in the resected tissue specimen. The dissection is completed by division of the breast tissue at the base of the ductal system. This final step in the dissection is done with digital palpation because exposure at the base of the breast wedge is limited. The extent of tissue resected is indicated by the dotted lines in both figures.

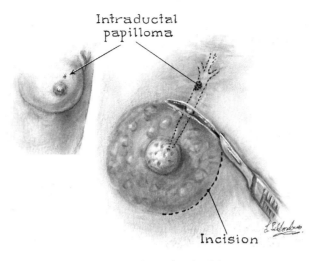

Fig 8-2.   Periareolar incision.

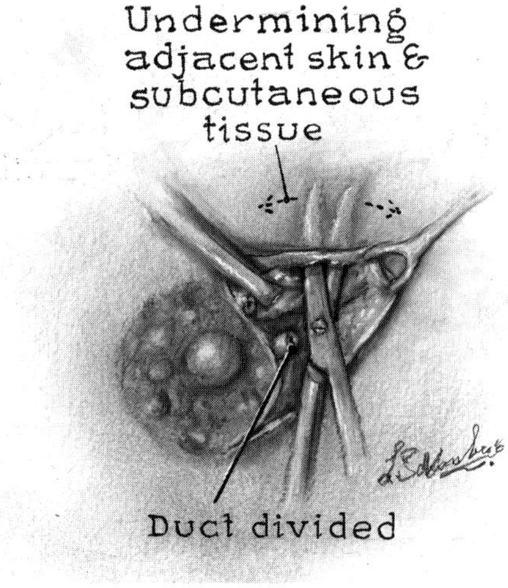

Fig 8-3.   Dissection of involved duct.

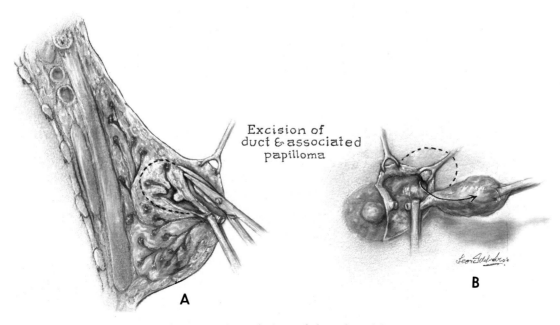

Fig 8-4.   Completion of ductal excision.

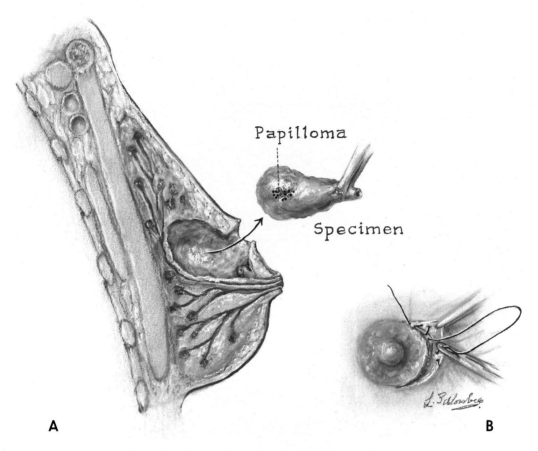

Fig 8-5. Excised specimen and incision closure.

Excised Specimen and Incision Closure (Figure 8-5)

As shown on the sagittal section in Figure 8-5, *A*, the tissue core of normal breast tissue and the involved ductal system are excised en bloc. The specimen can be opened and examined by the pathologist intraoperatively to confirm that the excised duct contains the papilloma. In most cases the intraductal papilloma appears as a soft, friable, reddish blue mass of variable size. Whether or not a papilloma is readily apparent, the entire excised specimen should be sent for pathologic evaluation. The remaining dead space is copiously irrigated, and hemostasis is achieved. As shown in Figure 8-5, *B*, the skin edges are reapproximated with a running subcuticular suture. Deep sutures are unnecessary and could distort the breast contour.

Postoperative Care

Following satisfactory recovery from anesthesia, the patient can be discharged from the outpatient surgical center. Continuous support with an elastic sports brassiere may reduce the ecchymosis and discomfort in the first few days after surgery. Postoperative pain is minimal and can generally be managed with oral analgesics. The incision heals in a week to 10 days. The resultant concavity in the region of the ductal excision is generally minimal and inconspicuous.

9

Excision of a Giant Fibroadenoma

Introduction

Giant fibroadenoma is a rare benign breast tumor that occurs predominantly in adolescent females. It is the most common cause of massive unilateral breast enlargement in this age group; complete excision is curative. The patient typically presents for treatment with marked breast asymmetry caused by a large breast mass of recent onset that has progressively increased in size. Characteristically a giant fibroadenoma is freely movable over the underlying chest wall. The borders of the tumor are usually well defined on physical examination. In Figure 9-1 a sagittal section of the breast shows a giant fibroadenoma in the inferior portion of the breast displacing and compressing the normal breast parenchyma superiorly.

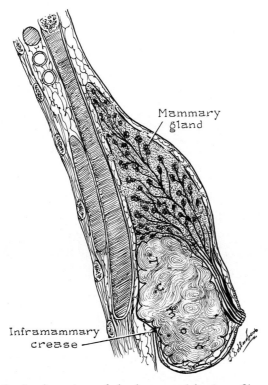

Mammary gland

Inframammary crease

Fig 9-1. Sagittal section of the breast with giant fibroadenoma.

If on physical examination the large breast mass is poorly circumscribed or is fixed to the underlying chest wall, an incisional biopsy should be performed first to exclude the presence of cytosarcoma phylloides or of soft-tissue sarcoma. These lesions require a more extensive resection of breast parenchyma and of surrounding soft tissue. Obviously such radical surgery, particularly in the adolescent age group, should be performed only when clearly indicated.

Indications

The presence of a giant fibroadenoma is an indication for its excision. Women of any age, particularly adolescents, are obviously upset by the presence of a large breast mass and the resulting appearance.

Contraindications

The surgeon must be certain that the lesion is not malignant. Inadvertent excision of a malignant tumor through an inframammary incision could result in extensive contamination of the chest wall and necessitate an extensive repeat operative procedure.

Complications

Bleeding and infection are potential complications because of the large space resulting from the extensive dissection.

Preoperative Preparation

Clinical evaluation supplemented on occasion by incision biopsy is sufficient for the diagnosis. For an older patient and for young patients in whom the diagnosis is not readily apparent, further evaluation should be considered. Removal of a giant fibroadenoma requires general anesthesia and a hospital stay of 2 to 3 days.

OPERATIVE PROCEDURE

Incision Placement (Figure 9-2)

This figure depicts the placement of the incision along the inframammary crease for excision of an extensive, well-defined tumor mass in the medial portion of the breast. This incision gives adequate exposure, and the scar is concealed.

Inframammary Incision (Figure 9-3)

After general anesthesia has been induced, the skin is cleansed and draped with the entire breast in the operative field. The breast is retracted superiorly to expose the inframammary crease. A skin incision lying in the inframammary crease is deepened through the subcutaneous tissue until the well-circumscribed tumor mass is encountered.

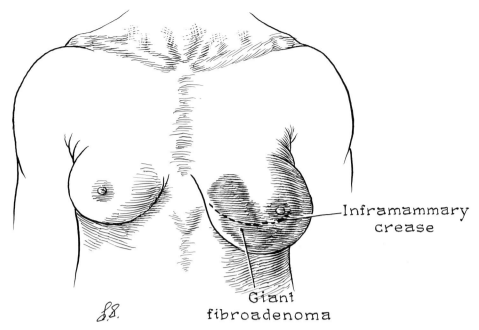

Fig 9-2. Incision placement.

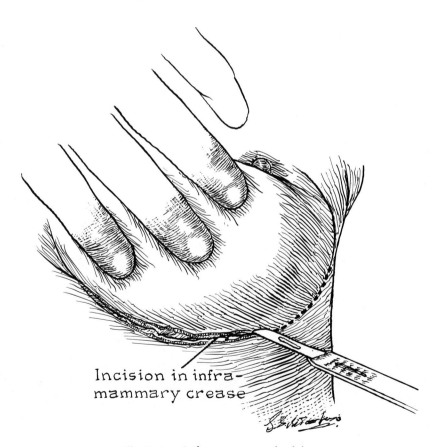

Fig 9-3. Inframammary incision.

Tumor Excision (Figure 9-4)

The surrounding normal breast tissue is sharply dissected from the well-circumscribed mass. A distinct tissue plane is easily identified between the mass and the normal breast parenchyma. Gentle traction on the edge of the tumor with an atraumatic clamp (as shown) allows manipulation of the tumor mass to facilitate visualization in the deepest part of the dissection field. The skin edges should be retracted to improve exposure. It is unnecessary to remove normal breast tissue surrounding the tumor mass. Following complete excision, the entire specimen is submitted for pathologic evaluation to confirm the clinical impression of a benign fibroadenoma.

Sagittal Section of Breast after Tumor Removal (Figure 9-5)

A large dead space remains, and meticulous hemostasis is required to prevent hematoma formation. A constant vacuum drain is inserted, and the wound is closed in a single layer with a running subcuticular suture. Deep sutures to obliterate the dead space are unnecessary and can distort the breast contour.

Postoperative Care

The patient is discharged when she is ambulatory and her pain can be controlled with oral analgesics. The drain is removed when accumulated fluid is less than 30 ml per 24 hours. An elastic support brassiere is worn for several weeks.

Postoperatively, the breast from which the tumor was removed may appear smaller than the other breast and have redundant skin. However, this circumstance rarely necessitates treatment because the breast will remold to its initial size and shape, ultimately resuming a symmetrical, satisfactory, cosmetic appearance.

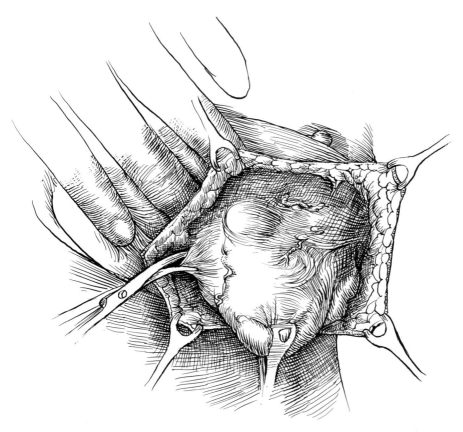

Fig 9-4.   Tumor excision.

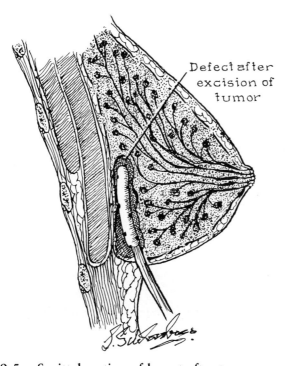

Defect after
excision of
tumor

Fig 9-5.   Sagittal section of breast after tumor removal.

10

Drainage of a Breast Abscess

Introduction

A breast abscess develops most frequently in lactating women and may involve any area of the breast or retromammary region. The most common infecting organisms are of the *Staphylococcus* or *Streptococcus* species. Mycobacterial infections are rare; however, they characteristically recur if the diagnosis is not established and if appropriate antibiotic therapy is not instituted at the time of drainage. Occasionally an inflammatory carcinoma mimics a breast abscess.

The patient with a breast abscess usually presents for treatment with a painful, tender, warm, erythematous mass that may be fluctuant. These classic signs of inflammation may be more subtle if the abscess is in a retromammary location. Aspiration is useful to establish the diagnosis and to obtain material for Gram stain and culture. Incision and drainage of the abscess followed by antibiotic therapy if indicated are curative in most cases. Biopsy of the abscess wall should be performed at the time of drainage to exclude malignancy.

Indications

The presence of a breast abscess is the indication for incisional drainage; the majority respond satisfactorily to this therapy. Delay in the diagnosis or in the implementation of appropriate treatment may result in excessive destruction of breast tissue because an established abscess will not resolve with antibiotic therapy alone.

Contraindications

There are no absolute contraindications to drainage of an abscess. Inadvertent treatment of an inflammatory carcinoma as a breast abscess can be avoided by skin biopsy when there is difficulty in distinguishing the two entities.

Complications

The major complication of breast abscess drainage is incomplete evacuation at the time of the initial operation. This complication can be avoided by making an incision of sufficient length to allow thorough exploration of the cavity and by manual disruption of all loculations within the cavity. A less frequent but important complication in lactating women is persistent milk drainage through the abscess cavity. This drainage may persist until lactation stops.

Preoperative Preparation

The tenderness associated with palpation of the affected breast precludes mammography. Needle aspiration of the mass with culture and Gram stain of the material is performed. Ultrasound may be useful for indeterminate cases, particularly when a retromammary abscess may be present. Drainage of the abscess is performed under general anesthesia; however, if the abscess is superficial, local anesthesia alone may suffice.

Sagittal Section of Breast with Abscess (Figure 10-1)

The patient is placed in a supine position. After induction of anesthesia, the skin is cleansed and the entire breast is draped in the operative field. Prominent edema of the skin usually overlies the mass. The abscess may extend in the breast tissue well beyond the region underlying the edematous skin. An incision parallel to Langer's lines is made directly overlying the area

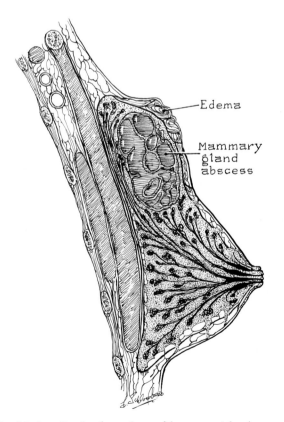

Fig 10-1. Sagittal section of breast with abscess.

of maximal induration and fluctuance. Specimens for aerobic and anaerobic cultures, as well as a Gram stain of the purulent drainage, are obtained as the abscess cavity is entered. If an unusual organism (i.e., mycobacteria, fungus) is suspected because of an atypical presentation, such as recurrent abscess formation or development of an abscess in an immunocompromised host, additional specimens for appropriate stains and cultures are also obtained.

Manual Disruption of Loculations (Figure 10-2)

As shown in Figure 10-2, **A,** the abscess cavity is manually evacuated, and all loculations are disrupted by inserting one or two fingers in the cavity and gently disrupting the thin-walled compartments of purulent material as they are palpated. Gentle probing of the cavity will not disrupt normal breast parenchyma beyond the extent of the abscess. The entire abscess cavity is copiously irrigated, and the cavity is palpated to detect the presence of any associated mass. If a mass is present, a biopsy procedure should be performed. A biopsy of the abscess wall should also be performed at this time.

The sagittal section shown in Figure 10-2, **B,** demonstrates a multi-loculated breast abscess. Although the surrounding breast parenchyma may be compressed by the abscess, parenchymal destruction is usually minimal.

Sagittal Section of Drain Placement in Breast (Figure 10-3)

After the abscess is evacuated, a soft rubber drain is placed in the cavity and brought out through the incision. The edges of the incision are loosely reapproximated; however, the edges should not be completely closed. The drain can be slowly retracted in the following days as the abscess cavity closes secondarily. Alternatively, for a large abscess, the cavity can be packed open and allowed to close entirely by secondary intent, with frequent packing changes.

Postoperative Care

Following incision drainage and local wound care, the abscess cavity usually closes within several weeks, with minimal cosmetic deformity.

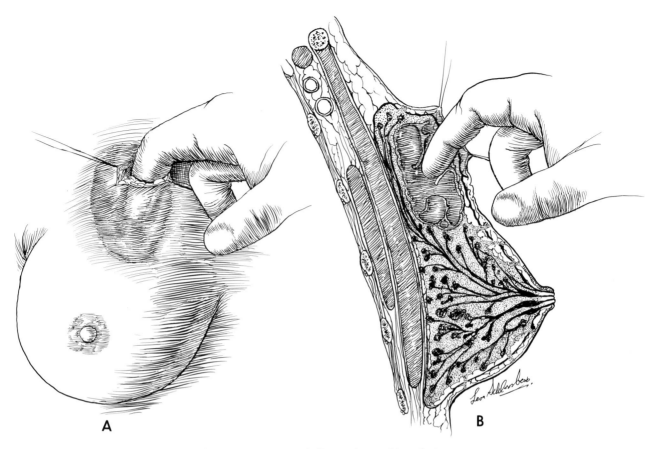

Fig 10-2. Manual disruption of loculations.

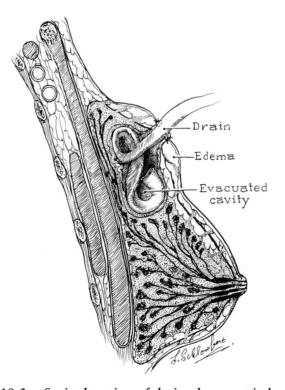

—Drain

—Edema

—Evacuated cavity

Fig 10-3. Sagittal section of drain placement in breast.

11

Subcutaneous Mastectomy

Introduction

The subcutaneous mastectomy procedure involves removal of 75% to 95% of the breast tissue, with preservation of the overlying skin and nipple-areolar complex and some of its underlying ductal tissue. Variable amounts of breast tissue are usually left in the axillary tail and on the skin flaps. The subcutaneous mastectomy differs significantly from the total mastectomy. In the total mastectomy, 95% to 98% of the breast, including the nipple-areolar complex and surrounding skin, is removed. Obviously, the subcutaneous mastectomy gives a more acceptable cosmetic result than the total mastectomy. These procedures are performed primarily for prophylaxis in the patient who is at risk for developing breast carcinoma. The choice between the two procedures should be made only after a thorough evaluation of the patient's risk factors and after the advantages and limitations of each procedure have been discussed with her.

Breast reconstruction usually is performed following subcutaneous mastectomy, and the results should be excellent because of the abundant, healthy chest wall skin. The reconstruction is most often done at the time of mastectomy, using either a tissue expander or an autogenous tissue flap. Less often, the breast reconstruction is delayed. The method of the reconstruction is determined on an individual basis and is discussed more fully in Part V.

Indications

Subcutaneous mastectomy is indicated for women at high risk for developing breast cancer, such as those with a strong family history of this disease or with progressive premalignant changes on successive biopsies. Extensive benign breast disease, which confuses the findings on physical examination and mammographic interpretation, may be an indication for subcutaneous mastectomy.

Contraindications

Subcutaneous mastectomy is not done in patients with invasive breast carcinoma. The procedure should not be performed in patients with mastodynia, which encompasses a variety of cyclical and noncyclical pain syndromes. Women with large breasts (over 1000 g of tissue per breast) are at substantial risk for skin necrosis following subcutaneous mastectomy. These patients are better treated by total mastectomy and replacement of the nipple-areolar complex as a free graft.

Complications

Early complications following subcutaneous mastectomy include bleeding, infection, and skin or nipple-areolar necrosis. Significant bleeding, requiring reoperation, occurs in fewer than 5% of patients.

Infection is uncommon following subcutaneous mastectomy alone. However, it occurs in approximately 10% of patients having reconstruction with an implant. Most infections are caused by staphylococcal species and can be treated successfully with antibiotics. Infection in the presence of an implant is a more serious complication because the prosthesis must be removed.

The risk of flap necrosis is increased in patients who smoke, have collagen vascular disease, have extremely large breasts, or have preexisting scars. A radially oriented incision, rather than an inframammary incision, should be used when more than 500 g of tissue is to be excised. If there are preexisting scars, the placement of the incision should be modified to minimize the risk of flap necrosis.

Preoperative Evaluation

A thorough history regarding familial breast carcinoma is obtained. Pathology reports from previous biopsies and prior mammographic studies should be reviewed. A mammogram is obtained if the patient has not had one within the past year.

The patient is thoroughly examined, in both the sitting and the supine positions, for the presence of palpable breast masses or adenopathy. The location and extent of scars from previous biopsies should be noted. The patient should be informed regarding the location of scars following the procedure, as well as the expected loss of breast and nipple-areolar sensation and the inability to lactate.

The methods of breast reconstruction should be discussed with the patient, and a decision should be made regarding the procedure to be used. Subcutaneous mastectomy is performed on an inpatient basis, with the patient under general anesthesia. Preoperative antibiotics are routinely administered.

OPERATIVE PROCEDURE

Subcutaneous Mastectomy

Incision Placement (Figure 11-1)

The midline of the sternum and the inframammary crease(s) are marked while the patient is in an upright position. The patient is then placed in a

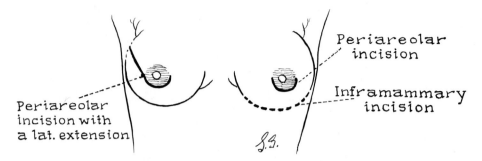

Fig 11-1.   Incision placement.

supine position with both arms abducted. After induction of general anesthesia, the patient is placed in a semisitting position. The skin of the entire chest, from clavicles to umbilicus, is included in the operative field. The skin is cleansed, the operative field is draped, and the planned incisions are marked.

An inframammary incision, a periareolar incision, or a periareolar incision with a lateral extension can be used for subcutaneous mastectomy, depending on the size of the breast and the presence of scars from previous biopsies. To reduce the risk of skin necrosis when scars are present, the incision should incorporate the scar or should minimize the amount of tissue beneath it.

An inframammary incision is most commonly used and is best for the patient with small breasts (less than 500 g of breast tissue). The incision is placed in the inframammary crease so that the scar will be hidden. A disadvantage of the incision is that removal of tissue in the superior portion of the breast is difficult.

A periareolar incision with a lateral extension is preferred if the patient has a scar in the superior portion of the breast. Because this incision roughly bisects the breast, it gives good exposure for the mastectomy and creates well-vascularized skin flaps. A periareolar incision with a lateral extension is occasionally used in patients with small breasts and large areolae.

Extent of Breast Tissue Excised (Figure 11-2)

The extent of the breast tissue to be excised is shown as the stippled area. The superior border of excision is the upper extent of palpable breast tissue. The medial extent is the lateral border of the sternum. The inferior extent is the inframammary crease, and the lateral extent is the midaxillary line.

Excision of Breast Tissue through an Inframammary Incision (Figure 11-3)

After an inframammary incision is made, the skin flap is developed in the plane between the subcutaneous fat and the breast tissue. However, in the area underlying the nipple-areolar complex the flap should be tailored to 5 to 7 mm thickness to maintain adequate circulation. The breast tissue then is retracted gently, and the electrocautery is used to dissect it from the underlying pectoral fascia. The edges of the resection should be feathered to avoid a visible ridge at the superior margin of the resection. Perforating

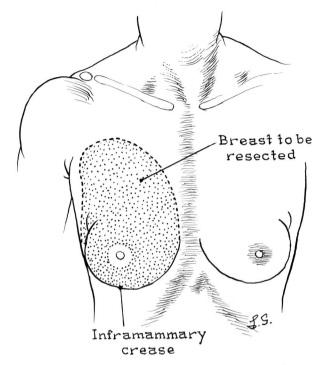

Fig 11-2. Extent of breast tissue excised.

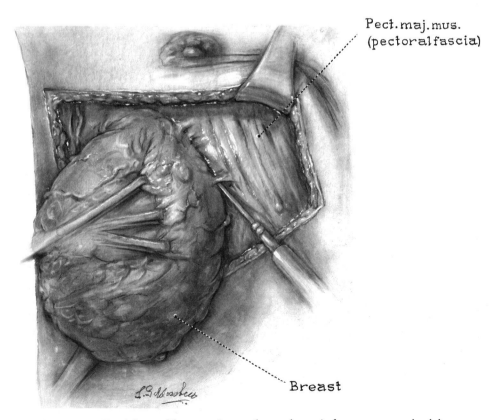

Fig 11-3. Excision of breast tissue through an inframammary incision.

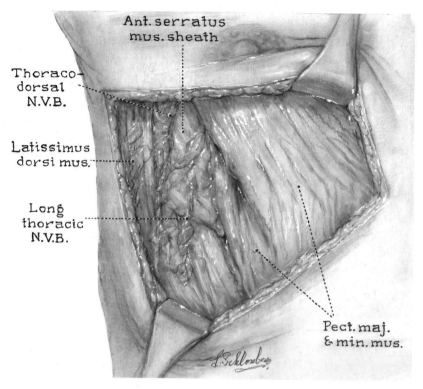

Fig 11-4. Subcutaneous mastectomy; operative field after surgery.

vessels emerging through the medial aspect of the pectoral fascia must be ligated and divided. The pectoral fascia is left attached to the muscle and will facilitate subsequent breast reconstruction.

The resection may be extended into the axillary space to excise the tail of Spence, but removal of axillary lymph nodes is not part of the subcutaneous mastectomy procedure. If the dissection proceeds laterally into the axillary space, the long thoracic nerve must be preserved throughout its course along the serratus anterior muscle. The thoracodorsal neurovascular bundle is also left intact. Further details regarding preservation of these nerves during dissection in the axilla are presented in Chapter 16 which describes the modified radical mastectomy procedure.

Subcutaneous Mastectomy; Operative Field After Surgery (Figure 11-4)

After the breast tissue has been excised, the pectoralis major muscle and the serratus anterior muscle are exposed. If the dissection is extended laterally to remove the axillary tail of the breast, the anterior border of the latissimus dorsi is seen. Complete hemostasis is achieved before reconstruction or wound closure can be performed.

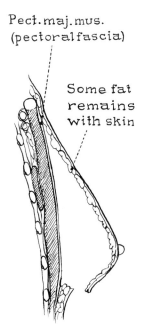

Pect.maj.mus.
(pectoralfascia)

Some fat
remains
with skin

Fig 11-5. Sagittal section of the chest after subcutaneous mastectomy.

Sagittal Section of the Chest after Subcutaneous Mastectomy
(Figure 11-5)

The pectoral fascia and underlying muscle, as well as the nipple-areolar complex, remain intact with a skin flap of fairly uniform thickness. For the occasional patient who will not undergo immediate reconstruction, the inframammary incision is closed in layers. The fascial layer is reapproximated with interrupted absorbable sutures, and the skin is closed with a running subcuticular suture. Drain placement is not necessary when the subcutaneous mastectomy procedure is performed without immediate reconstruction.

Postoperative Care

Following subcutaneous mastectomy alone, the patient usually requires only an overnight hospital stay for pain control. Following discharge she may resume light physical activity immediately and commence all regular activities within 2 to 3 weeks. The incisions are evaluated a week after surgery. When immediate reconstruction has been performed, the postoperative care is dictated by the type of reconstructive procedure.

Many patients undergo bilateral subcutaneous mastectomies because of high risk for breast carcinoma. Postoperatively, these women must continue with physical examinations and mammography at regular intervals. The risk of developing breast malignancy may have been substantially reduced; however, it has not been completely eliminated.

IV

Procedures for the Treatment of Breast Carcinoma

Breast carcinoma is a common disease in women of the United States of America. Approximately 100,000 new cases are reported annually. The majority of women with breast carcinoma are treated surgically; however, the extent of the operative procedures for carcinoma has changed substantially in the past two decades, and it continues to evolve.

The Halsted radical mastectomy was initially described in the late 19th century and was the most widely practiced operation for breast carcinoma until about 1970. Gradually, the modified radical mastectomy was more commonly used, and it soon replaced the radical mastectomy as the procedure chosen for all but a few patients with stage I or stage II breast carcinoma. Prospective randomized trials comparing radical mastectomy to modified radical mastectomy, in patients with localized invasive breast carcinoma, have demonstrated that the 5-year disease-free survival and overall survival are similar for appropriately selected patients treated with either procedure.

Recently the concept of breast conservation surgery for invasive carcinoma has gained widespread popularity. Breast conservation surgery accompanied by irradiation can produce rates of local disease control and overall survival comparable to those obtained with total or modified radical mastectomy. Several prospectively randomized trials have documented the comparability of treating patients with primary breast carcinoma by either segmental mastectomy, axillary dissection, and irradiation or by total mastectomy and axillary dissection.

Therefore breast conservation surgery, when used in conjunction with breast irradiation, has become a standard therapy for patients with invasive breast carcinoma. However, breast conservation alone for invasive carcinoma is associated with high rates of local recurrence.

It is essential that the surgeon be able to perform each of the currently accepted operations used in the treatment of patients with primary disease. No single procedure is appropriate for all patients. There may be more than one surgical approach that will provide satisfactory long-term disease control for the patient. The surgeon must be able to determine which treatment options are appropriate in a particular clinical situation. A procedure then can be selected after the options are thoroughly discussed with the patient and other physicians involved in the treatment plan.

The good long-term results obtained with breast conservation surgery in prospectively randomized trials can be achieved in clinical practice only if the guidelines for patient selection are carefully followed. Women who are candidates for breast conservation therapy should be evaluated preoperatively by the radiation oncologist who will be administering the treatment.

Many women desire breast reconstruction following mastectomy. A variety of these procedures are available. The surgeon performing the reconstruction should examine the patient and discuss with her the best type of reconstruction and the best timing for the procedure.

The treatment of in situ ductal carcinoma is more controversial than the treatment of invasive carcinoma. Tylectomy alone, tylectomy with radiation, and total mastectomy, have each been used in the treatment of this disease. However, tylectomy alone, when compared with tylectomy with radiation, appears to be associated with a higher rate of local recurrence. In situ lobular neoplasia is generally considered a marker of high risk for the subsequent development of breast carcinoma. The appropriate treatment of lobular neoplasia may include biopsy alone with careful long-term follow-up or bilateral total mastectomies, depending on the clinical situation.

Finally, the management of nonepithelial breast cancer has not been extensively studied. Breast sarcoma, melanoma, and lymphoma are managed on an individual basis, and the treatments are variable. The treatment for cystosarcoma phyllodes—the most commonly occurring nonepithelial breast malignancy—may range from local excision to total mastectomy.

12

Tylectomy

Introduction

For selected patients with invasive carcinoma of the breast, the removal of a segment of breast tissue fully encompassing the malignancy, combined with axillary dissection and radiation therapy, is an acceptable therapeutic alternative to modified radical mastectomy. The extent of the segmental resection necessary to achieve satisfactory local control has not been defined. Several conservative resection procedures have been described, including quadrantectomy, segmental mastectomy, lumpectomy, and tylectomy. Although these terms are sometimes used interchangeably, the procedures differ in relation to the extent of tissue removed. Quandrantectomy is the most extensive "conservative" procedure and involves resection of a full quadrant of the breast, including the skin, areola, parenchyma containing the carcinoma, and the underlying superficial fascia of the pectoralis major muscle. The procedure is performed through a radially oriented incision, and a relatively large portion of breast tissue is removed. Cosmetic results are variable, and some patients may require restorative breast reconstruction. In a segmental mastectomy a portion of the breast parenchyma encompassing the tumor is removed; however, the extent of tissue resection is not as well defined as it is for quadrantectomy. Tylectomy is defined as the excision of a portion of breast tissue incorporating the malignancy with a sufficient rim of normal breast parenchyma to ensure negative microscopic margins. Usually, at least 1 to 2 cm of normal-appearing breast parenchyma surrounding the malignancy is removed, although this amount may vary. By contrast, lumpectomy is the removal of gross tumor, with no attempt to excise the surrounding normal-appearing breast tissue. Carcinoma cells frequently involve the margin of resection following lumpectomy. Quadrantectomy results in the best local control rate; however, it gives the poorest cosmetic results. Lumpectomy alone produces the best cosmetic results but shows the highest rate of local recurrence. Tylectomy, the most widely accepted breast conservation procedure, generally can be performed with acceptable cosmetic results and with satisfactory local control.

Lesions less than 2 cm in diameter that are suspected to be carcinoma and nonpalpable lesions evident on mammography can be completely excised with a margin of normal tissue as a diagnostic biopsy. To ensure adequate examination of the margins, the entire tissue block should be inked and oriented before the specimen is incised by the pathologist. If the status of the margins is unclear, or if tumor is present at the resection margin, the entire biopsy site, including the scar, must be excised with a margin of normal tissue. To achieve satisfactory local control of invasive carcinoma, radiation therapy is given after breast conservation therapy.

Indications

For patients with established stage I or stage II breast carcinoma, tylectomy followed by radiation therapy is acceptable therapy, provided that resection margins free of disease can be obtained with satisfactory cosmetic result. Tylectomy is also indicated for the removal of small, nonpalpable, mammographically visualized lesions suspected to be carcinoma (see also Chapter 6, "Needle Localization Biopsy") and for the removal of palpable indeterminate masses.

Contraindications

At present breast conservation surgery is not performed for the patient with a large breast carcinoma, a multicentric or recurrent carcinoma, or a locally advanced carcinoma. Tylectomy is contraindicated in the treatment of patients with tumor adherent to the pectoralis major fascia or with tumor extending into the pectoralis major muscle. Tylectomy without adjuvant radiation therapy is inadequate treatment for invasive breast cancer. Therefore the inability to provide radiation therapy and the anticipated lack of patient compliance with radiation treatment are relative contraindications to tylectomy. In these situations a total mastectomy with axillary dissection is preferable.

Complications

Hematoma and wound infection are the early complications of tylectomy. Both can delay initiation of postoperative radiation therapy and adjuvant chemotherapy. Inadequate excision of a malignant tumor can result in persistent disease or local recurrence. Poor cosmetic results may occur in patients who have a large tumor in a small breast or in patients who have had repeated biopsies for benign disease before tylectomy.

Preoperative Preparation

A diagnostic biopsy may be planned as a tylectomy for the patient with a lesion that is suspect but who has not undergone a previous biopsy and who does not have a tissue diagnosis of carcinoma. In this setting the size of the palpable lesion or the approximate extent and location of the nonpalpable mammographic lesion determine the amount of tissue resection required for an adequate tylectomy procedure. If a diagnosis of invasive carcinoma is established intraoperatively, an axillary dissection may be performed.

For patients with an established diagnosis of carcinoma, tylectomy can be planned as the definitive surgical procedure, followed by adjuvant radiation therapy postoperatively. The radiotherapist should see the patient preoperatively. Tylectomy alone may be performed as an outpatient procedure; when it is performed with an axillary dissection, a postoperative hospital stay of several days is usually required.

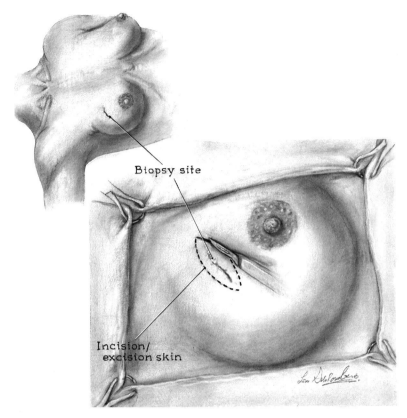

Fig 12-1.   Patient positioning; orientation of the tylectomy incision.

Although breast conservation procedures can be performed under local anesthesia, general anesthesia is often preferable and is always used when an axillary dissection is performed concurrently.

OPERATIVE PROCEDURE

Patient Positioning; Orientation of the Tylectomy Incision
(Figure 12-1)

This and subsequent figures demonstrate the tylectomy procedure in a patient with the diagnosis of carcinoma previously established by open biopsy. In the figures shown the diagnostic biopsy was performed several days before tylectomy. When a tylectomy is performed immediately following a diagnostic biopsy or shortly thereafter, a sterile adhesive dressing that fully occludes the biopsy site should be placed before the start of the procedure. This avoids contamination of the tylectomy incision by malignant cells extruded through the biopsy incision. The patient is placed on the operating table in a supine position. After general anesthesia has been satisfactorily induced, the breast, anterior chest wall, and axillary area are prepared and draped. The arm is prepared and draped in the operative field when an axillary dissection is anticipated. Otherwise, depending on the findings at frozen section, the operative field may be prepared and redraped and an axillary dissection performed after the carcinoma has been removed. An elliptical incision, fully encompassing the previous biopsy site, is oriented in a circumareolar or linear manner without compromising the adequacy of

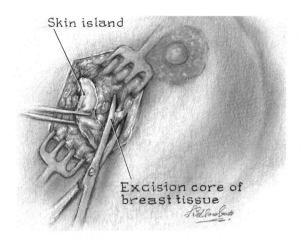

Skin island

Excision core of breast tissue

Fig 12-2. Tissue dissection.

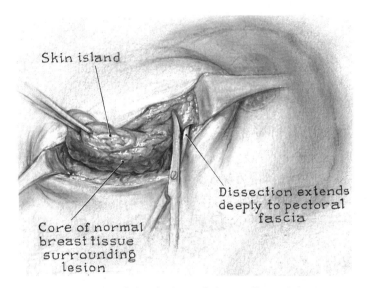

Skin island

Dissection extends deeply to pectoral fascia

Core of normal breast tissue surrounding lesion

Fig 12-3. Completion of tissue dissection.

the resection margins. Skin excision is required when a biopsy was previously performed or if the malignancy is located superficially. However, skin excision may not be necessary when tylectomy is performed as the initial biopsy procedure for a lesion deep in the breast.

Tissue Dissection (Figure 12-2)

The central core of tissue is grasped with a forceps, and retractors are placed at the skin margins. A malignancy that has previously undergone biopsy must be reexcised through unviolated, normal breast parenchyma so that the biopsy cavity and biopsy scar are removed en bloc, without entering the previous operative field. Macroscopic residual disease at the resection margin requires wound closure and resection of a wider block of tissue after the breast is reprepared and redraped and after new instruments are obtained to avoid contamination. If adequate resection is not feasible, the patient will require a total mastectomy for local tumor control.

70

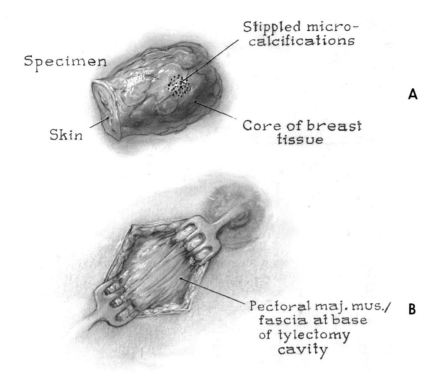

Fig 12-4. Excised specimen and wound closure.
Continued.

Completion of Tissue Dissection (Figure 12-3)

The breast tissue is sharply excised circumferentially, ensuring that the deepest margin is well beyond the tumor mass. This dissection may extend to the pectoralis major fascia. The tissue removed is sent to the pathologist after the specimen's deep margin has been marked with a suture (if necessary) so that it can be properly oriented. Depending on the preference of the radiotherapist, clips may be placed at the margins of resection to aid in planning radiation ports.

Excised Specimen and Wound Closure (Figure 12-4)

Figure 12-4, *A*, shows the appearance of a tissue block for a tylectomy performed after an open, incisional biopsy has been done to establish the diagnosis of carcinoma. The amount of tissue resected during a tylectomy varies considerably, depending on the clinical situation. The skin island shown here remains attached to the underlying breast tissue, and a margin of normal breast parenchyma fully surrounds the residual palpable mass and associated stippled microcalcifications. The specimen is sent immediately to the pathologist for inking of margins and preservation of part of the specimen for hormone receptors. The remainder of the specimen is processed for permanent sectioning. Frozen sectioning may be performed to evaluate the margins.

Figure 12-4, *B*, shows the appearance of the operative field following removal of the specimen. The tylectomy may extend to the pectoralis major fascia for removal of a lesion or a biopsy cavity deep in the breast. The site is copiously irrigated, and hemostasis is achieved. Drainage of the wound is not required.

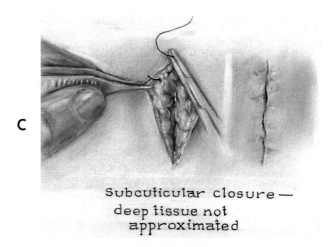

C

Subcuticular closure —
deep tissue not
approximated

Fig 12-4. Excised specimen and wound closure.

Deep sutures to reapproximate the breast tissue are unnecessary and may distort the contour of the breast. As shown in Figure 12-4, C, the skin is closed with a subcuticular technique, thus avoiding skin suture marks. If an axillary dissection is to be performed, the patient is appropriately draped and a separate incision is made. This procedure is discussed in detail in Chapter 14.

Postoperative Management

Patients may remain in the hospital for 2 or 3 days postoperatively if a concurrent axillary dissection is performed. For the patient undergoing tylectomy alone, outpatient surgery with same-day discharge is usually appropriate, unless an extensive tissue resection was performed. Patients should be advised postoperatively to wear an elastic sports brassiere 24 hours a day for the first few days to relieve discomfort and tension on the wound. Normal activities generally can be resumed the day after the procedure. Planned adjuvant radiation therapy and chemotherapy (if required) can usually be initiated within 2 to 3 weeks of surgery, when satisfactory wound healing is evident and if the final pathology report has confirmed that the tylectomy resection margins are free of tumor.

13

Iridium Needle Implant

Introduction

Postoperative irradiation to the breast following tylectomy consists of a 5- to 6-week course of external beam irradiation to the entire breast, with an additional boost of radiation to the excision site. The irradiation boost can be administered by external beam electrons produced by a linear accelerator or by temporary brachytherapy. Factors important in determining which type of irradiation boost to use include the total irradiation dose required (dependent on the size of the primary tumor and the status of the resection margins), the effects on normal tissue, local control of tumor growth, cost, and length of treatment.

The rationale for the use of electrons for boost treatment is that linear accelerators can produce electrons of various discrete energies. Because depth of penetration of electrons is energy dependent, this technique permits the delivery of irradiation to specific sites with concomitant sparing of normal tissues, such as the lungs and the heart. The electron therapy is delivered on an outpatient basis in five to ten treatments. Electron therapy is not uniformly available. The alternative method of treatment is temporary interstitial radioactive implants. Interstitial radioactive implants usually employ iridium-192 as the radioactive source. In most locations iridium-192 is available within 24 to 48 hours. Interstitial implants can deliver a defined dose of radiation therapy to a specific site, sparing the normal breast tissue. Time duration for implants ranges from 24 to 48 hours.

When tylectomy and iridium implantation are performed as a combined procedure, the hospitalization is usually not prolonged. This combined procedure is less expensive to the patient because it precludes a second hospitalization.

Indications

The use of interstitial iridium implants is generally limited to patients with stage I or stage II disease who have undergone tylectomy for removal of a primary breast carcinoma. The patient with a lesion deep in the breast parenchyma may be particularly well suited to receive boost treatment following tylectomy with interstitial implants rather than with external beam electrons.

73

Contraindications

This procedure is contraindicated in patients who are not candidates for conservative breast surgery, such as those with advanced malignancies or those with multicentric disease.

Complications

Complications associated with iridium needle implantation are minimal. Bleeding may occur at the sites of trocar placement, but it is usually self-limiting. Infection at the tylectomy incision or at the iridium implant sites usually responds to wound care and antibiotics. A specific complication of interstitial irradiation is the development of pneumonitis, which may occur when implants are placed deep in the breast parenchyma near the chest wall. A late complication of interstitial irradiation is subcutaneous fibrosis, which may be associated with a cosmetic deformity. Rib fractures in the proximity of the radiation field rarely occur.

Preoperative Preparation

Patients who undergo breast conservation surgery should have a preoperative consultation with the radiotherapist. General anesthesia is used for the procedure.

OPERATIVE PROCEDURE

Placement of the Iridium Needle Implant

Trocar Placement (Figure 13-1)

In Figures 13-1 to 13-5 the procedure for placement of a single row of implants is illustrated. When more than one row of implants will be used, all rows of trocars should be placed before any plastic tubing is advanced.

Iridium implant placement is generally performed immediately after the tylectomy is completed. The skin of the tylectomy incision is closed, and the patient remains under general anesthesia in the supine position. The entrance and exit sites for trocar placement are marked at 1.5-cm intervals on each side of the tylectomy incision so that the trocars will lie in a plane parallel to the chest wall. Hollow stainless steel trocars (16 gauge) are inserted into the breast at the entrance points and passed through the breast tissue to lie at the deepest margin of the tylectomy wound. They then are brought out through the skin on the opposite side of the tylectomy incision at the previously marked sites. These steps are repeated until all the trocars have been placed.

Advancement of Tubing through Trocars (Figure 13-2)

The trocars are sequentially replaced by lengths of hollow plastic tubing. Each plastic tube is firmly attached to a thin, solid plastic lead line. The diameter of the hollow plastic tube is slightly larger than the diameter of the trocar. In addition, the "stop," a slightly wider, solid section of plastic

74

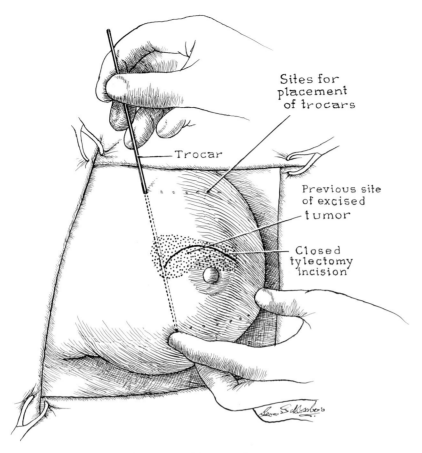

Fig 13-1.   Trocar placement.

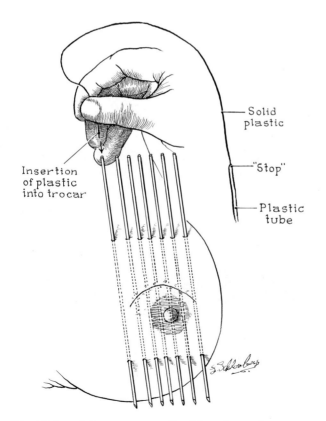

Fig 13-2.   Advancement of tubing through trocars.

between the lead line and the hollow tubing (shown here), ensures proper positioning of the hollow tubing at the blunt end of the trocar while preventing inadvertent advancement of the hollow tubing into the trocar, which could result in shearing.

The solid plastic lead is inserted, advanced completely through the trocar, and pulled out beyond the trocar, until the "stop" is properly positioned against the blunt end of the trocar. It is important that the lead be advanced through the blunt end, rather than the sharp end, of the trocar to avoid shearing the plastic components.

Tubing Advancement into Breast; Trocar Removal (Figure 13-3)

As shown in Figure 13-3, A, the plastic lead has been advanced through the trocar so that the position of the "stop" is maintained at the blunt end of the trocar. Traction is then maintained on the lead line so that, as the trocar is removed, the stop remains flush with the blunt end of the trocar. This will ensure that the hollow tubing will be properly positioned after the trocar has been completely removed, as shown in Figure 13-3, B. Each trocar is replaced by hollow tubing in the same manner.

Tubing Secured in Breast (Figure 13-4)

The tubing is secured at the distal end by crimping metal holders over the tubing at the skin surface, thus occluding the hollow tubing. The excess tubing beyond the crimped metal holders then can be cut off and discarded. At the proximal end the extra lengths of tubing outside the breast are left long to facilitate insertion of the radioactive iridium "ribbons." The positions of the hollow tubing are secured by metal holders placed over each length of tubing and secured to the skin.

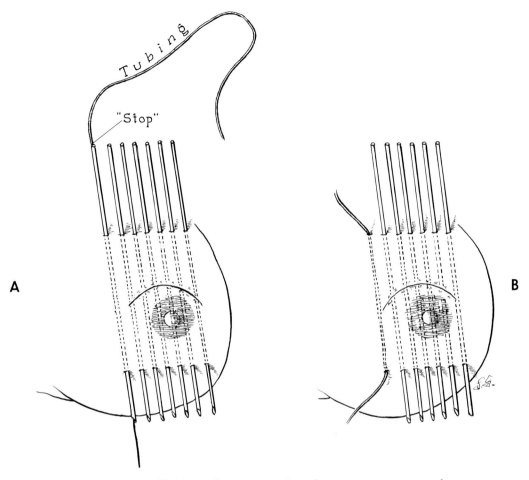

Fig 13-3. Tubing advancement into breast; trocar removal.

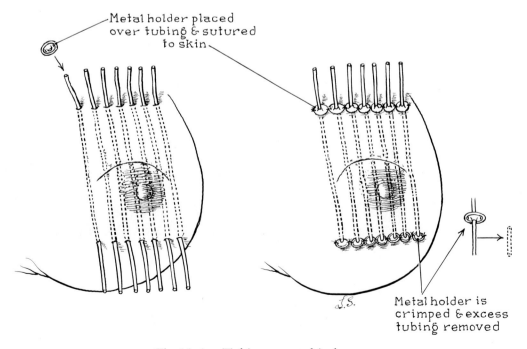

Fig 13-4. Tubing secured in breast.

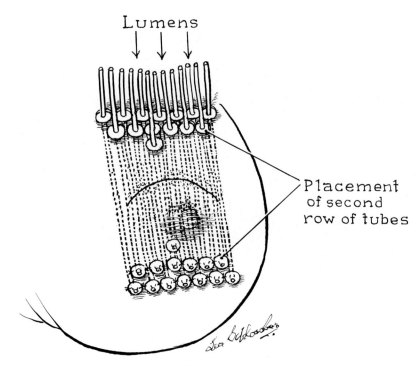

Fig 13-5.   Appearance of breast at completion of procedure.

Appearance of Breast at Completion of Procedure (Figure 13-5)

Multiple rows of tubing may be placed, depending on the location, the configuration, the size of the primary tumor, and the extent of tissue resection that was necessary for an adequate tylectomy. All of the tubing has been crimped inferiorly. In the superior portion of the breast the lumens of the hollow tubing remain patent, with the metal holders in place to secure their positions.

Postoperative Care

Following recovery from anesthesia, the patient is transferred to the radiation oncology department, where localized x-ray examinations are performed for computer isodose planning. The patient then is transferred to a private hospital room. The radioactive iridium is maintained in individual plastic "ribbons." Each ribbon length is determined from the localization x-ray examinations. These ribbons are inserted into the plastic tubing and secured by the metallic buttons. Placement of the ribbons into the patient's breast is usually performed 24 hours after the tylectomy and implant procedures. The implants remain in place for 24 to 48 hours depending on the irradiation dose needed. The implants are removed in the patient's hospital room following administration of a mild sedative.

14

Axillary Dissection

Introduction

Axillary dissection involves removal of the fatty tissue and lymph nodes from the axillary space. Usually 20 to 30 lymph nodes are present in the specimen. The node-bearing tissue within the axilla is divided into three levels. Level I lymph nodes are located in the tissue between the latissimus dorsi and the pectoralis minor muscle. Level II nodes are located beneath the pectoralis minor muscle, and Level III nodes are located medial to the pectoralis minor muscle. Level III nodes are generally accessible only by removing the pectoralis minor muscle or by dividing its tendinous insertion on the coracoid process. For patients with invasive carcinoma, who have no palpable axillary adenopathy, removal of level I and level II nodes is generally sufficient for accurate pathologic staging. This type of axillary dissection procedure is illustrated in this chapter. A more extensive axillary dissection, with removal of the pectoralis minor muscle and lymph nodes from levels I, II, and III, is routinely performed as part of the Patey modified radical mastectomy procedure and is illustrated in Chapter 16, "Modified Radical Mastectomy."

Axillary dissection may be performed immediately following tylectomy, using a separate incision. Axillary dissection may also be performed as a separate procedure. Often this is done when a satisfactory breast conservation procedure was accomplished at the time of diagnostic excisional biopsy of a small invasive carcinoma. Occasionally, a total mastectomy alone is performed for invasive carcinoma, and the axillary dissection is subsequently performed for staging purposes.

Indications

Axillary dissection is indicated in the primary management of women with stage I or stage II invasive breast carcinoma. The presence and extent of axillary nodal involvement have major prognostic significance in patients with breast carcinoma. Axillary nodal status also influences the need for adjuvant systemic chemotherapy.

Contraindications

Axillary dissection is often not necessary for women with stage 0 breast carcinoma because the incidence of axillary node involvement with in situ carcinoma is very low. Axillary dissection is also not routinely performed in patients with nonepithelial malignancies of the breast because a greater propensity for hematogenous rather than for lymphatic dissemination is present. However, axillary dissection may be indicated when clinically positive nodes are present.

Complications

Bleeding occurs infrequently and is usually caused by inadequate ligation of a branch of the axillary vein. Occasionally, reexploration is required to control bleeding and to evacuate a hematoma. Formation of a seroma is usually prevented by drain placement. Wound infection is infrequent and usually resolves satisfactorily with local wound care and systemic antibiotic therapy. Lymphedema is uncommon unless an extensive axillary dissection, including level III nodes, is performed or unless the axilla is irradiated postoperatively.

Three nerves are at particular risk for injury during the course of an axillary dissection. The intercostobrachial nerve traverses the axillary space and is often divided in the course of the axillary dissection. The resultant paresthesia in the medial aspect of the upper arm and the axilla is permanent. Division of the thoracodorsal nerve, with its associated vascular pedicle, generally precludes subsequent use of the latissimus dorsi muscle as a myocutaneous flap for breast reconstruction; however, the resulting functional deficit from division of this nerve is minimal. Division of the long thoracic nerve is a serious complication of axillary dissection because it produces a winged scapula, which is associated with significant cosmetic and functional deficits.

Preoperative Preparation

Appropriate selection of candidates for breast conservation surgery, which includes tylectomy and axillary dissection, is necessary to ensure satisfactory long-term therapeutic results. Careful clinical staging will avoid the inappropriate treatment of patients with locally advanced or metastatic breast carcinoma. The axillary dissection is performed on an inpatient basis, and general anesthesia is necessary.

OPERATIVE PROCEDURE

Incision Placement; Flap Development (Figure 14-1)

After general anesthesia is induced, the entire arm and shoulder are cleansed and draped in the sterile field so that the arm can be moved at the shoulder during the axillary dissection to facilitate exposure of the apex of the axilla.

Axillary dissection may be performed through a transverse or an oblique incision, as shown on the inset. The transverse incision starts just posterior to the anterior axillary fold and extends across the axilla to the posterior axillary fold. This incision provides excellent exposure and a minimally

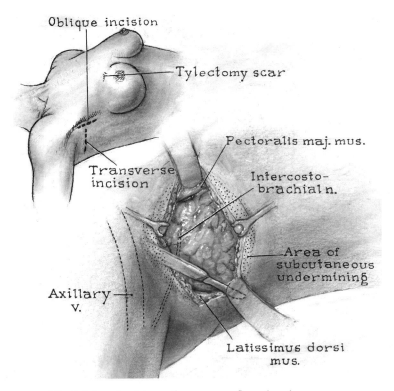

Oblique incision

Tylectomy scar

Pectoralis maj. mus.

Transverse incision

Intercosto-brachial n.

Area of subcutaneous undermining

Axillary V.

Latissimus dorsi mus.

Fig 14-1. Incision placement; flap development.

visible scar. Alternatively, an oblique incision parallel and just lateral to the edge of the pectoralis major muscle may be used. This incision also provides good exposure.

The incision is extended through the subcutaneous tissue to identify the lateral border of the pectoralis major muscle at the anterior aspect of the incision. Skin flaps (indicated by stippling) with a thin layer of subcutaneous tissue are raised by sharp dissection. The anterior border of the latissimus dorsi is identified through the extent of the operative field, superiorly to the level of the axillary vein and inferiorly for a few centimeters below the level of the skin incision. The latissimus dorsi muscle can be difficult to identify in obese patients because it is often small and underdeveloped. A large subcutaneous flap can be inadvertently raised by tunneling posteriorly in a plane superficial to the muscle when attempting to expose it. Palpation of the subcutaneous tissue lateral to the axilla may aid in the muscle's identification. The anterior border of the latissimus dorsi muscle is the lateral extent of the dissection. The intercostobrachial nerve traverses the axillary space superficially (shown here by the dashed lines). Whenever possible, this nerve should be preserved by skeletonizing it from the surrounding fatty tissue.

Exposure of Axillary Vein; Dissection of Apex of Axilla
(Figure 14-2)

The intercostobrachial nerve is shown here intact as it traverses the axillary space, fully freed from the axillary tissue. The axillary vein is identified posterior and lateral to the pectoralis major muscle. The clavipectoral fascia is exposed and then sharply incised along with the axillary sheath, as

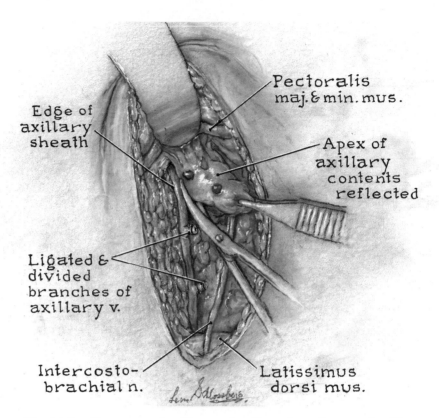

Fig 14-2. Exposure of axillary vein; dissection of apex of axilla.

it lies over the vein. The inferior border of the axillary vein forms the superior margin of the axillary dissection, and further exposure of the vein or dissection superior to it is unnecessary. The pectoralis major muscle and the underlying pectoralis minor muscle may be gently retracted medially to further expose the axillary vein. The arm can be abducted at the shoulder if necessary to facilitate exposure of the apex of the axillary dissection. The medial pectoral nerve (not shown here), along the border of the pectoralis minor muscle, may be visible and should be preserved. The interpectoral (Rotter's) nodes are not routinely included in an axillary dissection but could be included in the specimen by elevation of the pectoralis major muscle and by removal of the fatty tissue between the pectoral muscles. The fatty tissue in the axilla is cleared, starting superiorly at the most medial point of exposure of the axillary vein. The en bloc contents of the axilla are retracted laterally and inferiorly. Sharp dissection is initially used to clear the axillary vein inferiorly. The most superomedial axillary tissue is freed from the surrounding structures. If electrocautery is used, it must be done cautiously to avoid inadvertent nerve damage. The dissection along the axillary vein starts medially at the undersurface of the pectoral muscles and progresses laterally to the latissimus dorsi. The tissue at the apex of the dissection can be tagged with a suture as it is freed and is then gently retracted inferiorly and laterally. The numerous small branches of the axillary vein are ligated and divided as they are encountered. Ligation of visible lymphatic channels as they are identified may decrease lymphatic drainage postoperatively.

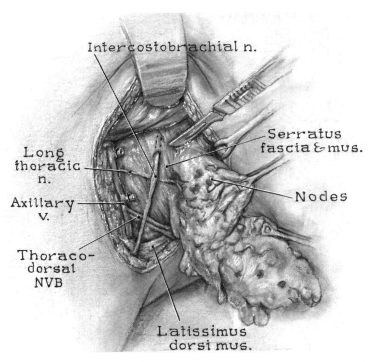

Intercostobrachial n.

Serratus
fascia & mus.

Long
thoracic
n.

Nodes

Axillary
V.

Thoraco-
dorsal
NVB

Latissimus
dorsi mus.

Fig 14-3. Identification and preservation of long thoracic nerve and thoraco-dorsal neurovascular bundle.

Identification and Preservation of the Long Thoracic Nerve and Thoracodorsal Neurovascular Bundle (Figure 14-3)

As the inferior border of the axillary vein is cleared, the long thoracic nerve, which lies posterior to the axillary vein, can be identified as it travels along the surface of the serratus anterior muscle. The nerve lies on the chest wall, and its early identification is facilitated by starting the dissection medially and progressing laterally. It is essential to take every precaution to preserve the long thoracic nerve. This is safely done by blunt dissection or cautious, sharp division of tissue that is posterior to the axillary vein. The nerve is located posterior to the point at which the intercostobrachial nerve exits the second interspace. After the long thoracic nerve is exposed, it is carefully protected for the remainder of the dissection. If necessary, it may be gently stimulated to confirm its identity. Repeated stimulation of the nerve is unnecessary and should be avoided. Lateral to the long thoracic nerve, additional tributaries to the axillary vein are ligated and divided as the inferior border of the axillary vein is cleared by a continued gentle inferior retraction of the tissue specimen.

The thoracodorsal nerve is identified as it courses with the thoracodorsal vessels in the axilla. This neurovascular bundle (NVB) should be skeletonized from the surrounding fatty tissue by sharp dissection. Occasionally the vessels or nerve may be ligated and divided if they are bound by bulky nodal disease; however, this usually is not necessary. The anterior border of the latissimus dorsi muscle is then fully exposed to the inferior margin of the operative field. After the inferior border of the axillary vein has been cleared along to

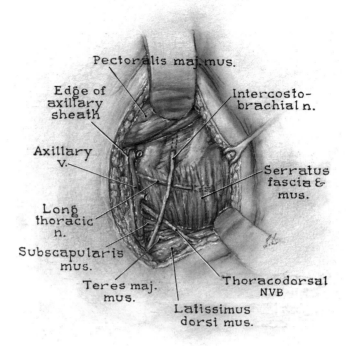

Fig 14-4.   Operative field after specimen removal.

the latissimus dorsi, the axillary contents are excised en bloc and freed from the floor of the axilla. The contents are dissected inferiorly to the lower margins of the operative field.

Operative Field After Specimen Removal (Figure 14-4)

The appearance of the operative field after removal of the specimen is shown here. The serratus anterior, with the long thoracic nerve coursing along its surface, forms the medial border of the axillary space. The skeletonized thoracodorsal nerve and vessels, as well as the intercostobrachial nerve, are clearly visualized. The underlying muscles, forming the floor of the axillary space, have been cleared of the node-bearing fatty tissue. The floor of the axillary space is formed predominantly by the teres major and subscapularis muscles. The wound is copiously irrigated with saline solution, and hemostasis is achieved with electrocautery, taking care to protect the preserved nerves.

Wound Closure (Figure 14-5)

A single, closed suction drain is placed in the axilla and brought out through a small stab wound in the skin. It is secured with a suture at its point of exit. The incision is closed in two layers, with the subcutaneous tissue reapproximated with interrupted absorbable sutures. The skin is closed with a running subcuticular suture. After adhesive strips are applied to the incision, the wound is covered with a dry gauze dressing.

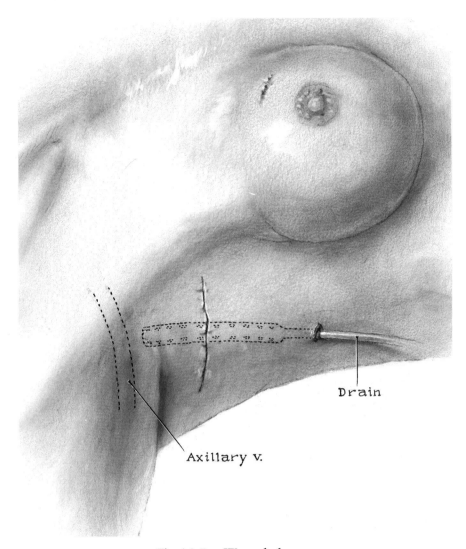

Fig 14-5. Wound closure.

Postoperative Care

The patient may be discharged from the hospital when she has recovered from the anesthetic and is able to ambulate and care for the drain. The drain is left in place until drainage decreases to less than 30 ml in 24 hours. Shoulder mobilization is started a few days after surgery and increased gradually as tolerated. There are no other specific activity limitations; however, all patients must be informed of appropriate precautions to prevent the development of lymphedema.

15

Total Mastectomy

Introduction

Total mastectomy is defined as removal of the breast with or without the underlying pectoralis major fascia. Because the lateral extent of the breast (tail of Spence) extends into the axillary space, a few level I axillary lymph nodes are often incorporated in the excised specimen. However, an axillary dissection is not part of the total mastectomy procedure.

Indications

Selected patients with intraductal carcinoma may be candidates for total mastectomy without axillary dissection because the incidence of axillary nodal metastases in these patients is less than 5%. Total mastectomy is also performed as palliative treatment in the patient with a large breast carcinoma that is associated with skin ulceration, pain, or extensive necrosis. A split-thickness skin graft is often required to close the wound.

Total mastectomy is also employed for a variety of relatively uncommon nonepithelial neoplasms. Primary sarcomas of the breast, low-grade (cystosarcoma phyllodes) and high grade (invasive sarcomas), are treated by total mastectomy if the tumor is not fixed to the underlying chest wall or the pectoralis fascia and muscle. Soft-tissue sarcomas metastasize primarily by hematogenous rather than by lymphatic routes; therefore axillary dissection is unnecessary if no palpable axillary adenopathy is present. A variety of rare lesions of the breast, both neoplastic (melanoma; dermatofibrosarcoma protuberans; lymphoma) and inflammatory (actinomycosis; tuberculosis, with chronic abscess and fistula formation) can also be effectively managed by total mastectomy.

Bilateral total mastectomies, with removal of the nipples and areolae, may be performed prophylactically in selected women at high risk for breast carcinoma. In this setting a total mastectomy is especially preferable to a subcutaneous mastectomy for the woman with a distorted nipple-areolar complex, major ptotic changes in the breast, or multiple scars that may impede circulation in the skin following subcutaneous mastectomy. The role of prophylactic surgery for breast carcinoma is discussed in Chapter 11.

Contraindications

Contraindications to the performance of a total mastectomy include fixation of the tumor to the pectoralis major muscle or fascia (these malignancies are best managed by radical mastectomy) or fixation of the tumor to the underlying chest wall (these malignancies are best managed by chest wall resection and radiation therapy). A relative contraindication to total mastectomy is neoplastic invasion of adjacent structures so that residual gross disease would remain following mastectomy. Occasionally, however, total mastectomy to debulk the malignancy is combined with other non-surgical forms of locoregional therapy (usually irradiation).

Complications

Total mastectomy as a palliative debulking procedure is often complicated by wound infection or dehiscence. However, the incidence of infection with this procedure in otherwise healthy patients is low. Bleeding from the flaps or chest wall postoperatively is uncommon.

Preoperative Preparation

Total mastectomy is performed under general anesthesia; however, in exceptional cases, when a severely debilitated patient requires a palliative mastectomy, local anesthesia with sedation may be used. Blood loss requiring transfusion is rare. Patients considering breast reconstruction are referred for plastic surgical consultation preoperatively.

OPERATIVE PROCEDURE

Incision Placement and Flap Development for Total Mastectomy
(Figure 15-1)

The patient is placed on the operating table in the supine position, with the arm abducted. After induction with general anesthesia, the operative field, including the region bounded by the supraclavicular fossa superiorly, the sternum medially, the costal margin inferiorly, and the posterior axillary fold laterally, is prepared and draped. Although axillary dissection is not performed, exposure for total mastectomy is facilitated by prepping and draping the entire axillary region and enclosing the arm in a sterile sheath. If a split-thickness skin graft is to be used, a donor site is sterilized and draped. When performing a skin graft, the operating surgeons must use fresh gowns and gloves, and the instruments must be separate from those used during the mastectomy to avoid inadvertent contamination of the graft donor site with breast carcinoma cells.

The inset shows the optimal placement of the incision for a total mastectomy (in this case with a tumor in the upper inner quadrant of the left breast). Skin incisions are placed in a transverse direction if possible to encompass an ellipse of skin with the nipple-areolar complex and a previous biopsy site (if present), with a 2- to 5-cm circumferential margin of normal

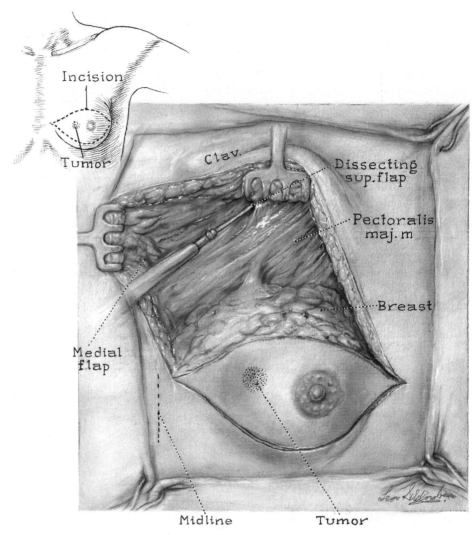

Fig 15-1. Incision placement; flap development.

skin. A transversely oriented, elliptical incision provides the best cosmetic result, with a scar on the chest wall well below the axilla. This incision is modified and extended as necessary to include any additional skin involved by tumor. If an incompletely healed biopsy incision is present, contamination with malignant cells can be avoided if the incision site is covered with an adhesive dressing before the mastectomy procedure is begun.

Skin flaps are developed in the subcutaneous planes superiorly to the clavicle and inferiorly to the upper border of the rectus abdominis muscle. The flaps are developed medially to the midline and laterally to the anterior border of the latissimus dorsi muscle. The flaps should be the same thickness and should be raised by sharp dissection with the scalpel or with the electrocautery. The assistant firmly retracts the upper skin flap with face lift retractors, and the operating surgeon retracts the breast tissue inferiorly. This facilitates identification of the appropriate plane for flap dissection, which is in the subcutaneous tissue immediately superficial to the fine layer of fascia overlying the breast. Periodically during the dissection the surgeon should palpate the developing flap to ensure that it is of proper and uniform thickness.

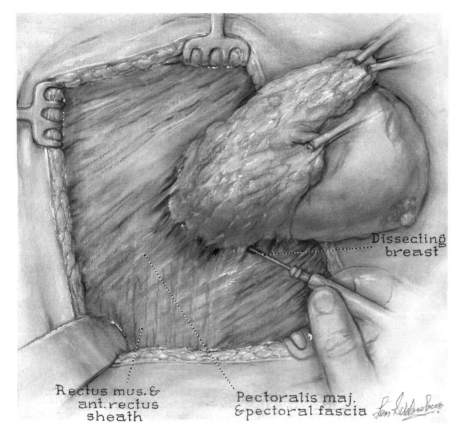

Fig 15-2. Dissection of breast from underlying chest wall musculature.

Dissection of Breast from Underlying Chest Wall Musculature
(Figure 15-2)

After developing the flaps, the entire breast is dissected free from the chest wall. Starting medially (when the mastectomy is performed for malignant disease), a plane is developed deep to the fascia of the pectoralis major muscle. Perforating branches of the internal mammary artery emerging through the underlying muscle must be carefully ligated on the chest wall before division. When performing a total mastectomy for nonmalignant disease, the surgeon may elect to develop a deep plane of dissection between the breast parenchyma and the superficial pectoral fascia (as shown), leaving the fascia in place overlying the muscle. This fascial layer facilitates alloplastic breast reconstuction.

The dissection proceeds laterally, and as the lateral border of the pectoralis major muscle is approached, the insertions of the serratus anterior muscle are identified and the dissection continues superficial to this plane. Caution must be exercised as the surgeon can inadvertently develop a plane deep to the superficial attachments of the serratus anterior muscle at this step in the procedure.

The dissection proceeds posteriorly and laterally into the axilla to the anterior border of the latissimus dorsi muscle. Then the dissection proceeds superiorly in the axilla to the inferolateral margin of the pectoralis minor muscle. In order to fully remove the axillary tail of Spence, the dissection must include tissue in the axilla anterior to the long thoracic nerve and the thoracodorsal neurovascular bundle.

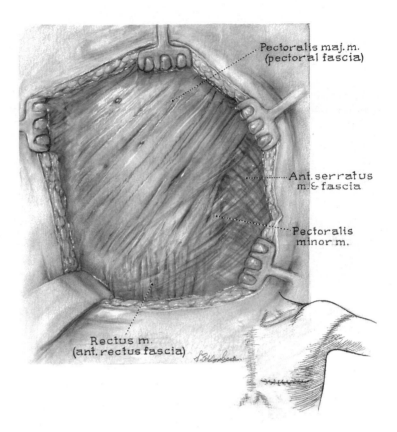

Fig 15-3.   Wound closure.

Wound Closure (Figure 15-3)

After the breast is completely removed, the wound is copiously irrigated with sterile saline solution and inspected for bleeding. The circulation to the flaps is assessed. A closed vacuum drain may be placed under the flaps and brought out through the skin in the axilla (not shown). If the skin can be primarily closed without undue tension on the flaps, this should be done with a two-layer closure. The subcutaneous tissue is reapproximated with interrupted absorbable sutures. The skin is closed with staples or with a subcuticular suture. Primary closure is feasible for most patients undergoing total mastectomy. In cases where skin grafting is required, the skin flaps are sutured to the underlying fascia and the remaining defect is covered with a split-thickness skin graft (not shown).

Postoperative Management

Following total mastectomy, patients usually may be discharged within 2 to 3 days. Activities should be advanced as tolerated. If drains have been placed, they are generally left until the 24-hour volume is less than 30 ml. For patients with locally advanced breast carcinoma, who have undergone palliative mastectomy because of the presence of an ulcerated lesion or an irradiated tissue bed, systemic antibiotics may be necessary and hospitalization may be prolonged.

16

Modified Radical Mastectomy

Introduction

The modified radical mastectomy is most often used for patients with stage I or stage II breast carcinoma. Two modified radical mastectomy procedures are used. The more commonly performed Auchincloss mastectomy consists of a total mastectomy with an axillary dissection. The Patey modified radical mastectomy consists of a total mastectomy and axillary dissection, with resection of the pectoralis minor muscle, allowing a more complete dissection of the axilla and removal of Rotter's nodes, which lie between the pectoralis major and pectoralis minor muscles. More axillary lymph nodes are removed in the Patey procedure; however, their removal brings about a greater risk of lymphedema. No data from prospective randomized controlled trials are available to indicate the superiority of one procedure over the other. The operative technique for the Patey procedure will be depicted with the Auchincloss modifications indicated in the text.

Indications

This operation is indicated in patients who have breast carcinoma confined to the breast and axilla, with no invasion of the pectoralis major muscle or fascia. Before performing a modified radical mastectomy, the surgeon should establish a tissue diagnosis of breast carcinoma and exclude the presence of distant metastases.

For patients with stage I and stage II disease, this procedure provides excellent local tumor control. For patients with locally advanced breast carcinoma (stage III), a modified radical mastectomy may be performed as part of a multimodality treatment program.

Contraindications

The presence of distant metastases precludes the performance of a modified radical mastectomy except in rare circumstances in which it may be the optimal palliative procedure. This procedure is contraindicated in patients if the carcinoma is attached to the pectoralis major fascia. Some surgeons have advocated a modified radical mastectomy with excision of an underlying wedge of fascia and muscle in such patients; however, a substantial risk exists for local recurrence. We recommend a radical mastectomy in this setting.

Complications

Hemorrhage resulting from inadequate ligation of the perforating vessels as they emerge medially through the pectoralis major muscle may require blood transfusion and reoperation. Meticulous attention to hemostasis and precise identification and ligation of these perforating vessels during the course of the procedure should minimize the likelihood of this complication. Modified radical mastectomy is associated with a low rate of wound infection. The majority of infections develop in conjunction with flap necrosis, which may result if the wound is closed with too much tension. Treatment consists of local debridement and administration of systemic antibiotics. The risk of flap necrosis can be minimized by proper incision design and by judiciously using skin grafts to cover a large defect. One of the most serious potential complications of modified radical mastectomy is injury to the long thoracic nerve, which supplies motor fibers to the serratus anterior muscle. The winged scapula deformity associated with injury to this nerve is unsightly and debilitating. It results from the inability of the serratus anterior muscle to pull the scapula forward when the patient attempts to raise the arm in front of the body. No reconstructive procedure is available to correct this deformity. The thoracodorsal and intercostobrachial nerves are also at risk of injury during axillary dissection; however, unlike the long thoracic nerve, either or both of these nerves can be sacrificed with minimal functional deficit. There are several reasons for preserving the thoracodorsal vessels and nerve. Division of the thoracodorsal nerve results in the loss of 50% of the bulk of the latissimus dorsi muscle, thus obviating its use for breast reconstruction following mastectomy. Division of the nerve and vessels also precludes subsequent use of the latissimus dorsi muscle as a flap for covering a chest wall defect. Finally, when autologous tissue reconstruction is performed, the thoracodorsal artery and vein are often the vessels of choice for anastomosis of a free flap in the chest.

The intercostobrachial nerve is frequently divided as it exits the chest wall into the axillary fat, and the resultant sensory deficit consists of paresthesia in the medial aspect of the upper arm and the axilla. An adequate axillary dissection can be difficult to perform without division of this nerve; however, the nerve should be identified and preserved when possible. The patient should always be informed preoperatively of this potential sensory deficit that may be permanent following the procedure. Brachial plexus injury following a modified radical mastectomy is usually attributable to hyperabduction of the arm at the shoulder. It is manifest most often postoperatively as an ulnar nerve palsy. Careful attention to patient positioning and arm manipulation during the procedure minimizes this risk. An unusual complication of modified radical mastectomy is lymphedema caused by the extensive disruption of normal lymphatic channels that drain the arm. Frequently this is encountered following radical mastectomy (see Chapter 17). Seroma formation, the subcutaneous accumulation of lymphatic fluid, usually can be avoided by postoperative drainage of the axillary space and chest wall skin flaps. If this complication develops after drain removal, it can be managed on an outpatient basis by repeated aspiration.

Preoperative Preparation

Patients treated for breast carcinoma must be fully informed regarding the various therapeutic possibilities. The option of immediate or delayed reconstruction should be addressed with the patient, and the opportunity for consultation with a plastic surgeon should be offered. Previous biopsy sites should be well healed. The procedure is performed with the patient under general anesthesia.

OPERATIVE PROCEDURE

Incision Placement for Modified Radical Mastectomy (Figure 16-1)

The position of the patient before beginning the skin cleansing and draping is shown. The dashed lines demarcate the planned skin incision for the mastectomy. The stippled area above and below these lines denotes the extent of the skin flaps that will be developed. The incision is usually slightly oblique, and it should be made with margins that are at least 2 cm from the edge of the previous biopsy site. Larger margins are rarely necessary and could compromise the primary closure of a planned reconstructive procedure. In this illustration, strips of adhesive are on the previous biopsy site to approximate the wound edges. The adhesive should be removed before beginning the preparation of the skin and before draping the breast. (If immediate reconstruction is to be performed, the midline of the sternum and both inframammary creases are marked while the patient is upright and before anesthetic induction.) The use of a nonparalytic agent should be discussed with the anesthesiologist. Such an agent may facilitate identification of the long thoracic nerve during the axillary dissection procedure. After general anesthesia is induced, the skin of the breast, chest wall, axilla, and adjacent neck and upper abdomen is prepared in a standard manner with the patient in a supine position. The skin of the left arm, shoulder, and posterior and lateral portion of the back should be prepared last. The arm

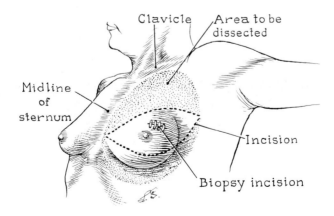

Fig 16-1. Incision placement.

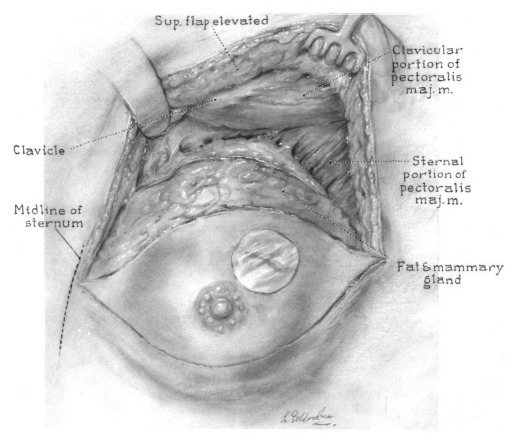

Fig 16-2. Development of the superior skin flap.

is prepared and then lowered onto a sterile field after being enclosed in a sterile drape. The arm should be left free to be maneuvered during the procedure if necessary. The arm should not be abducted beyond 90 degrees on an armboard to avoid the risk of brachial plexus injury. It is often helpful to place a rolled drape under the shoulder to elevate the upper torso and to provide better exposure to the breast and axilla. The entire prepared area then is draped in a standard fashion, and the patient is positioned for surgery. Once the operative field is completely draped, the previous biopsy site is covered with sterile adhesive drape. This can be done by cutting a disk of adhesive of sufficient size to completely cover the previous skin incision so that any fluid or cells extruded from the incision site will be contained. This prevents tumor cell seeding of the mastectomy field during manipulation of the breast.

Development of the Superior Skin Flap (Figure 16-2)

After the skin incision is made and extended through the subcutaneous tissue, the flaps are developed. In contrast to the thin flaps that were advocated in the classic Halsted radical mastectomy, most surgeons now prefer to create flaps with some residual fat and subcutaneous tissue attached. Most patients today (compared with those undergoing mastectomy in Halsted's day) have smaller carcinomas that are usually detected at an early stage, and local recurrence is a minimal risk. Furthermore, many patients are candidates for immediate or delayed reconstruction, and it is important that the skin

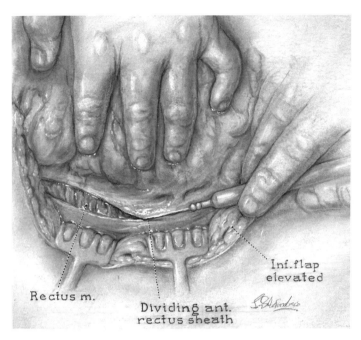

Fig 16-3. Development of the inferior skin flap.

flaps be thick enough to provide acceptable covering of a prosthesis. However, curative resection is of paramount importance throughout the procedure. Complete resection of the carcinoma must not be compromised for considerations of breast reconstruction and cosmetic appearance. Usually, the superior flap is elevated first. It is important to define the anatomically correct plane for flap dissection in the subcutaneous tissue. The absolute thickness of the flap varies among individuals, depending on body habitus and on the amount of subcutaneous fat present. However, in any given patient the flap should be of uniform thickness and include skin and subcutaneous tissue only. Blood loss is minimal when skin flaps of appropriate thickness are developed in the correct plane. Although a scalpel can be used during this part of the procedure, the electrocautery may be preferable because it provides for a drier field and a more rapid dissection of tissues. It is important that the assistant maintain steady upward traction on the skin edges as the dissection proceeds.

The superior border of the operative field is the clavicle. As this landmark is approached, the breast tissue becomes attenuated and may completely disappear, leaving a bare portion of pectoralis major fascia for a few centimeters below the clavicle. The dissection should be continued until a complete margin of pectoralis muscle and fascia borders the superior portion of the field. The pectoral fascia is incised along the upper margin of the dissection to expose the underlying pectoralis major muscle. Hemostasis is achieved, and a moist laparotomy sponge is placed between the flap and the underlying muscle.

Development of the Inferior Skin Flap (Figure 16-3)

The inferior skin incision is extended through the subcutaneous tissue until the proper plane of dissection is identified. As the plane is developed, the operating surgeon retracts the breast superiorly with one hand while dissecting the skin flap with the other. The assistant surgeon retracts the flap at a 90-degree angle from the plane of dissection to minimize the risk of the surgeon's cutting through the skin. The dissection is continued until the rectus abdominis fascia is reached. However, the breast may extend inferiorly only to overlie the fascia of the pectoralis major muscle rather than the rectus sheath. As the dissection of the inferior flap is completed, circumferential isolation of the breast tissue on the underlying fascia is nearly complete. At this point of the operation some surgeons choose to begin removing the breast tissue and fascia from the chest wall. Alternatively, the axillary dissection may be done first with subsequent removal of the breast. In the following illustrations the breast is removed first, followed by axillary dissection. The beginning of the dissection is shown in the bottom of this figure, as the fascia of the rectus abdominis muscle is divided.

Identification of the Latissimus Dorsi Muscle (Figure 16-4)

The fascia of the anterior rectus sheath is divided inferiorly, and the incision is extended laterally and superiorly over the serratus anterior muscle to the axillary region. The anterior border of the latissimus dorsi muscle is identified and cleared to the level of the superior flap dissection. Note the position of the surgeon's left hand in retracting the breast tissue superiorly and medially. Rake retractors are used to elevate both the superior and inferior flaps perpendicular to the plane of dissection when exposing the anterior border of the latissimus dorsi. The latissimus dorsi muscle may be quite small and underdeveloped, particularly in an obese woman, and if it is not identified, the subcutaneous tissue superficial and lateral to it can inadvertently be extensively undermined. Palpation of the tissue in this region is a useful way to identify the latissimus dorsi muscle when it cannot be readily visualized.

Sagittal Section of the Breast with Skin Flaps (Figure 16-5)

This sagittal view of the breast and chest wall defines the anatomy at this point of the dissection. Note the skin flaps with subcutaneous fat and the superior (clavicle) and inferior (anterior rectus sheath) margins of the dissection. The breast containing the tumor is shown with the overlying full-thickness skin lying centrally between the superior and inferior incisions. The anterior rectus sheath has been divided inferiorly, and the pectoralis fascia has been divided superiorly.

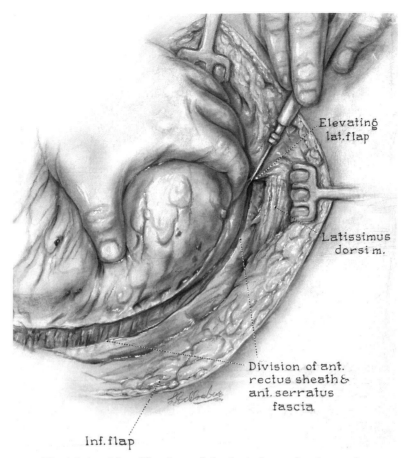

Fig 16-4.   Identification of the latissimus dorsi muscle.

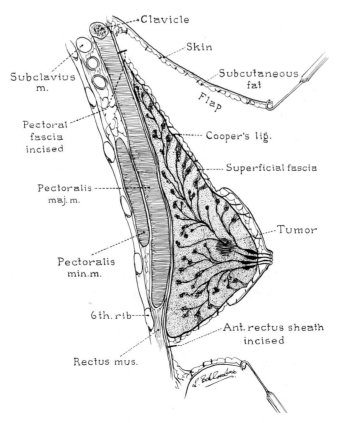

Fig 16-5.   Sagittal section of the breast with skin flaps.

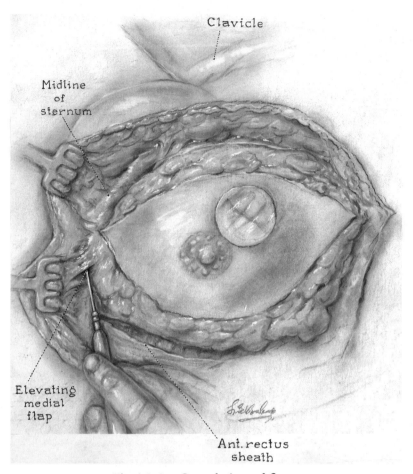

Fig 16-6.   Completion of flaps.

Completion of Flaps (Figure 16-6)

The dissection of the breast and the underlying fascia from the chest wall is begun at the most medial extent of the dissection and proceeds laterally. As the superior and inferior flaps are completed medially, the breast, with the underlying pectoralis fascia, is isolated circumferentially. Note the placement of the retractors medially and the continued use of the electrocautery as the dissection of the breast off the chest wall is started medially. Alternatively, a scalpel may be used to dissect the breast and underlying fascia from the pectoralis major muscle.

Removal of the Breast and Underlying Pectoralis Fascia from the Chest Wall (Figure 16-7)

As the dissection proceeds laterally, two or three perforating vessels in the medial part of the field must be identified, clamped, ligated, and divided. The breast and fascia are retracted laterally and dissected off the pectoralis major muscle. The breast must be kept under constant traction with the surgeon's hand or with instruments, such as the Allis clamps illustrated here. The electrocautery may be used during this part of the dissection. The surgeon must be aware of the location of the carcinoma within the breast and the proximity of the tumor, or the previous biopsy cavity, to the deep margin of the dissection. The breast is gently palpated to confirm the location of the biopsy cavity or tumor, and the adequacy of the deep resection margin

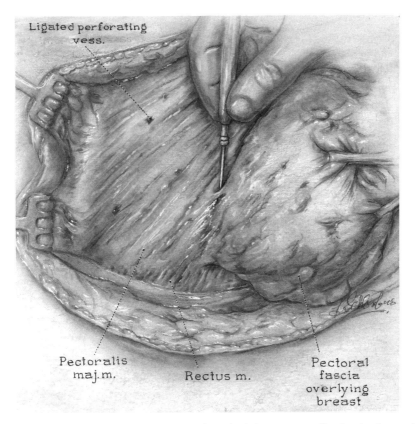

Fig 16-7. Removal of the breast and underlying pectoralis fascia from the chest wall.

is assessed. If the malignancy is cut across or the previous biopsy site entered, seeding of the wound with malignant cells may occur, with a high likelihood of tumor recurrence postoperatively. If it becomes apparent during the dissection between the pectoralis fascia and the muscle that the carcinoma is adherent to or immediately adjacent to the pectoralis fascia, the decision must be made to excise a portion of the pectoralis major muscle surrounding the carcinoma or to convert the procedure to a radical mastectomy and remove the entire pectoralis major muscle.

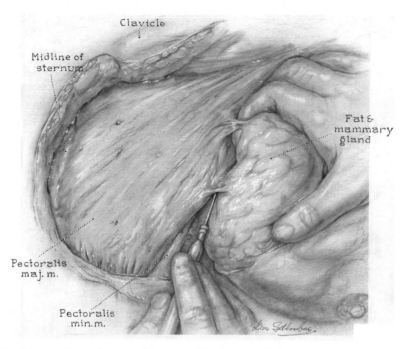

Fig 16-8. Completion of breast dissection off the anterior chest wall.

Completion of Breast Dissection off the Anterior Chest Wall (Figure 16-8)

In this figure the breast and underlying fascia have been dissected off the pectoralis major muscle to its lateral border, and the edge of the underlying pectoralis minor muscle can be seen. As the dissection of the breast off the chest wall is completed, the entire axilla becomes exposed as the surgeon continues the dissection and the assistant retracts the breast laterally. At this point in the dissection, it may not be necessary to retract the breast because it will remain laterally displaced under its weight.

Exposure and Division of the Pectoralis Minor Muscle (Figure 16-9)
(This step is omitted in the Auchincloss modified radical mastectomy)

The dissection of the axilla is the most time-consuming aspect of the modified radical mastectomy and must be done meticulously. To begin the axillary dissection, the pectoralis major muscle is retracted medially to expose the deep pectoral fascia, which is sharply incised transversely, exposing the pectoralis minor tendon and the medial pectoral neurovascular bundle (NVB). This bundle is ligated and divided distal to the origin of the branches that supply the pectoralis major muscle. The medial and lateral anterior thoracic nerves are contained in the more proximal part of this bundle and must be preserved to avoid atrophy of the pectoralis major muscle. The tendinous attachment of the pectoralis minor muscle to the coracoid is elevated by a forefinger and divided with a scalpel or with the electrocautery (shown here).

Resection of the Pectoralis Minor Muscle (Figure 16-10)
(This step is omitted in the Auchincloss modified radical mastectomy.)

The pectoralis minor muscle, containing the closely attached Rotter's lymph nodes, is retracted inferiorly and laterally. With gentle retraction the

100

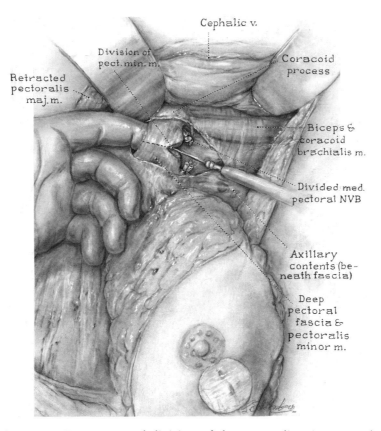

Fig 16-9. Exposure and division of the pectoralis minor muscle.

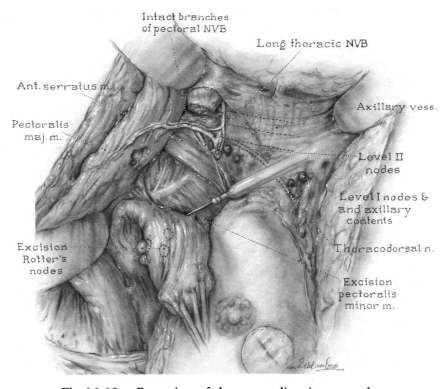

Fig 16-10. Resection of the pectoralis minor muscle.

muscle is resected from the uppermost ribs. During this step, care is taken to avoid inadvertent entry into the pleural space. This step in the procedure is especially hazardous if the patient is extremely thin. The intact branches of the medial pectoral neurovascular bundle supplying the retracted pectoralis major muscle can be seen more fully at this point. The long thoracic nerve in the superomedial aspect of the axilla close to the serratus anterior muscle also can be seen at this stage of the dissection. The relationship of the detached pectoralis minor muscle and Rotter's nodes to the associated level I and level II lymph nodes is shown.

Axillary Dissection (Figure 16-11)

(This step and the remaining description of the procedure are applicable to both the Auchincloss and the Patey modified radical mastectomies.)

The axillary vein represents the superior border of the dissection, and the resection of axillary tissue begins superomedially in the apex of the axilla and continues inferolaterally. This part of the dissection can be done with the scalpel or scissors. The soft tissue and lymph nodes inferior to the axillary vein are mobilized inferiorly and laterally. All neurovascular structures below the axillary vein are sacrificed, except for the long thoracic nerve and the thoracodorsal NVB. The identification of the long thoracic nerve can be confirmed by direct stimulation, resulting in contraction of the serratus anterior muscle. The thoracodorsal nerve (shown here) is always preserved unless it is adherent to bulky nodes. The intercostobrachial nerve is shown divided, and the medial remnant of the nerve can be seen at the inferior edge of the medial retractor of the pectoralis major muscle. However, the nerve should be skeletonized and preserved when possible, depending on the extent of its involvement with the axillary lymph node tissue.

As the dissection progresses, the fatty tissue containing the axillary lymph nodes and the breast are reflected inferiorly and the tissue block continues to serve as a natural retractor. The inferior extent of the axillary dissection is the point at which the latissimus dorsi muscle directly overlies the lateral chest wall.

Cross Section View of Patey Modified Radical Mastectomy (Figure 16-12)

This cross section of the breast and chest wall defines the anatomy at this point of the operation. From the midline in the superior portion of this figure the elevated medial skin flap is seen. The retracted pectoralis major muscle is lateral to this. In the inferior portion of the figure are the lateral skin flap and the latissimus dorsi muscle. The dissection plane is deep to the pectoralis minor muscle and continues superficial to the long thoracic nerve and the thoracodorsal nerve (along the arrows and dotted line) as the dissection is completed. The entire block of soft tissue, muscle, and lymph nodes is removed, passed from the operative field, and given to the surgical pathologist.

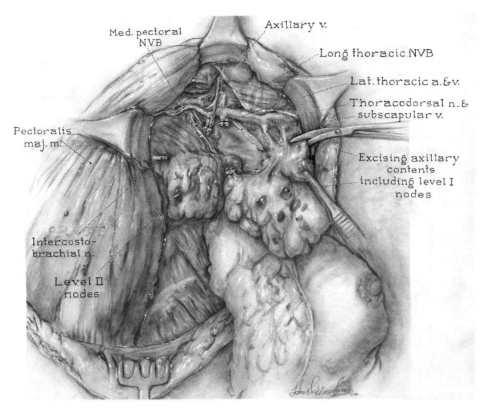

Fig 16-11. Axillary dissection.

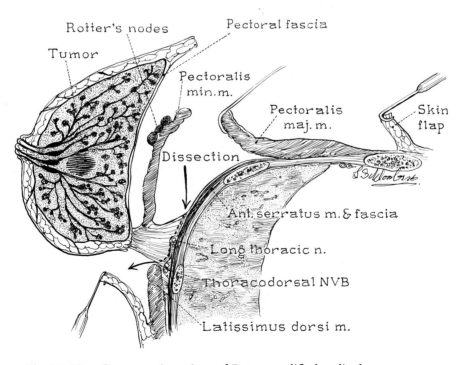

Fig 16-12. Cross section view of Patey modified radical mastectomy.

Operative Field after Completion of Mastectomy and Axillary Dissection (Figure 16-13)

The operative field is shown after the breast and soft tissue have been removed. The clavicle defines the superior margin of the resection, and the presternal fascia is shown at the most medial extent of the field. The inferior margin of the field shows the rectus abdominis muscle and its interdigitation with the pectoralis major muscle. The pectoralis major muscle spans the serratus anterior muscle as it extends superiorly to insert into the humerus. The skeletonized axillary vein and its branches, as well as the divided intercostobrachial nerve, the intact thoracodorsal neurovascular bundle, and the intact long thoracic nerve, are depicted. The subscapularis muscle, the teres major muscle, and the latissimus dorsi muscle are shown in the superolateral portion of the field, forming the posterior wall of the axillary space.

Wound Closure (Figure 16-14)

Upon completion of the procedure, the wound is irrigated and suction drains are placed under the flaps, exiting inferiorly through separate incisions in the axilla. The subcutaneous tissue is reapproximated with absorbable sutures, and the skin is then closed with a running subcuticular suture. If the skin is under excessive tension, the superior and inferior flaps can be further mobilized. Rarely, a split-thickness skin graft may be necessary for wound closure, if a large portion of the skin overlying the breast was removed. A sterile dressing is applied, and the patient is sent to the recovery room.

Postoperative Management

Following a modified radical mastectomy the suction drains are left in place until the 24-hour drainage is less than 30 ml per drain. Patients may be discharged within 3 to 4 days if the skin flaps are viable and if no infection is evident. Activities should be advanced as tolerated. If postoperative complications do not occur, chemotherapy, if indicated, can begin 2 weeks after surgery. Immediate alloplastic breast reconstruction does not prolong the hospital stay. However, autogenous tissue reconstruction may require a hospitalization of 7 to 10 days. Most patients can return to light work in 2 weeks following mastectomy, even if immediate reconstruction has been performed. The recovery time, following a modified radical mastectomy and reconstruction with an autogenous tissue flap, is typically 4 to 6 weeks.

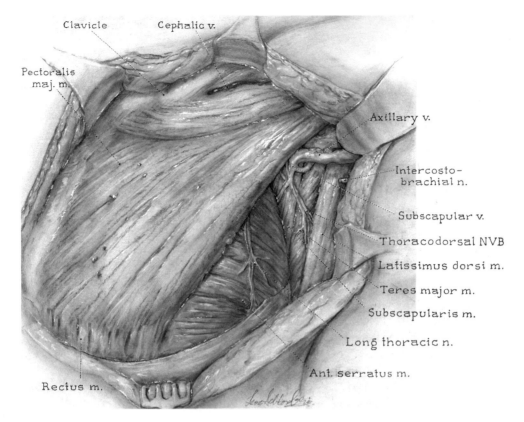

Clavicle
Cephalic v.
Pectoralis maj. m.
Axillary v.
Intercosto-brachial n.
Subscapular v.
Thoracodorsal NVB
Latissimus dorsi m.
Teres major m.
Subscapularis m.
Long thoracic n.
Ant. serratus m.
Rectus m.

Fig 16-13.   Operative field after completion of mastectomy and axillary dissection.

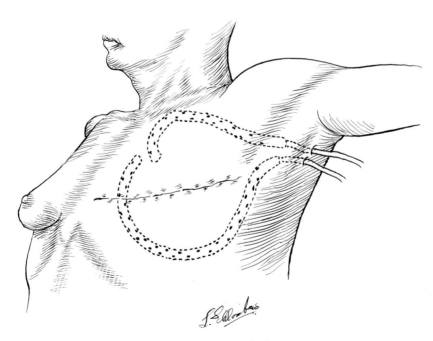

Fig 16-14.   Wound closure.

17

Radical Mastectomy

Introduction

Radical mastectomy refers to the en bloc removal of the breast and overlying skin, the pectoralis major and minor muscles, and the axillary soft tissue and lymph nodes. The operation as it is currently performed was first described by William Halsted at the end of the 19th century. It remained the standard surgical therapy for virtually all patients with breast carcinoma until 25 years ago. Since then, a greater emphasis has been placed on less radical procedures. Today most patients with breast carcinoma are treated either by tylectomy, combined with axillary dissection and regional radiation therapy, or modified radical mastectomy.

Indications

Radical mastectomy is the operation of choice for cases in which the primary tumor invades the pectoralis major muscle. Radical mastectomy is also indicated in patients with a primary tumor deep in the breast parenchyma, where the pectoralis major muscle has been penetrated during biopsy. In addition, radical mastectomy may be performed as part of multimodality therapy for selected patients with stage III breast carcinoma, following induction chemotherapy.

Contraindications

Radical mastectomy is contraindicated in patients with distant metastatic disease. In addition, the presence of skin ulceration, peau d'orange, fixed axillary nodes, or invasion of the underlying chest wall by tumor indicate locally advanced disease that is incurable by surgery.

Complications

Perioperative complications include hemorrhage, pneumothorax, flap necrosis, wound infection, nerve injury, and lymphedema. Significant hemorrhage requiring transfusion and, in some cases, reexploration can result from incomplete identification and ligation of perforating vessels on the chest wall. Occasionally, a hematoma may develop under the skin flap or in the axillary space and require reexploration for evacuation. Pneumothorax is an uncommon complication that should be considered in any patient who has undergone a radical mastectomy and who develops symptoms of respiratory insufficiency. This is usually seen in thin women with poorly developed chest wall musculature. It results from inadvertent laceration of the parietal plura during dissection of the pectoralis major muscle off the chest wall. Wound infection is uncommon following radical mastectomy. Infection is usually caused by staphylococcal organisms and is associated with flap necrosis caused by undue tension of the suture line at wound closure. The wound infection usually responds to local debridement and the administration of systemic antibiotic therapy.

The long thoracic nerve, the thoracodorsal nerve, the intercostobrachial nerve, and the brachial plexus are at risk for injury during a radical mastectomy. The complications associated with injuries to these nerves have already been discussed in Chapter 16.

Lymphedema is seen more frequently after a radical mastectomy than after a modified radical mastectomy or an axillary dissection. When radiation therapy is used following radical mastectomy, lymphedema is even more likely to occur because of extensive disruption of the normal lymphatic channels that drain the upper extremity. When manifest in the early postoperative period, arm elevation usually results in significant improvement of symptoms. As collateral lymphatic flow develops, the lymphedema of the early postoperative period may completely resolve. When lymphedema persists postoperatively, the functional and cosmetic deficits are significant. A graded pressure stocking sleeve and arm elevation when the patient is at rest are important. After a radical mastectomy all patients must be advised to wear gloves in order to protect the arm and hand from even minor injury. Because of the persistent impaired lymphatic drainage, an otherwise minor injury to the upper extremity can result in the development of severe lymphangitis. Lymphangiosarcoma is a rare late sequela of chronic arm lymphedema. The mean time interval between mastectomy and presentation of lymphangiosarcoma is about 10 years.

Postoperative drainage of the axillary space and chest wall skin flaps will minimize the development of a seroma. Seroma formation after drain removal is managed by fluid aspiration on an outpatient basis.

Preoperative Evaluation

Preoperatively, the patient must be counseled regarding treatment options available for breast cancer. An appropriate evaluation to rule out metastatic disease should be performed before a radical mastectomy. The patient should be told of various reconstructive procedures. She should have the option of consultation with a plastic surgeon to discuss immediate or delayed reconstruction before definitive breast cancer surgery. The procedure is performed under general anesthesia on an inpatient basis. The use of a nonparalytic anesthetic agent during the axillary dissection to facilitate long thoracic nerve identification should be discussed with the anesthesiologist before the start of the procedure.

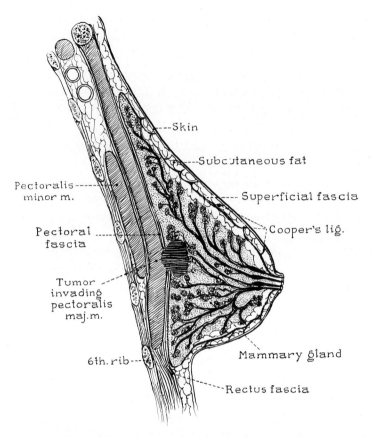

Fig 17-1. Sagittal section of the breast; carcinoma invading pectoralis major muscle.

OPERATIVE PROCEDURE

Radical Mastectomy

Sagittal Section of the Breast; Carcinoma Invading the Pectoralis Major Muscle (Figure 17-1)

This view of the breast shows a primary breast carcinoma deep in the breast parenchyma invading the underlying pectoral fascia and pectoralis major muscle but without invasion of the deeper chest wall musculature. For patients with such lesions and with stage I or stage II primary breast carcinoma, a radical mastectomy is the procedure of choice.

Radical Mastectomy Incision (Figure 17-2)

The patient is placed in the supine position on the operating table, and general anesthesia is induced. The skin is prepared with sterile solution, and the area is draped, exposing the chest, neck, and arm. The arm is generally placed in a sterile sleeve in the operative field so that it may be repositioned during the procedure. If a tissue diagnosis of carcinoma has not been established, a biopsy is performed under standard conditions. Once the diagnosis of breast carcinoma is confirmed, the skin is closed and the area is reprepared and draped for the definitive procedure. The biopsy site is covered by an occlusive adhesive dressing. The arm is abducted on an arm board at an angle not exceeding 90 degrees. The sites of the planned skin incisions from which the superior and inferior flaps will be developed are marked with a

108

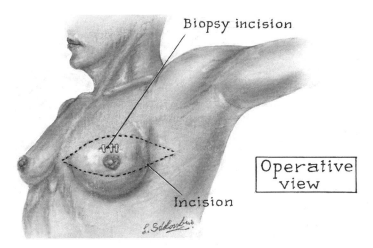

Fig 17-2. Radical mastectomy incision.

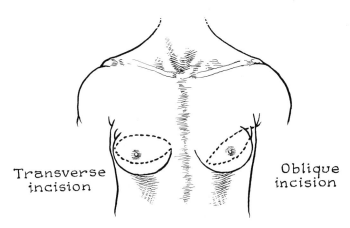

Fig 17-3. Incision modifications.

transversely oriented ellipse, extending to the lower sternum in the midline and beyond the anterior axillary fold laterally (shown). The dashed lines denote the planned incision for the radical mastectomy procedure. The nipple-areolar complex and a margin of at least 2 cm of normal skin around the biopsy site are included in the ellipse of skin to be removed.

Incision Modifications (Figure 17-3)

The planned incision may be modified to a more obliquely oriented incision to obtain an adequate margin of normal tissue around the tumor. The classic radical mastectomy described by Halsted, which involves a vertically oriented incision extending to the clavicle, is rarely necessary. This incision involves excessive skin removal and necessitates an additional incision on the chest if reconstruction is performed.

The orientation and width of the skin island to be excised are dictated by the location and size of the tumor and by the need for adequate exposure to complete the resection. Typical incisions are shown; however, incision placement should be individualized and must not be compromised by plans for reconstruction. The general surgeon and the plastic surgeon should discuss the appropriate incision for patients desiring reconstruction.

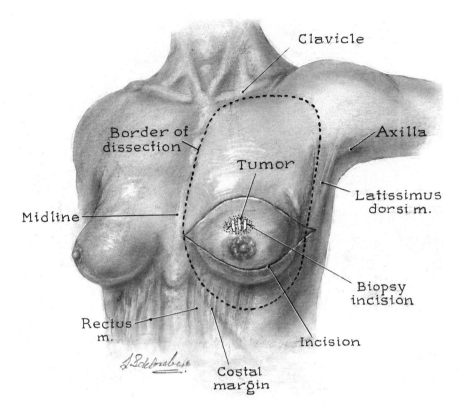

Fig 17-4. Extent of flap elevation.

Extent of Flap Elevation (Figure 17-4)

The extent of the dissection for flap elevation is demonstrated here. Flaps are raised superiorly to the level of the clavicle, medially to the midline of the sternum, inferiorly to the rectus abdominis sheath, and laterally to the anterior border of the latissimus dorsi muscle. Adhesive strips, if present, should be removed before the skin is prepared and before the operative field is draped. Before the skin is incised, any recent biopsy site should be covered with a sterile circular patch of adhesive drape (shown in subsequent figures in this chapter).

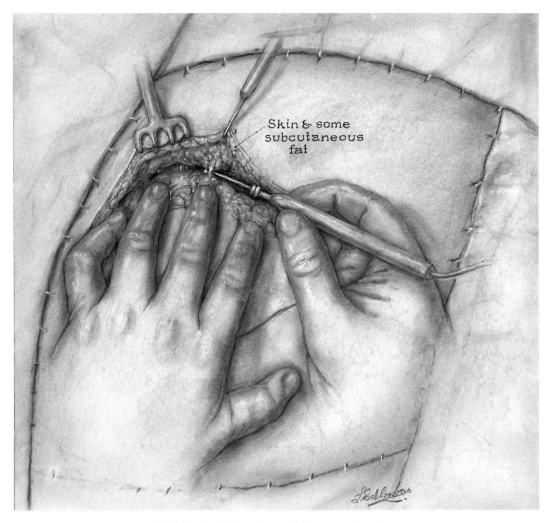

Skin & some
subcutaneous
fat

Fig 17-5.   Elevation of the superior flap.

Elevation of the Superior Flap (Figure 17-5)

After the skin is incised, the superior flap is developed, using the scalpel
or the electrocautery. The electrocautery is generally preferable because much
less blood is lost than when the scalpel is used. Also, flaps of uniform thickness can be more easily developed. However, slightly more serous drainage
occurs in the postoperative period when the electrocautery is used. A plane
of dissection is developed immediately superficial to the breast parenchyma,
leaving a thin layer of subcutaneous tissue on the undersurface of the flap.
An assistant maintains upward traction on the edges of the flap with skin
hooks or facelift retractors. The surgeon maintains countertraction on the
underlying breast. Consistent upward traction on the flap perpendicular to
the field of dissection greatly assists the surgeon in developing an optimal
plane in the subcutaneous tissue. It is equally important for the surgeon or
an assistant to maintain a steady, downward traction on the breast.

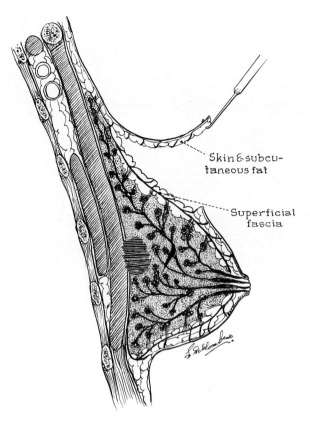

Fig 17-6.   Sagittal section of the breast; superior flap elevated.

Sagittal Section of the Breast; Superior Flap Elevated (Figure 17-6)

The plane of dissection for the superior flap is illustrated in this section. An optimal dissection leaves a thin layer of subcutaneous fat on a well-vascularized skin flap.

Completion of the Superior Flap (Figure 17-7)

The undermined superior flap is of uniform thickness and extends to the clavicle superiorly and to the midline of the sternum medially. After the flap and underlying chest wall are inspected to ensure that hemostasis is adequate, a moist laparotomy pad is placed beneath the superior flap and attention is directed to development of the inferior flap.

Elevation of the Inferior Flap (Figure 17-8)

The inferior flap is developed in a similar manner. Upward traction is maintained on the skin edges perpendicular to the plane of dissection by an assistant, while countertraction is maintained by the surgeon who is retracting the breast superiorly. Sharp dissection is used to develop the plane in the subcutaneous tissue superficial to the underlying breast parenchyma. The lower flap is developed to the sternum medially and to the rectus sheath on the upper abdominal wall inferiorly. The lateral extent of the inferior flap (not shown here) is the anterior border of the latissimus dorsi muscle. With the completion of the lower flap the circumferential margins of the dissection have been completed, and the surgeon is prepared to begin the resection of the breast and associated muscles and soft tissues.

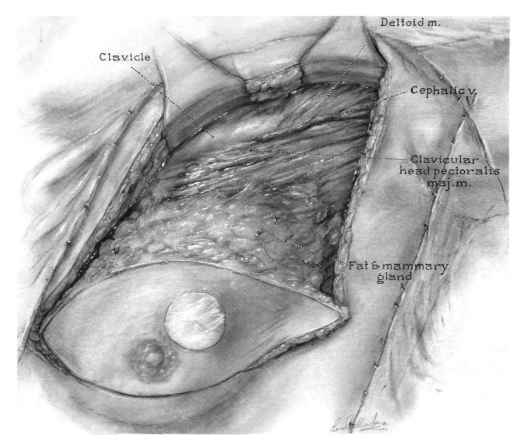

Fig 17-7. Completion of the superior flap.

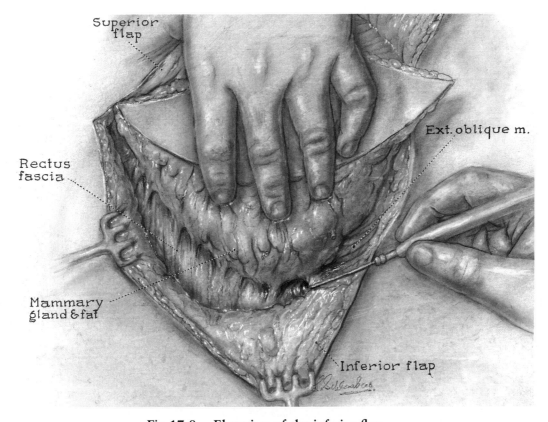

Fig 17-8. Elevation of the inferior flap.

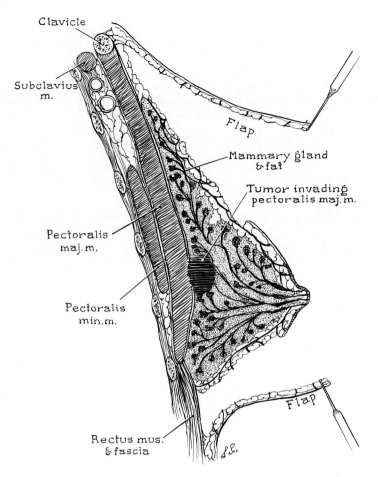

Fig 17-9. Sagittal section of the breast with superior and inferior flaps.

Sagittal Section of the Breast with Superior and Inferior Flaps
(Figure 17-9)

This sagittal section of the breast and chest wall shows the upper margin of dissection of the superior flap at the clavicle and the lower margin of dissection of the inferior flap at the rectus abdominis fascia.

Cross Section of the Breast with Superior and Inferior Flaps
(Figure 17-10)

This cross section illustrates the medial and lateral extent of the dissection at this point in the operative procedure. The medial extent of the dissection overlies the sternum, and the lateral extent overlies the latissimus dorsi muscle. The block of tissue being removed includes the breast, the pectoralis major muscle, the pectoralis minor muscle, and the soft-tissue contents of the axilla. The long thoracic nerve lies immediately superficial to the serratus anterior muscle. The thoracodorsal neurovascular bundle lies in close proximity to the latissimus dorsi muscle. It enters the muscle about 10 cm below the axillary vein.

Elevation of the Medial Flap (Figure 17-11)

Dissection of the breast and underlying pectoralis muscles off the chest wall is completed medially. The superior and inferior flap margins are fully developed along the sternum with the electrocautery.

114

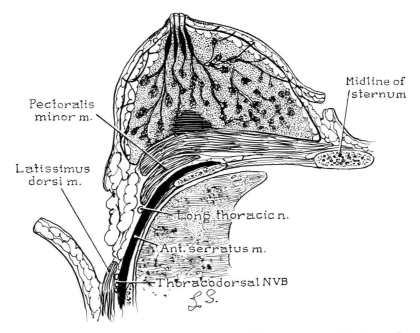

Fig 17-10. Cross section of the breast with superior and inferior flaps.

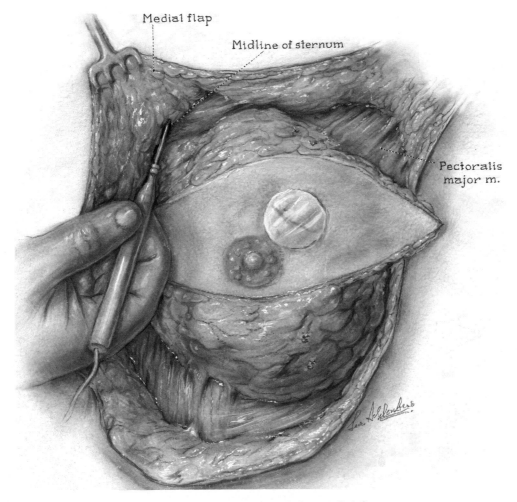

Fig 17-11. Elevation of the medial flap.

115

Dissection of the Lateral Border of the Pectoralis Major Muscle (Figure 17-12)

Attention is then directed to the axilla; the lateral edge of the pectoralis major muscle is freed by sharp dissection. The axillary vein, enclosed in the pectoral fascia and the axillary sheath, is exposed. The anterior border of the latissimus dorsi muscle, exposed during elevation of the inferior flap laterally, is shown. The axillary vein is the superior margin of the axillary dissection. The anterior border of the latissimus dorsi muscle marks the lateral extent of the dissection. The muscle border can be more fully exposed as a small flap is elevated laterally with the electrocautery.

Division of the Pectoralis Major Tendon (Figure 17-13)

The superior flap is retracted to the shoulder to expose the insertion of the pectoralis major muscle tendon onto the humerus. The cephalic vein defines the margin between the pectoralis major muscle and the deltoid muscle. The fibers of the deltoid and the pectoralis muscles are manually separated, and the tendinous insertion of the pectoralis is defined circumferentially. The pectoralis major muscle is sharply divided through its narrow tendon of insertion onto the humerus. Care is taken to protect the underlying axillary sheath during this part of the procedure. The divided muscle edge, which remains attached to the humerus, must be carefully inspected for bleeding. The clavicular origins of the pectoralis major muscle then are divided, and the muscle is retracted inferiorly. Division of the costal and sternal origins is started. They are exposed by downward retraction of the divided pectoralis major muscle.

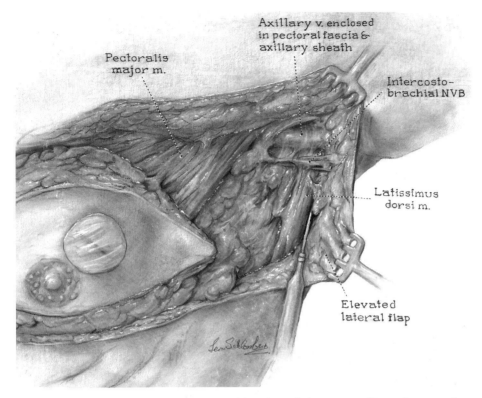

Fig 17-12.   Dissection of the lateral border of the pectoralis major muscle.

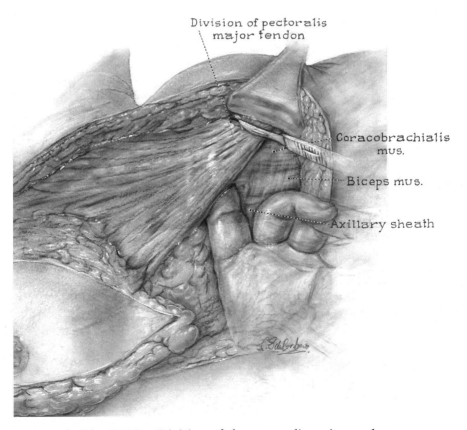

Fig 17-13.   Division of the pectoralis major tendon.

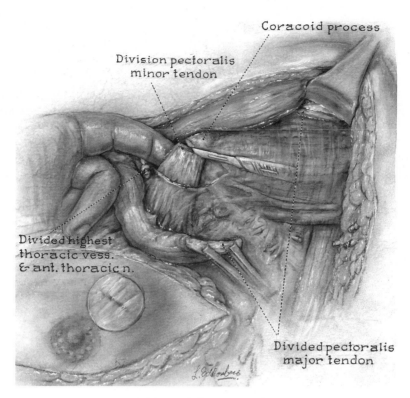

Fig 17-14. Division of the pectoralis minor muscle.

Division of the Pectoralis Minor Muscle (Figure 17-14)

The divided pectoralis major muscle is retracted inferiorly, usually with Allis clamps, to expose the underlying clavipectoral fascia. Beneath this fascia lies the pectoralis minor muscle, which inserts into the coracoid process of the scapula. The neurovascular bundle on the undersurface of the pectoralis major muscle is exposed, ligated, and divided. The pectoralis minor muscle is circumferentially isolated and then divided through its tendinous insertion.

Exposure of the Axillary Contents (Figure 17-15)

Downward traction on the pectoralis major and minor muscles exposes the axillary bed. The superior boundary of the axillary dissection is the axillary vein, which is covered by a thin layer of fascia, with its medial portion just beneath the clavipectoral fascia. This fascia is sharply incised along the inferior border of the vein. Branches of the axillary vein are individually isolated, ligated, and divided. The lateral and medial pectoral neurovascular bundles are isolated and divided while the pectoralis major and minor muscles are being retracted inferiorly. The anatomic locations of the level I and level III lymph nodes and Rotter's nodes, located between the pectoralis major and minor muscle, are illustrated. Level II nodes, which lie beneath the pectoralis minor muscle, are not shown in this illustration.

Axillary Dissection (Figure 17-16)

The dissection of the axillary contents begins in the apical region where the cephalic vein joins the axillary vein. This procedure should be performed by sharp dissection. Hemostasis must be maintained as the soft tissues are removed from the axillary vein. At this point the long thoracic nerve can be

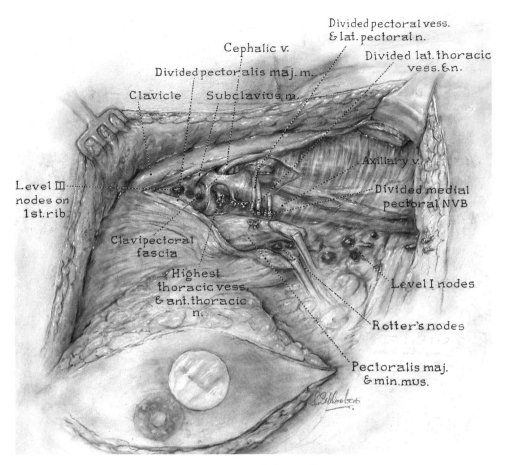

Fig 17-15. Exposure of the axillary contents.

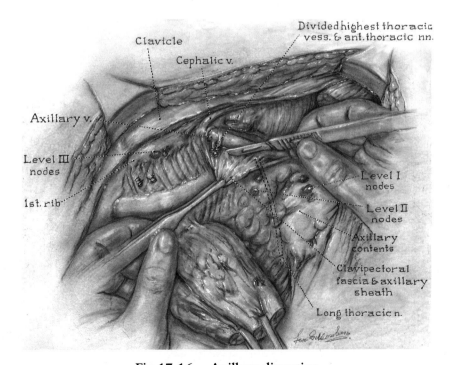

Fig 17-16. Axillary dissection.

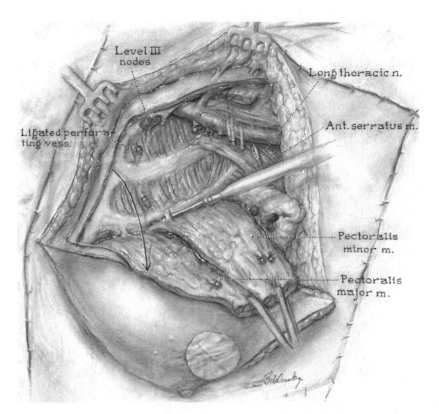

Fig 17-17. Division of costal origins of the pectoralis muscles.

visualized medially and posteriorly, close to the chest wall. The nerve can be identified high in the axilla by gentle palpation along the chest wall while the overlying soft tissue is retracted laterally. The nerve can be traced along the surface of the serratus anterior muscle. It is imperative that the nerve be identified and preserved throughout its course. Stimulation of the nerve with a nerve stimulator will elicit the characteristic contraction of the serratus anterior muscle as long as the patient is not paralyzed. This can be helpful in definitive identification of the nerve. Once the nerve has been identified, the remainder of the axillary contents is cleared en bloc by sharp and blunt dissection. The thoracodorsal neurovascular bundle is generally preserved while the axillary contents are cleared laterally to the anterior border of the latissimus dorsi muscle. The intercostobrachial nerve (not shown here) courses across the axilla after it emerges from the second intercostal space and is generally divided during the axillary dissection.

Division of Costal Origins of the Pectoralis Muscles (Figure 17-17)

The remaining attachments of the pectoralis minor and major muscles to the underlying ribs, as well as any remaining sternal origins for the pectoralis major muscle, are sharply divided as the specimen is retracted inferiorly. Again, care must be taken to identify and ligate the perforating branches of the internal mammary arteries, which are most prominent as they emerge medially in the first four intercostal spaces. The intact long thoracic nerve is shown exposed as it courses along the serratus anterior muscle.

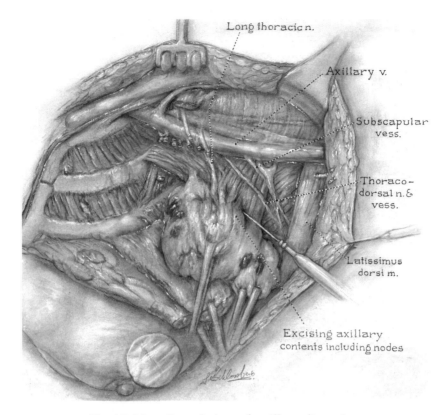

Long thoracic n.

Axillary v.

Subscapular vess.

Thoraco- dorsal n. & vess.

Latissimus dorsi m.

Excising axillary contents including nodes

Fig 17-18. Completion of axillary dissection.

Completion of Axillary Dissection (Figure 17-18)

As the pectoralis muscles are retracted inferiorly, the axillary dissection is completed to the anterior border of the latissimus dorsi muscle laterally. This muscle was previously exposed during the development of the inferior flap. Although the thoracodorsal vessels and nerves may be divided and ligated, if necessary, to adequately remove axillary nodal tissue, they are generally preserved as they course inferiorly and posteriorly to the latissimus dorsi muscle. The inferior extent of the axillary dissection is the point at which the latissimus dorsi muscle directly overlies the lateral chest wall. The subscapularis, teres major, and latissimus dorsi muscles form the posterior wall of the axillary dissection as the adipose tissue and lymph nodes are cleared.

The en bloc specimen is continually retracted inferiorly with division of the remaining muscular origins from the ribs so that the pectoral muscles are completely detached from the chest wall. The inferior and lateral borders of the pectoralis major muscle interdigitate with the muscle fibers of the serratus anterior muscle. Careful scrutiny of the serratus anterior muscle avoids inadvertent division of its fibers while the pectoralis major muscle is detached from the underlying chest wall.

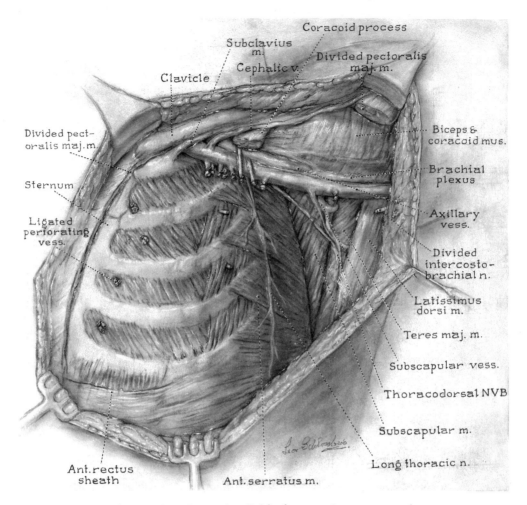

Fig 17-19. Operative field after specimen removal.

Operative Field After Specimen Removal (Figure 17-19)

The entire specimen, including breast, pectoralis major and minor muscles, and contents of the axilla, as well as the interpectoral nodes, is passed off the table to the surgical pathologist.

The operative field is carefully inspected for bleeding. Particular attention is directed to the perforating vessels on the chest wall, the skin flaps, the divided pectoral vessels, and the branches of the axillary vein. The intact long thoracic nerve is viewed, coursing along the serratus anterior muscle. The thoracodorsal nerve, artery, and vein are also shown intact in the axillary space anterior to the teres major and subscapular muscles. The distal stump of the divided intercostobrachial nerve is shown anterior to the latissimus dorsi muscle.

At the end of the procedure two closed suction drains are placed and brought out through small incisions in the axilla below the incision. One drain is generally placed under the superior flap, and one is placed in the axilla. The incision is closed primarily in two layers, as long as flap circulation is not compromised by excessive tension. If flap viability is questionable, fluorescein should be administered intravenously and the flaps should be examined with a Wood's ultraviolet light. If a large area of skin has been excised, a split-thickness skin graft may be necessary for wound coverage. When wound closure is completed, the operative site is dressed with sterile gauze and the patient is sent to the recovery room.

Postoperative Management

Following a radical mastectomy the suction drains are left in place until the 24-hour drainage is less than 30 ml. Patients are carefully monitored for signs of bleeding early postoperatively. Patients may be discharged within 4 to 7 days, depending on the amount of wound drainage, if the skin flaps are viable, and if evidence of infection is not present. The upper extremity should be kept elevated, and hand exercises should be encouraged to minimize swelling. Compression therapy should be initiated if signs of lymphedema develop. Skin sutures are removed on the seventh postoperative day. Activities should be advanced as tolerated. If no further complications occur, chemotherapy, if indicated, can begin 2 weeks after surgery. Particularly in older, physically inactive women, a frozen shoulder can develop if full mobilization of the arm is not achieved expeditiously. Early involvement of a physical therapist should be considered in the postoperative care of many patients following a radical mastectomy. It is far easier to prevent the development of a frozen shoulder than to improve the patient's condition once this complication has developed.

V

RECONSTRUCTIVE PROCEDURES

Reconstructive breast surgery following mastectomy is being practiced with increasing frequency because of increased patient awareness, wider acceptance by general surgeons, and improved results. Excellent cosmetic results have been achieved. Current reconstructive procedures and recent developments in myocutaneous flap transfer or transposition, tissue expansion, immediate reconstruction, creation of a nipple-areolar complex, and creation of an inframammary crease have greatly enhanced the surgeon's ability to replace the missing breast. The chapters in this section describe these reconstructive procedures in detail.

Although any woman undergoing a mastectomy should be considered for breast reconstruction, not all patients are suitable candidates. In general the breast carcinoma should be under control, locally and systemically, before reconstruction is begun, and the patient should be well adjusted psychologically, with a reasonable life expectancy. An absolute contraindication to breast reconstruction is ulceration of the chest wall skin—an occasional complication of radiation therapy and a challenging problem for the surgeon. The use of myocutaneous flap coverage in the treatment of radiation ulcers is also described in this section.

In recent years the development and subsequent progressive advances in tissue expansion and autogenous tissue flaps have made immediate reconstruction at the time of mastectomy more feasible. The evolution of tissue expansion techniques and tissue expander materials has enabled surgeons to obtain excellent results. The recent introduction of anatomically designed "tear drop" tissue expanders allows for the creation of a more naturally contoured breast mound, unlike the spherical breast resulting from the use of traditional expanders and implants. At the same time an increasing experience in autogenous tissue flap development has improved the surgeon's ability to reconstruct a breast with distant tissue at the time of mastectomy. Given the wide range of procedures available, the surgeon can perform immediate reconstruction for almost any patient.

The case for delayed reconstruction has been based primarily on the presumption that increased viability of chest wall flaps and the availability of more pliable tissue results in complete wound healing. Also, a definitive knowledge of the patient's pathologic diagnosis and nodal status and the need to complete adjuvant chemotherapy or radiation therapy have favored the delayed technique. However, with the advent of newer methods of tissue expansion and autogenous tissue transfer or transposition, immediate reconstruction frequently can be performed in association with administration of chemotherapy. Currently, delayed reconstruction is indicated if the patient desires it, if risk factors or logistic considerations preclude immediate reconstruction, or if the patient needs postoperative radiation therapy.

The three major goals of breast reconstruction are to (1) recreate the breast mound; (2) establish symmetry with the opposite breast; and (3) recreate the nipple-areolar complex. Two or more operations over a number of months are usually required to complete all steps of the reconstruction process.

The staging procedures vary for each patient and depend on the number of operations necessary to achieve symmetry. The reconstructed breast mound and the modified contralateral breast will assume permanent shape approximately 3 months after reconstruction, whether surgery is immediate or delayed. To achieve the best esthetic outcome, nipple-areolar reconstruction should only be performed after both breasts have adopted their final contour. An attempt to perform more than one procedure at a time increases the probability of error in positioning or shaping thereby compromising the cosmetic result. Although the risk of asymmetry exists even when procedures are staged, the likelihood is reduced because the surgeon has to deal with fewer variables.

If immediate reconstruction is chosen, the first stage involves creating a breast mound with a tissue expander, an implant, or an autogenous tissue flap. Adjustments to the size and shape of the contralateral breast, replacement of a tissue expander with a permanent implant, or modification of a tissue flap would be done as second-stage procedures. Nipple-areolar reconstruction would be performed in the third stage.

Delayed reconstruction should be done only after the mastectomy site has completely healed and the edema has resolved. In the first stage of delayed reconstruction a breast mound is created by inserting a tissue expander or by transferring a myocutaneous flap from a distant site. It can be difficult to predict the final contour of the reconstructed breast mound at this stage, so contralateral breast modifications are generally postponed, allowing time for the breast mound to assume a more permanent size and shape. Nipple-areolar reconstruction is usually performed as a second-stage procedure, and small adjustments can be made to either breast for symmetry. However, if the contralateral breast must be significantly modified during the second stage, the nipple-areolar reconstruction is best delayed until a third stage. Occasionally, additional procedures may be required subsequently to revise scars, adjust the inframammary crease, or remove a tissue expander fill port.

The simplest means of local tissue reconstruction involves placement of an implant beneath the pectoralis major muscle to create the breast mound. An extension of this principle consists of placement of a tissue expander in a totally submusculofascial pocket with postoperative volume adjustment. An important advantage of tissue expansion is that the patient can participate in determining the size of the final breast mound. Placing a tissue expander immediately after mastectomy allows for the reconstruction of a larger breast than could be achieved with implant insertion alone. Furthermore, the tissue expansion technique can be combined with a local flap advancement from the upper abdomen to create a natural-appearing inframammary crease and breast ptosis.

A myocutaneous flap is used for reconstruction when (1) local tissue is relatively deficient or the pectoralis major muscle is absent; (2) the surgeon needs to match the reconstructed breast with a large or ptotic contralateral breast; (3) the chest wall has been irradiated and has become fibrotic or ulcerated; or (4) the patient prefers the use of autogenous tissue.

If tissue from a distant site is required, the two myocutaneous pedicle flaps with the highest reliability are the latissimus dorsi flap and the rectus abdominis flap. Each flap has distinct advantages, which are discussed in the chapters in this section. An alternative flap reconstruction procedure involves microvascular surgery and the transfer of free tissue from either the gluteus maximus or the lower rectus abdominis myocutaneous units. Microsurgery is also used when vascular augmentation of a transverse rectus abdominis myocutaneous (TRAM) pedicle flap is required to ensure adequate tissue volume for reconstruction of a large breast mound or for filling an extensive chest wall defect. Although the role of microvascular surgery in breast reconstruction is still evolving, the techniques described in this section are employed with increasing frequency and are extremely useful in appropriately selected cases.

Reconstruction of the nipple-areolar complex is a highly specialized procedure that has recently undergone major technical advances. Reestablishing the nipple-areolar complex completes the breast reconstruction and, ideally, converts a mere breast mound into an anatomic structure that closely matches its natural counterpart.

Establishing symmetry with the opposite breast is essential to a successful reconstruction, and it must be considered an integral component when the surgical plan is first developed. To achieve symmetry, the normal breast often requires modification. As with reconstruction of the resected breast, a patient's preference regarding the opposite breast will influence selection of the reconstructive method used. For example, if a patient's remaining breast is quite large and she is unwilling to have it reduced, a myocutaneous flap, a free flap, or a pedicle flap is the only procedure that will ensure sufficient volume to match the remaining breast. Part VI of this text describes the cosmetic procedures—augmentation, mastopexy, and reduction—that are most often used to attain symmetry with the reconstructed breast.

18

Tissue Expansion

Introduction

Reconstruction of the breast mound is readily performed by inserting a tissue expander or a permanent implant. These prostheses are used when local tissue is adequate for reconstruction and when no specific indications for using vascularized autologous tissue are evident. The technique of initial tissue expansion has largely replaced immediate reconstruction with a permanent implant. Tissue expansion provides greater versatility and allows the patient to be involved in deciding the size of the breast mound. Essentially, the process combines stretching and migration of local tissue as the expander is enlarged. When the desired size of the breast mound is achieved, the tissue expander is replaced with a permanent implant. The anatomically configured textured tissue expander produces a normally shaped breast mound that is soft and natural in appearance and texture. With this method of reconstruction the tissues gradually expand, thereby limiting excessive pressure on the skin flaps and minimizing the risk of ischemia and skin necrosis. These skin complications occur more often with the immediate placement of a permanent implant.

Breast reconstruction by tissue expansion is relatively quick and is associated with a low complication rate, yet it can produce an excellent esthetic result in properly selected patients. The expander can usually be inserted through the mastectomy incision, avoiding the need for additional incisions. Tissue does not need to be harvested from a distant donor site, so the morbidity associated with flap transfer is avoided. The expander does not mask or interfere with the detection of recurrent tumor. Tissue expansion can be safely completed while the patient receives chemotherapy. Tissue expansion does not preclude the future use of a myocutaneous flap.

This reconstruction technique typically requires two or more stages for completion. The expander usually produces a breast mound that is rounder than normal so the creation of an inframammary crease may be necessary to improve the breast contour. Most patients also elect to undergo reconstruction of the nipple-areolar complex. These adjunctive procedures (discussed in later chapters) are important refinements of reconstruction that can transform a breast mound into a natural-appearing breast.

Tissue expansion can be used to create a breast mound at the time of mastectomy or at a later date. Immediate reconstruction offers the potential psychologic benefit of diminished emotional trauma caused by the loss of the breast. The tissues appear to expand more easily when reconstruction is immediate rather than when it is delayed. Sufficient expansion to produce a satisfactory breast mound usually can be accomplished within 4 to 6 weeks following mastectomy. When the procedure is delayed, 3 months must be allowed for the mastectomy wound to heal completely, for the scar to mature, and for the skin and subcutaneous tissue to become soft and pliable.

The results with delayed reconstruction are best when the skin flaps are well vascularized. The tissue expander can be placed in either a subcutaneous or a submusculofascial location. However, if the skin and subcutaneous tissue flaps appear too thin to adequately pad and protect the prosthesis, a submusculofascial pocket should be used.

Indications

The procedure is most often performed after total, modified radical, or subcutaneous mastectomy, when the pectoralis major muscle and nerves and the anterior axillary fold have been preserved. Tissue expansion should be used only when the procedure will produce a symmetrical breast mound. For some patients this may require mastopexy or reduction mammoplasty of the contralateral breast, reducing its size, because tissue expansion will not necessarily produce a large breast mound.

Contraindications

Tissue expansion is contraindicated in the patient who has a contaminated wound or in the patient who has excessively tight or thin skin. Patients who have grafted skin on the chest wall or those who have undergone radiation therapy of the anterior chest wall are also not good candidates for tissue expansion because irradiated skin and muscle are fibrotic, poorly vascularized, and inelastic. An attempt to expand irradiated tissue frequently leads to necrosis of a portion of the chest wall skin and to extrusion of the expander. Even if expansion can be completed successfully in the patient with radiation-damaged skin, the resultant breast mound is almost always undesirably firm and spherical. Reconstruction with autologous, vascularized tissue is preferable for these patients.

Reconstruction with tissue expansion alone is usually contraindicated following radical mastectomy because there is either insufficient muscle to cover the tissue expander or insufficient skin to create a breast mound. These patients require an autologous flap procedure for reconstruction. Relative contraindications to tissue expansion include an atrophic or denervated pectoralis major muscle, an absent anterior axillary fold, or the need to match a contralateral breast that is large, or ptotic, or both. A latissimus dorsi flap combined with placement of a tissue expander produces a much more satisfactory result in these cases.

Complications

Early complications of tissue expansion include bleeding, infection, extrusion of the prosthesis, and delayed healing. Bleeding that necessitates reexploration of the chest wound is uncommon. In immediate reconstruction the incidence of infection is less than 5% when the tissue expander is placed in a submusculofascial pocket. However, the risk of infection increases significantly when the expander is positioned subcutaneously. Placement of the expander in the submusculofascial position also provides a well-padded, richly vascularized environment, where the risks of extrusion and capsular contracture are minimized. In addition, should skin necrosis subsequently develop, the tissue expander will be protected by muscle and the need for implant removal will be minimized. Wound infection usually responds to incision, drainage, local wound care, and antibiotics if the infection is confined to the superficial wound. Although the expander does not have to be removed as long as it remains covered by healthy tissue, it must be removed if the prosthetic pocket becomes infected. After the infection has resolved and the tissues have softened, the expander can be reinserted and expansion begun again. Extrusion is uncommon unless the chest wall tissue is inadequate for coverage or the tissue has been previously irradiated. If extrusion occurs, the expander must be removed. Additional tissue then may need to be brought to the chest wall for adequate prosthetic coverage after the wounds have healed and the tissues have softened.

Uneven tissue expansion is an occasional problem. When it occurs, the upper part of the chest wall usually expands more than the lower part and produces a full, superiorly displaced breast. This complication occurs more commonly with a submusculofascial implant than with a subcutaneous implant. Rarely, poor breast contour can result from improper pocket design. If uneven expansion or contour irregularities cannot be corrected by either pocket revision or capsulectomy, the addition of tissue from a latissimus dorsi or a rectus abdominis myocutaneous flap may be required to correct the deformity.

Sometimes, the tissue expander can be improperly positioned too superiorly, too inferiorly, or too laterally. Superior displacement is easily corrected by inferior dissection with pocket enlargement and further release of muscles overlying the expander. An expander positioned too far inferiorly can be revised with inferior capsulorrhaphy and creation of a new inframammary crease. Lateral displacement results from insufficient detachment of the pectoralis major muscle medially, an overly large pocket laterally, or a combination of these two problems. Insufficient detachment of the pectoralis muscle is corrected by further medial dissection, and lateral displacement caused by too large a pocket is corrected by lateral capsulorrhaphy. Replacement of a smooth implant with a textured one can also help correct displacement because the adherence of surrounding tissues to the textured surface helps maintain the implant in an appropriate position.

Capsular contracture, which produces a round, firm, and occasionally painful breast, has been a troublesome complication of implant placement. However, the growing use of implants with textured surfaces has significantly reduced the frequency of this condition. The rate of capsular contracture, when smooth-walled expanders are replaced by smooth permanent implants, is 30% to 40%. However, the rate of contracture formation, when textured expanders are replaced by textured implants, is only 5% to 10%. The use of steroids and antibiotics has not been shown to diminish the incidence of contracture. Massage of textured implants is contraindicated because it impedes the implant's adherence to the surrounding tissue. Repositioning a subcutaneous implant in the submuscular position will frequently eliminate the problem of contracture formation. Otherwise, removal of the implant and reconstruction with autologous tissue from a rectus abdominis flap or, occasionally, a superior gluteal free flap may be necessary.

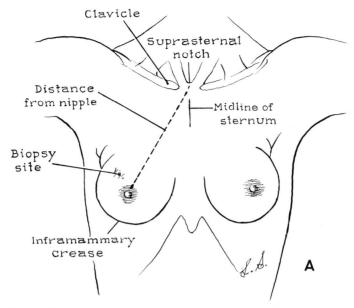

Fig 18-1. Preoperative marking, and patient positioning. *Continued.*

Preoperative Evaluation

At the initial preoperative consultation, a thorough medical history is obtained and pathology and mammogram reports are reviewed. During the physical examination the location of any scars from prior biopsies should be noted. The size, shape, and degree of ptosis of the opposite breast should also be assessed. Reconstruction with local tissue will produce good results only when a symmetrical appearance can be achieved. Before proceeding with reconstruction, the surgeon must be sure that the patient understands the demands of the staged operations and possesses realistic goals about the outcome. Furthermore, the patient should be psychologically prepared to deal with potential complications. Blood loss is minimal with this procedure, so autologous blood donation is not necessary. Perioperative antibiotic prophylaxis is used.

OPERATIVE PROCEDURE

Placement of a Tissue Expander I: Submusculofascial Placement

Preoperative Marking, and Patient Positioning (Figure 18-1)

For immediate reconstruction, as shown in Figure 18-1, *A,* the midline of the sternum and both inframammary creases are marked before the mastectomy procedure, while the patient is in an upright (sitting) position. The distance between the nipple and the suprasternal notch is measured and recorded for future reference. After marking, the patient is placed in a supine position, general anesthesia is induced, and the planned mastectomy is performed, with the wound left open at the completion of the procedure. Immediate reconstruction can be performed while the patient is still in the standard mastectomy position.

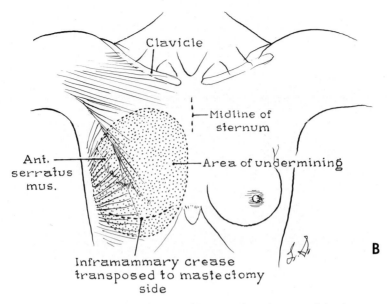

Fig 18-1.   Preoperative marking, and patient positioning.

For delayed reconstruction, as shown in Figure 18-1, *B*, the contralateral inframammary crease serves as a guide for determining the correct location of the reconstructed inframammary crease, which is marked as shown. Then, a line 2 or 3 cm below that level on the mastectomy side is marked to define the inferior limit of the pocket dissection. To construct a properly positioned breast mound and to compensate for the recruitment of abdominal tissue as expansion occurs, the dissection is extended slightly lower than the level of the desired inframammary crease. After marking, general anesthesia is induced, and the patient is placed in a semisitting position with both arms abducted at a 90-degree angle.

Chest Wall Appearance After Modified Radical Mastectomy (Figure 18-2)

The appearance of the chest wall, after a modified radical mastectomy has been performed, is depicted here. The skin flaps are retracted to expose the pectoralis major and the serratus anterior muscles.

The procedure for creation of the submusculofascial pocket at the time of delayed breast reconstruction is similar to the procedure that will be illustrated for immediate reconstruction. However, for delayed reconstruction the skin and subcutaneous tissue first must be elevated from the serratus anterior and pectoralis major muscles. The raised flaps extend over the lateral aspect of the pectoralis major muscle and the medial portion of the serratus anterior muscle, so that the muscle borders are visualized the way they would be immediately following mastectomy.

Identification of the Pectoralis Minor Muscle (Figure 18-3)

It is important to avoid inadvertent elevation of the pectoralis minor muscle with the pectoralis major muscle during dissection of the submusculofascial pocket. Therefore elevation of the pectoralis major muscle should begin in its midportion and superior to its origins from the lowermost ribs.

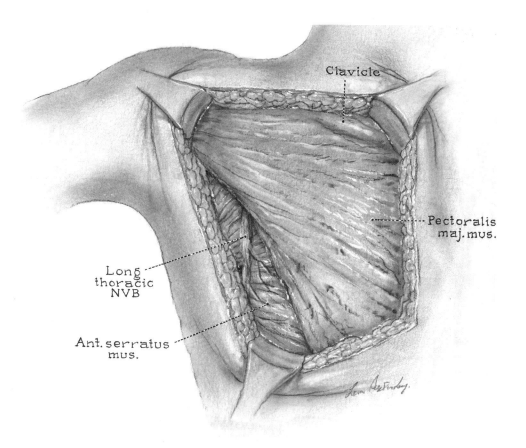

Fig 18-2. Chest wall appearance after modified radical mastectomy.

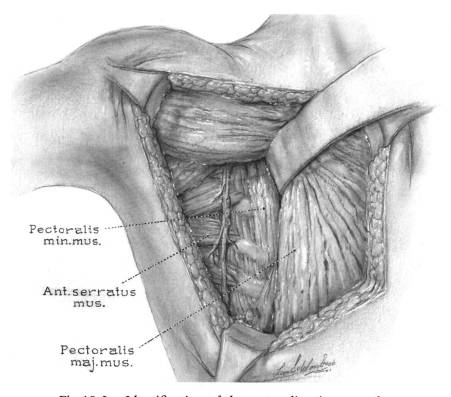

Fig 18-3. Identification of the pectoralis minor muscle.

The plane between the pectoralis major muscle and the pectoralis minor muscle is readily identified by retracting the lateral border of the pectoralis major muscle medially, just below the anterior axillary fold.

Elevation of the Pectoralis Major Muscle (Figure 18-4)

Elevation of the pectoralis major muscle starts superolaterally and progresses inferomedially. The superior portion of the submusculofascial pocket is created by dissection with a finger or blunt instrument to elevate the pectoralis major off the chest wall, ribs, and pectoralis minor. The dissection is extended to just beneath the clavicle superiorly and to the pectoralis major muscle's origin from the sternum and ribs medially and inferiorly. The inferior fascial attachments between the serratus anterior and the pectoralis major muscles are intact at this point in the dissection.

The medial and inferior origins of the pectoralis major muscle then are divided, using the electrocautery with a long insulated tip. The medial perforating vessels, as they pierce the pectoralis major muscle, are carefully coagulated and divided as they are identified. As the medial fibers of the muscle are divided just superior to their origins from the lower ribs, a layer of subcutaneous fat will become visible. The remaining superficial portion of the muscle should be left attached to this subcutaneous fat so that a layer of tissue covers the prosthesis. The pocket's medial margin should be at least 1 or 2 cm lateral to the midline of the sternum to prevent tenting of the presternal skin. It is particularly important to maintain this medial margin during bilateral reconstruction. After completion of the medial dissection, the inferior origins of the pectoralis major are detached from the ribs. This dissection is most safely performed by starting laterally and proceeding medially along the anterior surface of each rib to free the fibers at their origins. Some of the fibers are loosened easily with blunt dissection, and other, more firmly attached fibers are divided with the electrocautery. Injury to the intercostal muscles or inadvertent entry into the pleural space is avoided by limitation of the dissection to the anterior surface of the rib. In elderly and thin individuals the inferior portion of the pectoralis is often attenuated and may be easily perforated. Care must be taken to keep this area intact during elevation so that the tissue expander will be completely covered.

If during mastectomy the dissection extends beyond the origin of the pectoralis major muscle, the medial and inferior attachments should not be divided during the immediate reconstruction, or the tissue expander will be exposed medially and inferiorly. (This precaution does not apply to patients undergoing delayed reconstruction.) It is preferable to leave the muscle attached but still proceed with expander insertion and subsequent inflation rather than risk muscle retraction and implant exposure after division of the attachments. The pocket can later be enlarged medially to revise the position of the breast mound.

The dissection progresses beneath the rectus fascia as the inferior margin of the pectoralis major is reached. Blunt dissection is used to elevate the rectus fascia for a distance of 2 or 3 cm below the inframammary crease. Dissection further inferiorly will produce a pocket that is too large to permit the nipple to be centered on the reconstructed breast mound. Although the malposition can be corrected, it would require an additional operation.

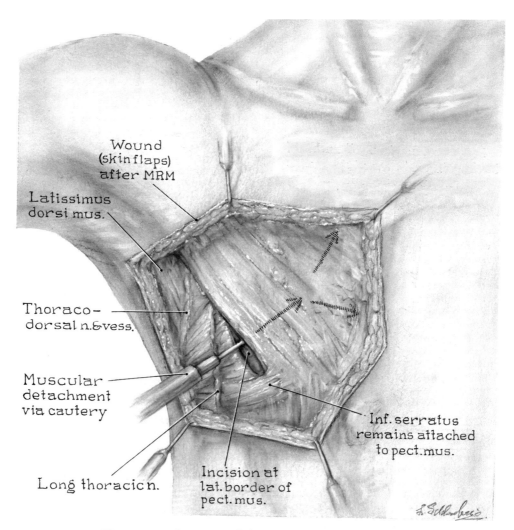

Wound
(skin flaps)
after MRM

Latissimus
dorsi mus.

Thoraco-
dorsal n.&vess.

Muscular
detachment
via cautery

Long thoracic n.

Incision at
lat. border of
pect. mus.

Inf. serratus
remains attached
to pect. mus.

Fig 18-4. Elevation of the pectoralis major muscle.

Elevation of the Serratus Anterior Muscle (Figure 18-5)

Elevation of the serratus anterior muscle begins superiorly and lateral to its attachment to the ribs. The superior slips are detached, and then a finger is inserted to elevate the muscle to its point of origin on the ribs. The muscle fibers are divided by the electrocautery starting superiorly and proceeding inferiorly. Dissection of the pocket and elevation of the serratus anterior muscle extends laterally to the midaxillary line. The serratus anterior is elevated inferiorly to the level of the inframammary crease. Dissection is carried superiorly only as far as there is sufficient muscle bulk at the medial margin of the serratus to be sutured to the lateral border of the pectoralis major. The long thoracic nerve, which usually has been exposed during mastectomy, must be carefully protected during elevation of the serratus. A combination of the serratus anterior and pectoralis major muscles will provide a continuous musculofascial layer for adequate prosthesis coverage at closure. After the serratus anterior has been completely elevated, hemostasis in the pocket is achieved. A sizing implant is then inserted beneath the pectoralis major to assess the pocket size and contour. The pocket is carefully inspected and palpated, and any detected irregularities are modified before insertion of the tissue expander.

Insertion of the Tissue Expander, and Positioning for Immediate Reconstruction (Figure 18-6)

Before insertion the tissue expander is deflated and flattened. The expander is positioned beneath the pectoralis major muscle. Its inferior margin is at or just below the level of the inframammary crease, and its medial margin is at the medial margin of the pocket, 1 or 2 cm lateral to the midline of the sternum. The tissue expander must lie flat after it is properly positioned. If crumpled or folded, it will not occupy a space large enough to produce a properly shaped breast mound. The pocket will collapse around a folded expander and inhibit normal expansion, resulting in a breast mound of limited volume and distorted shape. If skin and muscle are sufficient to accommodate some inflation of the expander, saline solution is instilled to prevent the expander from crumpling.

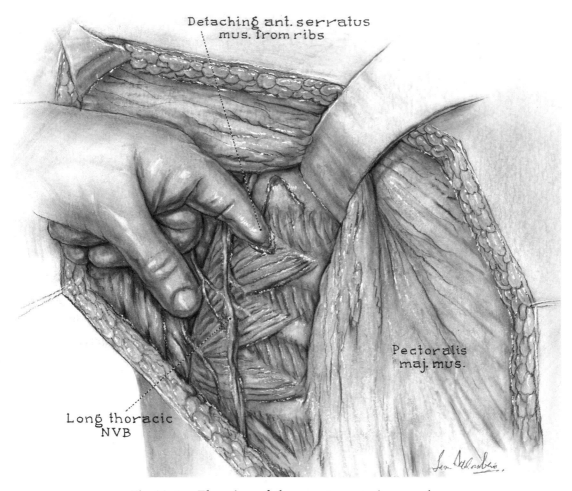

Fig 18-5.   Elevation of the serratus anterior muscle.

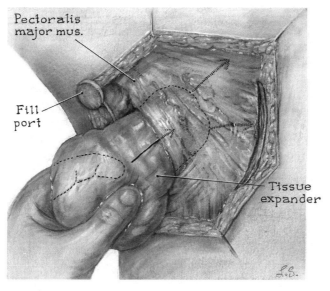

Fig 18-6.   Insertion of the tissue expander, and positioning for immediate reconstruction.

137

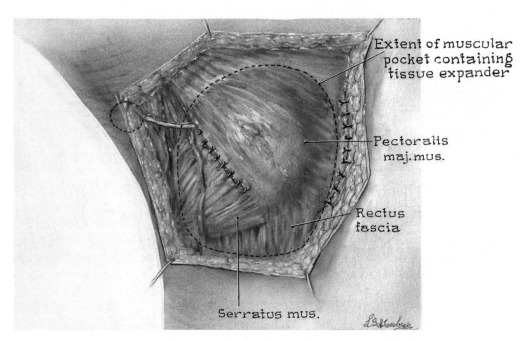

Fig 18-7. Muscle closure and positioning of the fill port.

Muscle Closure, and Positioning of the Fill Port (Figure 18-7)

Once the tissue expander is properly positioned in the submusculofascial pocket, the lateral border of the pectoralis major muscle is sutured to the medial border of the serratus anterior muscle with an absorbable suture, so that the expander is completely covered with muscle.

When an expander with a remote fill port is used, the port is positioned in a location that will result in minimal scarring. It may be placed outside the implant pocket but close enough so that it can be removed from inside the pocket when the expander is converted to a permanent implant. Placement of the port near the axilla (as shown) is also an option because it permits removal through a separate incision that will leave a well-camouflaged scar. The fill port may also be positioned so that it can be removed through either an old biopsy site or the mastectomy scar.

The fill port must be positioned close enough to the skin to permit easy identification by palpation. If not placed in an accessible spot, the port may be so difficult to palpate in obese individuals that an ultrasound or x-ray examination will be needed to locate it. In addition, the fill port should be securely positioned, using sutures to prevent rotation. Postoperative correction of a rotated fill port can be difficult, and needle injection of saline solution through a malpositioned port is awkward. Problems of port placement are avoided when a tissue expander with a built-in fill port is used.

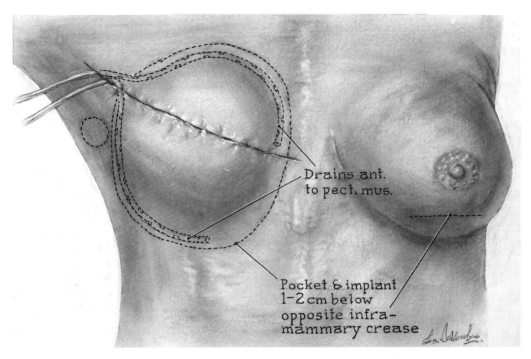

Fig 18-8.   Insertion of drains, and wound closure.

Insertion of Drains, and Wound Closure (Figure 18-8)

Two constant vacuum drains are placed beneath the skin flaps, one superiorly and medially and the other inferiorly and laterally. They are brought out through the incision (as shown) or through separate incisions in an area of the axilla where the scars will be minimally visible. A drain is also placed in the axilla if an axillary dissection has been performed.

The chest wound is closed with a layer of interrupted absorbable sutures, followed by a running layer of fine subcuticular sutures. A sterile bandage of nonadherent gauze covered by a dry dressing is then applied. A pressure dressing is not used, and care is taken to avoid direct placement of tape on the skin flaps.

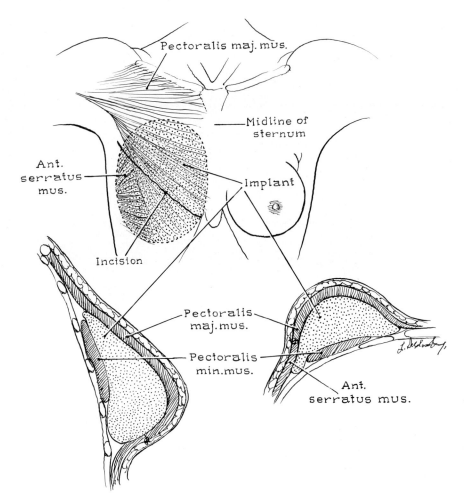

Fig 18-9. Final position of the submusculofascial prosthesis.

Final Position of the Submusculofascial Prosthesis (Figure 18-9)

After submusculofascial placement, the prosthesis overlies the pectoralis minor muscle on the chest wall. The tissue expander is fully covered superficially by the serratus anterior and by the pectoralis major muscles, as shown on the cross section and sagittal section illustrations.

Placement of a Tissue Expander II: Subcutaneous Placement

Final Position of the Subcutaneous Tissue Expander (Figure 18-10)

Marking for subcutaneous placement of the prosthesis proceeds, as illustrated in Figure 18-1, for placement of the submusculofascial prosthesis. The margins of the flaps raised for placement of the subcutaneous prosthesis are similar to the margins of the skin flaps raised for a modified radical mastectomy. The inferior border of the pocket is 2 to 3 cm below the inframammary crease, the medial border is 1 to 2 cm lateral to the sternal midline; the lateral border is at the midaxillary line; the superior border is several centimeters below the clavicle. After the implant is properly positioned and flat, without being crumpled or folded, the fill port is positioned and the wound is closed as illustrated in Figure 18-8. Drains are routinely used following subcutaneous placement of the prosthesis. After subcutaneous

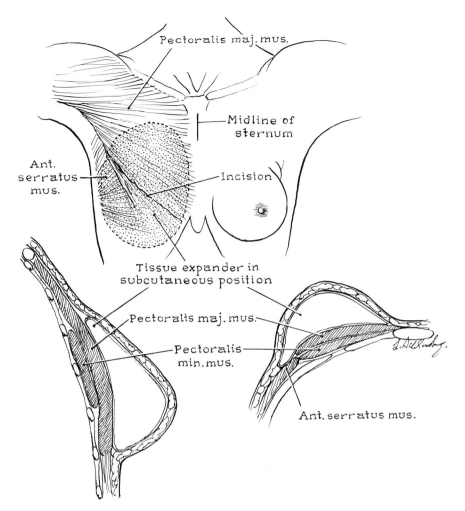

Fig 18-10.   Final position of the subcutaneous tissue expander.

placement the tissue expander overlies the serratus anterior and the pectoralis major muscles. Superficially, the tissue expander is covered only by subcutaneous tissue and skin (shown here on the cross section and sagittal section illustrations).

Postoperative Care and Tissue Expansion

Following the placement of a tissue expander for immediate reconstruction, patients who can manage the drains at home may be discharged after 2 or 3 days. Placement of a tissue expander for delayed reconstruction may require only overnight hospitalization. Drains are removed when the volume is below 30 ml a day. Patients can shower when all drains have been removed. Most women can return to normal activities within a few weeks, depending on the individual patient and the physical demands of her life and occupation.

Tissue expansion is usually begun on the fifth to seventh day and then repeated at weekly intervals until a breast mound of satisfactory dimensions has been created. However, expansion should begin earlier in patients who have excess skin. If the skin is allowed to fold and heal in its unexpanded position, wrinkles or creases may result, which are difficult to correct when expansion is initiated.

19

Creation of an Inframammary Crease

Introduction

The goal of the inframammary crease procedure is to create a well-defined and symmetrical inframammary fold that gives the reconstructed breast mound a natural appearance. This can be established most easily by advancing a skin flap superiorly from the upper abdominal wall. This skin flap then is attached to the periosteum of a selected rib at the same time that skin from the breast mound is advanced inferiorly and sutured to the abdominal wall flap. This simple technique uses local skin of homogeneous color and texture. Creation of an inframammary crease is a second-stage procedure and should be postponed until reconstruction with tissue expansion has been completed and the tissues are soft and pliable. Typically, a time interval of 3 months or more following the most recent operative procedure is appropriate.

The technique described here is used following reconstruction with placement of an implant. Rarely, it is necessary to create a new inframammary crease following autologous tissue reconstruction. This is generally done by suction lipectomy and is not described here.

Indications

The creation of an inframammary crease is indicated when breast reconstruction by tissue expansion or implant insertion has resulted in an abnormally low inframammary crease (as shown in the right breast in Figure 19-1). An absence of ptosis in the reconstructed breast, a contralateral breast with moderate ptosis, or an abnormally spherical breast contour following reconstruction are also indications for creation of a new inframammary crease.

Contraindications

Creation of an inframammary crease is generally contraindicated in the patient who has undergone a reconstructive procedure (insertion of either

142

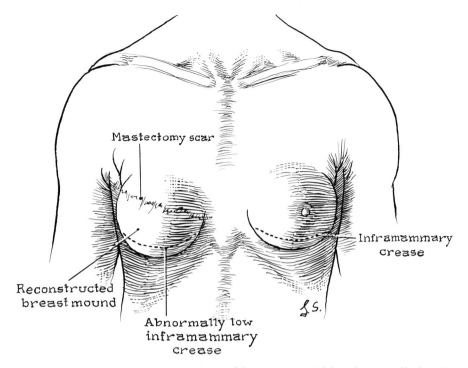

Fig 19-1. Asymmetric appearance of breasts caused by abnormally low inframammary crease on reconstructed right breast mound.

an implant or tissue expander) within less than 3 months. An inframammary incision made during this period of wound maturation can result in necrosis of a portion or of all the tissue between the inframammary incision and the mastectomy incision. Prior radiation therapy also increases the risk of flap necrosis.

Complications

The complications associated with creation of an inframammary crease include bleeding, infection, and recurrence of the deformity if the upper abdominal wall flap becomes detached from the rib. The risk of tissue necrosis between the inframammary incision and the mastectomy scar has been mentioned. In addition, a cosmetic deformity causing asymmetry of the breasts can result from a malpositioned inframammary crease.

Preoperative Preparation

The creation of an inframammary crease may be performed as an outpatient procedure under general anesthesia. Prophylactic antibiotics are routinely administered for this procedure because an implant is in place.

OPERATIVE PROCEDURE

Preoperative Marking (Figure 19-2)

The inframammary crease of each breast is marked (as shown by the dashed lines). The marking for the contralateral inframammary crease is used as the guide for marking and properly placing the new inframammary crease. The position of the new inframammary crease is marked while the patient is upright because the level of the marking changes when the patient is in a supine position with the arms abducted. After the proper level for the revised crease is defined, the skin is crosshatched an equal distance inferior and superior to the crease mark, until a crescent shape is outlined. The area within this crescent represents the dermal edges of the skin flaps that will be advanced. In the midportion of the crescent the crosshatched area should be between 2 and 6 cm in height. Toward the medial and lateral ends of the inframammary fold the crescent should be approximately 1 cm in height. The length of the crescent is determined by the distance the abdominal flap will need to be advanced to elevate the inframammary crease to a level symmetrical with the opposite breast. When the marked inframammary crease is incised horizontally, a breast flap and an upper abdominal flap will be created within the crosshatched area. To complete the marking, the skin to be undermined is outlined and then stippled on the upper abdominal wall. The width of the stippled area needs to be approximately 1½ times the width of the skin area that will be advanced superiorly.

Creation of an Inframammary Crease; Anatomy (Figure 19-3)

Pertinent tissues involved in creation of an inframammary crease include the ribs, the existing inframammary crease, the upper abdominal skin, and the anterior rectus fascia. During the procedure the skin and subcutaneous tissues of the upper abdomen must be elevated at the level of the rectus fascia. The portion of the abdominal flap lying within the marked crescent will be deepithelialized, advanced superiorly, and attached to the periosteum of a rib. The breast mound flap then will be advanced inferiorly and attached to the upper abdominal flap at the level of the inframammary crease.

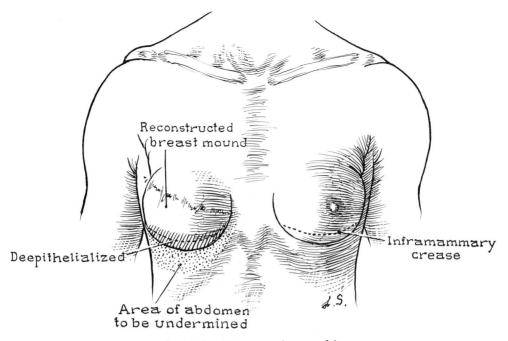

Fig 19-2. Preoperative marking.

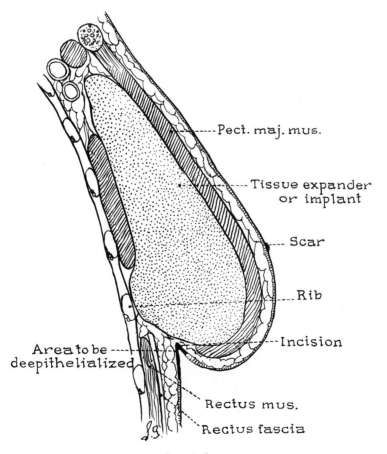

Fig 19-3. Creation of an inframammary crease: anatomy.

Removal of the Breast Implant, and Attachment of the Abdominal Flap (Figure 19-4)

Following proper marking and induction with general anesthesia, the patient is placed in a semisitting position on the operating table. After preparation and with both breasts in the operative field, the marked inframammary crease in the middle of the crosshatched crescent is incised as a full-thickness skin incision. The central portion of the incision is then deepened through the subcutaneous tissue to the periprosthetic capsule. The tissue expander or implant is removed and the pocket irrigated with povidone-iodine solution. Next, the skin and subcutaneous tissue overlying the upper abdominal wall are elevated at the level of the rectus fascia and undermined to the limits of the stippled area shown in Figure 19-2. An appropriate rib (or ribs) is identified for attachment of the advanced upper abdominal flap. Depending on the skin flap's angle and the curvature of the rib cage, more than one rib may be used. Once the most appropriate rib is identified, the periosteum is exposed. The upper abdominal flap is advanced by gently pulling it toward the exposed rib periosteum at or just above the intended location of the new inframammary crease. The breast flap is gently pulled inferiorly onto the upper abdominal flap to assess the final appearance of the crease. The point at which the flaps overlap is marked and the portion of the upper abdominal flap that will be buried and attached to the rib is deepithelialized (marked by a heavy black line in Figure 19-4). A dozen or more nonabsorbable sutures are then placed to fix the dermal edge of the upper abdominal flap to the rib periosteum.

Replacement of the Implant, and Attachment of the Breast Flap (Figure 19-5)

As shown in this sagittal section the permanent implant is reinserted and properly positioned. If a smooth prosthesis or expander had been used during the first stage of breast reconstruction, the capsule should be excised and a textured implant inserted in its place. A constant vacuum drain should be inserted (not shown) in the breast pocket and brought out through a small incision in the axilla to minimize accumulation of serum. Next, the superior breast flap is advanced downward to cover the implant and meet the upper abdominal flap. The edge of the breast flap is sutured directly to the abdominal flap after the abdominal flap has been securely attached to the periosteum at the level of the inframammary crease.

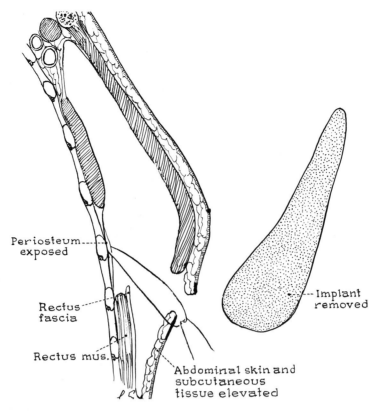

Fig 19-4. Removal of the breast implant, and attachment of the abdominal flap.

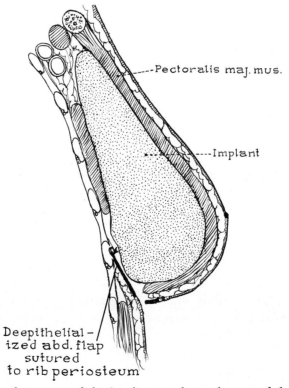

Fig 19-5. Replacement of the implant, and attachment of the breast flap.

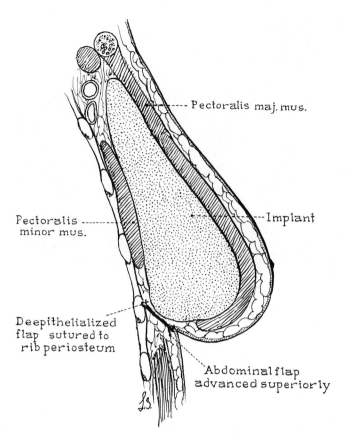

Fig 19-6.   Wound closure.

Wound Closure (Figure 19-6)

This section shows the final position of the abdominal flap sutured to the rib periosteum and the breast flap sutured to the abdominal flap to create a well-defined, properly positioned inframammary crease.

The wound is closed with a layer of interrupted absorbable sutures followed by a running subcuticular layer. This combination of sutures will securely affix the joined portions of the breast flap and the advanced upper abdominal flap at the level of the inframammary crease. A sterile dressing of nonadherent gauze and tape is then applied.

Postoperative Care

The patient is discharged following satisfactory recovery from anesthesia. The dressing and drain are removed after 4 or 5 days. The patient should wear a lightly supportive brassiere continuously for at least 2 weeks. She will feel some tightness at the point where the two flaps are joined that usually subsides within 6 to 8 weeks. Although the inframammary crease may seem exaggerated at first, the tissue in the inferior half of the breast mound will soften, stretch, and conform to a more natural shape within 6 months. In addition, gravitational forces will direct the implant inferiorly to produce a ptotic-appearing breast mound. This shifting of the breast mound also helps to hide the scar in the inframammary crease. As shown in Figure 19-7, a satisfactory cosmetic result is generally obtained with this procedure.

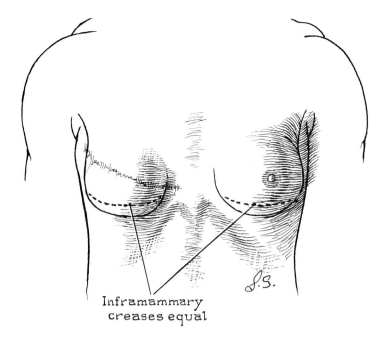

Inframammary
creases equal

Fig 19-7.   Symmetrical appearance following creation of an inframammary crease on the right breast mound.

20

Latissimus Dorsi Flap

Introduction

The latissimus dorsi muscle represents a versatile source for a reliable myocutaneous flap for breast and chest wall reconstruction. A portion of the muscle, or the entire muscle with a skin island, can be transposed to recreate a breast mound, fill a specific defect, or cover a breast implant. Because the latissimus dorsi is large and has a long vascular pedicle with a 120-degree arc of rotation, the flap can be used on almost any area of the anterior chest wall. A skin island may be oriented in any direction over the underlying muscle flap. The skin will remain firmly attached to the muscle by multiple perforating vessels, arising from branches of the thoracodorsal artery, and cutaneous nerves, which pass through the muscle into the overlying skin.

Transposition of the latissimus dorsi muscle is associated with a minimal functional deficit. The latissimus adducts and medially rotates the arm. However, if all other shoulder muscles are intact, they will duplicate all important functions of the arm that would involve the latissimus dorsi, except for one. This function is best described as the posterior "push off." An individual pushes forward with the hands positioned behind the back, as in snow skiing. The latissimus contributes to formation of the posterior axillary fold; however, the teres major provides most of the contour of the fold. Thus little if any cosmetic deformity other than the scar results from transposition of the latissimus and its tendon of insertion to the anterior chest.

Elevation of the muscle and dissection of the vascular pedicle is facilitated by the remarkably constant anatomy, which is illustrated in detail in Figures 20-1 through 20-6. As shown in Figure 20-1, the origins and insertion of the latissimus dorsi muscle are best illustrated in the posterior oblique view. The latissimus originates from the spines of the lower six thoracic vertebrae, the posterior layer of the lumbodorsal fascia, the iliac crest, and the lower four ribs and extends toward the axilla. It is a large, triangular muscle that covers the lower half of the thorax and lumbar region. The muscle fibers spiral as they converge toward the inferior tip of the scapula and then insert into the intertubercular groove of the humerus. The latissimus dorsi is thinnest (approximately 1 cm) at its lower fascial origins. As it approaches its insertion, the muscle thickens to approximately 2 to 2.5 cm. Superiorly in the axilla, the latissimus dorsi is just lateral and inferior to the teres major. Because fibers of the latissimus spiral around and beneath the teres major, a distinct plane between the two muscles may be difficult to

150

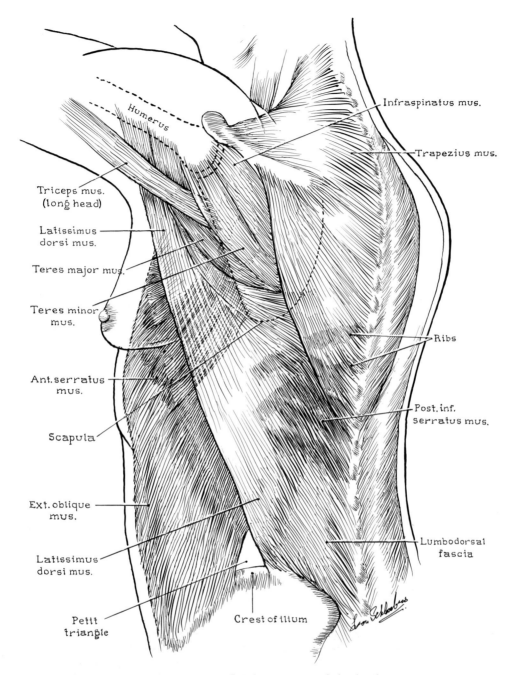

Triceps mus.
(long head)

Latissimus
dorsi mus.

Teres major mus.

Teres minor
mus.

Ant. serratus
mus.

Scapula

Ext. oblique
mus.

Latissimus
dorsi mus.

Petit
triangle

Humerus

Infraspinatus mus.

Trapezius mus.

Ribs

Post. inf.
serratus mus.

Lumbodorsal
fascia

Crest of ilium

Fig 20-1. Superficial anatomy of the back.

visualize. Farther posteriorly, its superior border lies immediately inferior to the tip of the scapula. The muscle's medial superior region lies deep to the most inferior portion of the trapezius muscle.

Anteriorly, the latissimus dorsi overlies the serratus anterior muscle. Near its obliquely oriented inferior margin, the serratus anterior is attached to the latissimus dorsi by a fibrofatty bridge (not shown). In the center of the back the latissimus is immediately above the rib cage. Further inferiorly and toward the midline of the back, the latissimus overlies the serratus posterior inferior muscle. The lumbodorsal fascia and paraspinal muscles are deep to the posterior border of the latissimus. At its anterior and inferior margin, the latissimus dorsi overlies the external oblique muscle. A pertinent point is the muscle's connection to the lumbodorsal fascia. This fascia must be recognized and carefully divided during elevation, or the paraspinal muscles may be injured.

As shown in Figure 20-2, the primary blood supply for the latissimus dorsi muscle are the thoracodorsal artery and vein. In this figure the latissimus dorsi and the trapezius muscles, as well as the lumbodorsal fascia, have been partially resected to better illustrate the vascular supply to the latissimus dorsi muscle and to the deep back structures. The thoracordorsal artery, which has a diameter of about 2 mm, enters the muscle on its deep surface, 10 or 12 cm below the axillary artery, and runs approximately 2 or 3 cm inside the muscle's anterior border. Several centimeters before entering the latissimus dorsi, the thoracodorsal artery branches to the serratus anterior muscle. This collateral serratus branch courses along the superficial surface of the serratus anterior and has a rich anastomosis with several intercostal arteries (not shown). When the thoracodorsal pedicle is ligated or damaged by radiation, flow reverses in the serratus branch and becomes the primary arterial flow to the latissimus dorsi. The collateral serratus branch can serve as a main blood supply or a secondary blood supply for flap transposition if necessary. However, the flap's arc of rotation is decreased when this collateral serratus branch is used as the dominant vascular pedicle. Paraspinal perforating vessels, which emerge through the erector spinae muscles, provide a secondary blood supply to the latissimus dorsi muscle. However, these vascular branches are not useful in transposing the muscle for breast reconstruction.

The thoracodorsal nerve provides motor function to the latissimus dorsi. It is derived from the lower cervical roots of the posterior cord of the brachial plexus. It runs parallel to, and enters the muscle with, the vascular pedicle. Sensation to the skin of the back is segmental in origin, and the sensory nerves must be divided when the flap is elevated. Dividing the sensory nerves results in a skin island on the breast mound that is insensate.

Figures 20-3 through 20-6 illustrate in cross section the regional anatomy, particularly the relationship of the thoracodorsal vessels to the surrounding muscles and nerves. As shown in Figure 20-3, at the level of T3, the latissimus dorsi muscle inserts in the intertubercular groove of the humerus by way of a fibrous tendon that is several centimeters long. Immediately anterior to the insertion point is the coracobrachialis muscle. Anterior to that are the pectoralis major muscle and its tendon. Lateral to the coracobrachialis and posterior to the lateral extent of the pectoralis muscle lies the short head of the biceps muscle. Posterior to the latissimus tendon is the teres major. At the level of insertion of the latissimus dorsi tendon the thoracodorsal nerve, artery, and vein are located in the axillary fat, several centimeters posterior to the tendon. The neurovascular structures that are closest to the latissimus tendon at this level are the brachial plexus and the axillary vessels.

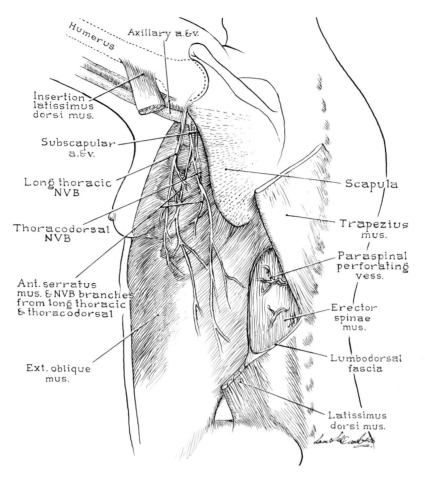

Fig 20-2. Neurovascular anatomy and deep structures of the back.

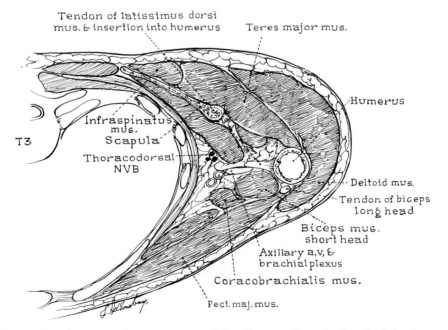

Fig 20-3. Cross section anatomy of the chest wall at the level of the insertion of the latissimus dorsi into the humerus.

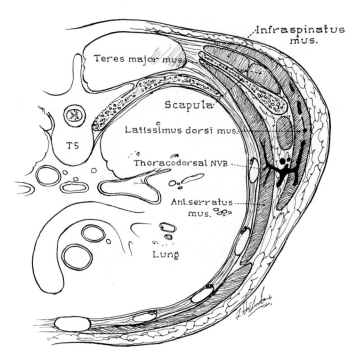

Fig 20-4. Cross section anatomy of the chest wall 10 cm below the axilla at the level of T5.

As shown in Figure 20-4, approximately 10 cm below the axilla at the level of T5, the thoracodorsal artery and vein course medial to the latissimus dorsi muscle and enter its deep surface. Before entering the latissimus, the thoracodorsal trunk gives off arterial and venous branches to the serratus anterior muscle. These collateral branches lie on the anterior surface of the serratus anterior and can be used as a landmark to identify the thoracodorsal pedicle. At this level the latissimus dorsi is located superficially, immediately beneath the subcutaneous fat, and overlies the tip of the scapula, the teres major muscle, and the inferior portion of the infraspinatus muscle.

Figure 20-5 illustrates the midportion of the back at the level of T7; the latissimus dorsi spreads out to form a large, flat, sail-shaped muscle, which is thicker at its anterior margin and thinner toward its posterior margin. The serratus anterior muscle lies beneath most of the anterior portion of the latissimus dorsi. Posteriorly the latissimus dorsi spreads over the teres major and paraspinal muscles. At about the level of the seventh rib, the thoracodorsal artery and vein arborize into multiple branches and send off numerous perforating vessels into the subcutaneous tissue and skin. This arborization of blood vessels allows the latissimus to be divided into separate segments, should that be necessary. More important, because of this extensive vascular network, a skin island extending 4 or 5 cm beyond the anterior margin of the latissimus dorsi will survive.

As shown in Figure 20-6 at the level of T9, the arborization of blood vessels extends inferiorly and is distributed throughout the muscle. At this level the muscle is located superficially and is attenuated posteriorly as it becomes continuous with the lumbodorsal fascia. In summary, the constant anatomy and the rich blood supply facilitate use of the latissimus dorsi flap for a wide spectrum of purposes, including breast reconstruction.

154

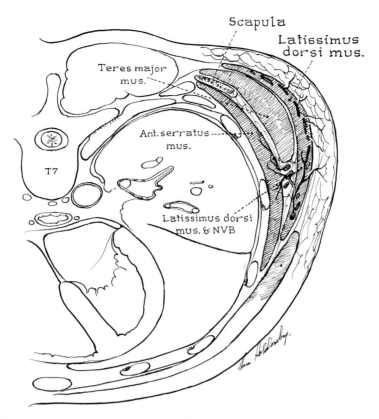

Fig 20-5. Cross section anatomy of the chest wall at the level of the seventh vertebra.

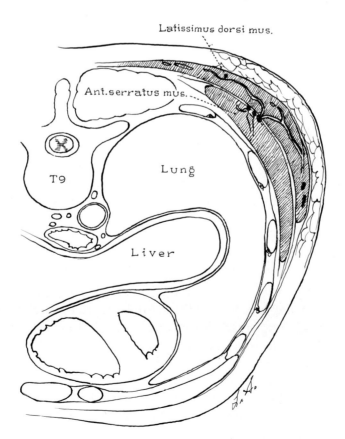

Fig 20-6. Cross section anatomy of the chest wall at the level of T9.

The design of most latissimus dorsi flaps in breast reconstruction incorporates an elliptical skin island with a length that is approximately three times its width. The scar from a transversely oriented skin island, as illustrated in Figure 20-7, *A*, is easily hidden with a swimsuit or bra, although the medial portion of the scar will be visible with a neckline cut low in the back. A flap with a transversely oriented skin island will have a large amount of muscle lying superior to the skin island when the flap is inset on the anterior chest wall. It therefore adds padding to the upper portion of the reconstructed breast mound. A transversely oriented skin island is easily inset into an oblique or transverse chest wall incision.

The scar from an obliquely oriented skin island, as illustrated in Figure 20-7, *B*, is hidden by a low-cut neckline; however, it is usually visible beneath a bra or swimsuit. A flap with an obliquely oriented skin island has roughly equal amounts of muscle above and below the inset skin island. If a particularly large skin island is needed, the obliquely oriented skin should be centered near the anterior border of the muscle, where the blood supply to the muscle and the overlying skin is most abundant. As with the transverse orientation, a flap designed with an obliquely oriented skin island can easily be inset into an oblique or transverse chest wall incision.

Because the flap can be inset in any direction on the anterior chest, the actual orientation of the skin island on the latissimus dorsi muscle is determined by the location and orientation of the mastectomy scar, the areas of the anterior chest wall that need muscle padding, the presence of grafted or radiation-damaged skin, and the patient's preference regarding scar location on the back.

The latissimus dorsi myocutaneous flap has significant disadvantages. This flap rarely provides sufficient bulk to produce an adequate breast mound. Volume may be added by the insertion of an implant or tissue expander, with all the attendant risks of a breast prosthesis. Furthermore, the posterior trunk skin is a poor match for the color and texture of the anterior chest skin, so the darker skin island associated with a latissimus flap often is noticeable. Removal of a large skin island can produce a depression in the contour of the back and a prominent scar. Finally, because sensation to the skin of the back is segmental in origin, the sensory fibers are divided when the flap is elevated and the skin island of the breast mound is insensate. Despite these disadvantages the latissimus dorsi provides a durable and reliable flap for a wide range of reconstructive purposes.

Indications

The latissimus dorsi flap may be used for reconstruction, generally with an implant, following modified radical or total mastectomy. This flap is also the best option for reconstruction following a radical mastectomy if contraindications are present for a pedicled or free TRAM flap. The latissimus dorsi flap can be more safely transposed and is less sensitive to hypothermia than the TRAM flap, so it may be preferred in patients with significant risk factors for TRAM flap transposition. In addition, this flap is useful for covering radiation ulcers of the chest wall, and the flap may be used as an alternative reconstructive option if another approach has failed. Finally, the

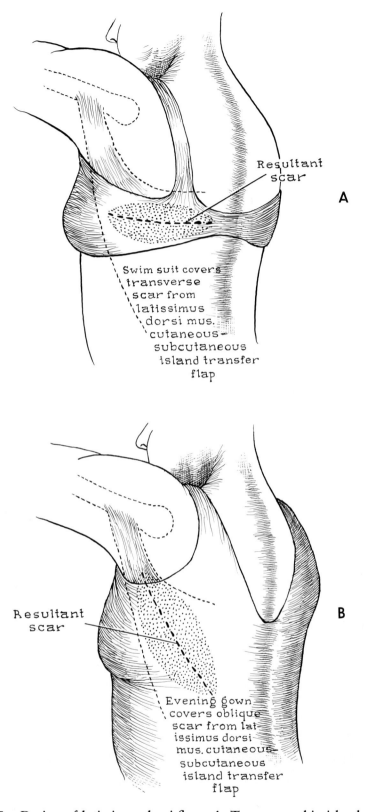

Fig 20-7. Design of latissimus dorsi flaps. A, Transverse skin island.
B, Oblique skin island.

latissimus dorsi muscle can be used as an autologous implant, without a skin island, to supplement a deficient pectoralis major muscle or to create an anterior axillary fold.

Contraindications

Transposition of a latissimus dorsi flap requires several hours of surgery and general anesthesia, and it may not be well tolerated in individuals with significant medical problems. A previous thoracotomy with division of the latissimus dorsi muscle precludes transposition of this myodermal unit for breast reconstruction. However, the proximal portion of the muscle may still be used to create an anterior axillary fold or to fill an infraclavicular depression. Division of the thoracodorsal nerve, which may occur during axillary dissection, results in atrophy of the latissimus dorsi. However, denervation does not prohibit muscle transposition if sufficient residual muscle is present for reconstruction. Also, axillary radiation does not preclude transposition of the latissimus dorsi as a pedicle flap.

Complications

Bleeding is rare if meticulous hemostasis is maintained during flap elevation. However, seroma formation in the donor site is a common early complication of the procedure and occasionally requires surgical drainage for resolution. The most common infectious complication is cellulitis, resulting from *Staphylococcus aureus*. A prominent scar on the back is usually the result of excessive tension on the incision at closure, which would occur when an excessively wide skin island is harvested. Necrosis, delayed healing, and complete loss of a latissimus dorsi flap are extremely rare because of the muscle's excellent blood supply. When flap loss does occur, it usually involves only a portion of the transposed muscle.

Preoperative Evaluation and Preparation

The patient's general medical condition and suitability for the procedure are carefully assessed. The shape and size of the remaining breast are measured, and a decision is made to match or modify the remaining breast. The suitability of the latissimus dorsi muscle for reconstruction must be established preoperatively. This is easily done in the thin individual by instructing the patient to place her hand on her hip and push down. The anterior edge of the contracted latissimus dorsi can be readily palpated if the innervation to the muscle is intact. If the muscle is denervated, it is likely that the entire thoracodorsal pedicle has been interrupted and the remaining secondary blood supply will limit the muscle's arc of rotation. Physical examination may be more difficult in obese individuals. For these patients, electromyography can be used to assess innervation and computed tomography will demonstrate the muscle bulk.

The patient must be well hydrated before surgery, and antibiotic prophylaxis is routinely administered. Some surgeons advocate intravenous corticosteroids before surgery or administration of intraoperative steroids and vasodilators to stabilize cell membranes and diminish swelling.

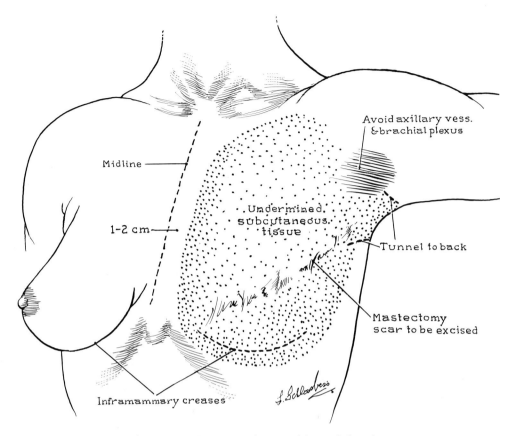

Fig 20-8. Preoperative marking of the chest.

OPERATIVE PROCEDURE

Preoperative Marking of the Chest (Figure 20-8)

With the patient in an upright position, before anesthetic induction, the contralateral inframammary crease is marked and a corresponding line is drawn on the side of the chest wall where the mastectomy was performed. If the mastectomy scar is low and transverse or oblique, as shown, the scar is excised with the chest wall incision. The anterior chest wall dissection and the creation of the anterior portion of the tunnel to the back are performed through this incision. The final positioning of the flap is determined after it is transposed to the anterior chest wall and with the patient in a semisitting position.

The ideal location for the skin island is low and oblique on the breast mound so that the inferior margin of the scar is incorporated in the inframammary crease and an optimal cosmetic appearance is achieved. If the mastectomy scar is medial and vertical, it is ignored, and a new chest incision is planned so that the lower margin of the skin island will be at the level of the new inframammary crease. This incision will be made 1 or 2 cm above the line corresponding to the opposite inframammary crease because the chest tissue retracts inferiorly after it is incised. The skin island is planned to fill the skin defect, which may be substantial for patients who have a skin graft or severe radiation damage, and to provide sufficient tissue bulk to create a breast mound that is symmetrical with the contralateral breast in terms of size, position, and contour. The area that will be undermined during

159

elevation of the chest skin flaps and creation of the breast pocket is delineated by stippling. The site for the subcutaneous tunnel from the back to the chest is located so that injury to the axillary vessels and the brachial plexus is avoided.

Preoperative Marking of the Back, and Positioning the Patient (Figure 20-9)

With the patient in a sitting position, the borders of latissimus dorsi muscle and the planned skin island are outlined. The outline of the skin island and muscle can be traced on x-ray film or paper and the tracings placed on the anterior chest wall to ensure that the planned flap transposition will provide appropriate skin replacement and muscle bulk to produce an adequate breast mound. The marking of the subcutaneous tunnel for transposition of the flap to the anterior chest is also completed.

After general anesthesia is induced, the patient is placed in a lateral position so that the surgical team can have simultaneous access to both the anterior chest and the back. The arm is abducted, as shown in this figure, with the elbow flexed and supported on a well-padded, right-angle arm support. The arm must remain in a relaxed position, free of pressure or traction, during flap elevation. A urinary bladder drainage catheter is inserted, and a pillow is placed between the legs with the hips flexed. The hips are padded and the lower torso is secured in position.

In this position the anterior chest wall dissection and elevation of the latissimus flap can be performed without repositioning the patient. If two teams are operating simultaneously, one can create the breast pocket while the other elevates the flap. If a single surgeon is performing the entire reconstruction, the anterior chest wall dissection is done first.

Positioning the patient with such a large surface area exposed can lead to hypothermia; therefore the patient is placed on a warming blanket, and the operating room is kept warm. After positioning, the patient is prepared and draped with the chest wall and the back in the same sterile field.

Anterior Chest Wall Dissection (Figure 20-10)

This figure illustrates the anterior chest wall dissection in a patient who had a modified radical mastectomy, with some atrophy of the pectoralis major muscle. After the chest incision has been made, the skin and subcutaneous tissues are elevated off the underlying chest wall to create a pocket for the muscle flap insertion. An implant will be placed beneath the flap. The dissection for the pocket extends medially to within 1 or 2 cm lateral to the midline of the sternum; inferiorly to the location of the proposed inframammary crease; and laterally to the midaxillary line. The superior margin of dissection is determined by the extent of padding needed in the infraclavicular area. If none is needed, the dissection extends to just below the clavicle. If an infraclavicular hollow is present and if padding is required in this region, the dissection is extended to the clavicle. Care must be taken to avoid injury to the brachial plexus and the axillary vessels during dissection in the axilla. The chest wall dissection proceeds in a similar manner following a radical mastectomy. If the anterior axillary fold is absent because of removal of the pectoralis major muscle, the pectoralis major tendon stump must be identified and exposed so that the latissimus dorsi can be attached to it.

160

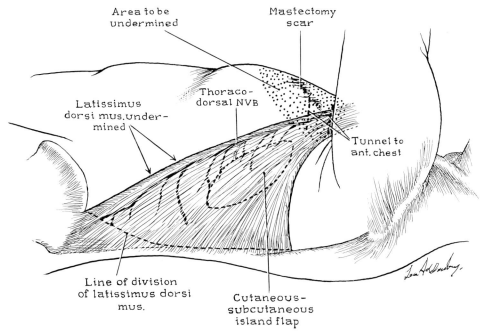

Fig 20-9.   Preoperative marking of the back, and positioning of the patient.

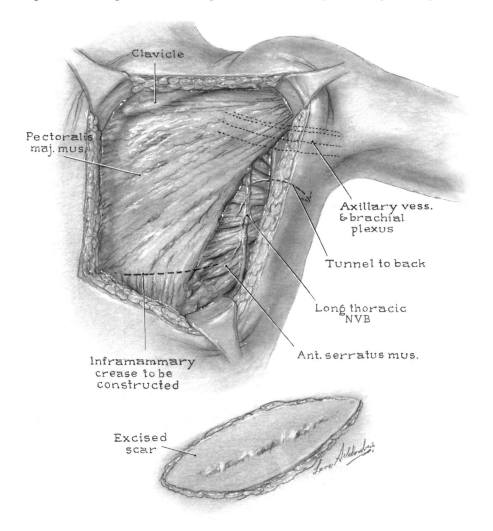

Fig 20-10.   Anterior chest wall dissection.

After the chest wall skin flaps have been elevated, a subcutaneous tunnel is created by sharp and blunt dissection from the anterior chest to the anterior border of the latissimus dorsi muscle. Through this tunnel the flap will be transposed from the back to the breast pocket. The opening must be sufficiently large to permit passage of the surgeon's hand and the entire flap during surgery and also to accommodate the edema that develops postoperatively. After completion of the anterior chest wall dissection, the wound is packed with a moist laparotomy sponge.

Skin Island Incision for Flap Elevation (Figure 20-11)

Flap elevation is started by incising the marked skin island. The incision on the back should be beveled 45 degrees away from the marked ellipse of skin, making the base of the skin territory wider than its surface. Inclusion of additional perforating vessels by beveling the skin at this angle will maximize the blood supply to the skin island and provide a larger paddle of subcutaneous tissue overlying the muscle. The skin edges retract so that subcutaneous fat beyond the territory of the skin island remains on the muscle. Failure to properly bevel the flap results in a narrow pedicle of subcutaneous tissue between the muscle and skin, causing a diminished blood supply to the skin island. After the skin island has been incised and properly beveled, the incision is extended down to the surface of the muscle. If no skin island is required, an obliquely oriented incision of sufficient length is made over the latissimus dorsi muscle to obtain adequate exposure for muscle elevation.

Superficial Dissection: Latissimus Dorsi Flap (Figure 20-12)

Skin flaps overlying the portion of the latissimus dorsi that are to be used for transposition are elevated at the level of the musculofascial plane around the skin island. The extent of the skin and subcutaneous tissue elevation required for transposing the entire muscle is shown here by the dashed line and stippling. After the skin flaps are raised, the anterior and superior borders of the latissimus dorsi and the lumbodorsal fascia, serving as landmarks for safe flap elevation, can be identified readily and exposed. Superficial dissection overlying the superior extent of the latissimus dorsi must be high enough posteriorly to allow free rotation of the muscle to the anterior chest wall.

If the latissimus tendon is to be transposed to recreate an anterior axillary fold, the dissection must proceed even higher to gain adequate length for attachment to the pectoralis major tendon.

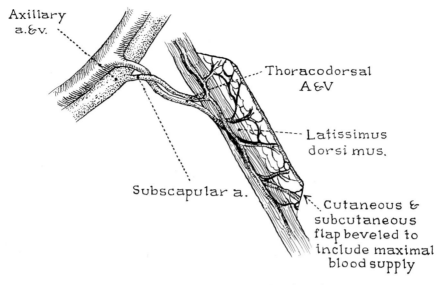

Axillary a.&v.

Thoracodorsal A&V

Latissimus dorsi mus.

Subscapular a.

Cutaneous & subcutaneous flap beveled to include maximal blood supply

Fig 20-11.   Skin island incision for flap elevation.

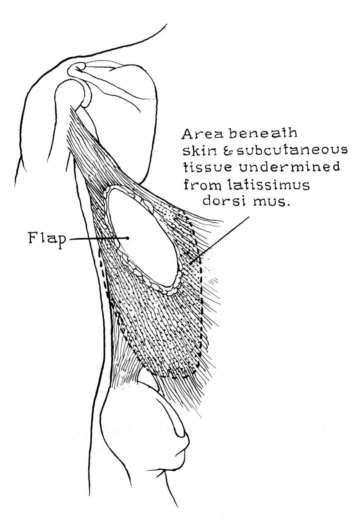

Area beneath skin & subcutaneous tissue undermined from latissimus dorsi mus.

Flap

Fig 20-12.   Superficial dissection: latissimus dorsi flap.

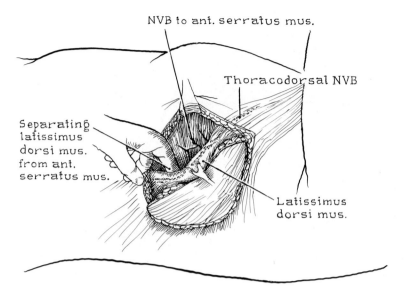

NVB to ant. serratus mus.

Thoracodorsal NVB

Separating
latissimus
dorsi mus.
from ant.
serratus mus.

Latissimus
dorsi mus.

Fig 20-13. Elevation of the anterior border of the latissimus dorsi.

Elevation of the Anterior Border of the Latissimus Dorsi (Figure 20-13)

After the skin flaps have been developed and the muscle borders identified, the latissimus dorsi is elevated. First, the anterior border of the latissimus dorsi, overlying the serratus anterior muscle, is raised and the thoracodorsal neurovascular bundle is identified and exposed. To identify the main thoracodorsal pedicle, the collateral branch of the thoracodorsal artery and vein that supply the serratus anterior are identified on that muscle's surface and then traced proximally. Early identification and exposure of the thoracodorsal neurovascular pedicle reduce the likelihood of inadvertent injury to the vessels, which could compromise the success of the flap transposition. The anterior border of the latissimus dorsi muscle then can be safely elevated by gentle retraction on the muscle edge and blunt dissection with a finger to fully free the anterior border.

Elevation of the Superior Border of the Latissimus Dorsi Muscle (Figure 20-14)

After the thoracodorsal vascular pedicle has been identified and the anterior portion of the latissimus dorsi elevated, a finger is inserted posteriorly beneath the muscle, just inferior to the tip of the scapula. By sharp and blunt dissection the superior portion of the muscle is raised off the underlying chest wall. The superior border of the latissimus dorsi is elevated, starting posteriorly and progressing anteriorly with the electrocautery to separate the muscular interdigitations from the teres major. The latissimus dorsi can be separated bluntly from the lower margin of the trapezius muscle.

Elevation of the Posterior and Inferior Borders of the Latissimus Dorsi (Figure 20-15)

Posteriorly and inferiorly the latissimus dorsi is detached by electrocautery from the lumbodorsal fascia, the ribs, and the iliac crest as shown by the dotted line. Care must be taken to avoid injury to the paraspinal muscles

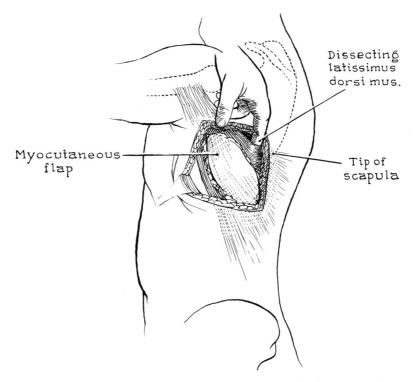

Fig 20-14.   Elevation of the superior border of the latissimus dorsi.

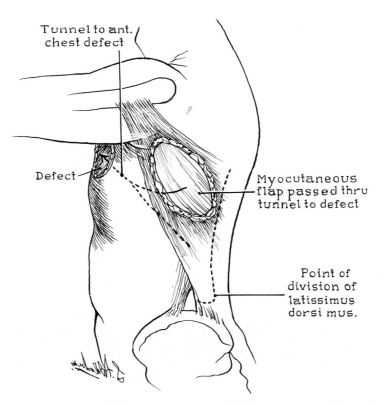

Fig 20-15.   Elevation of the posterior and inferior borders of the latissimus dorsi.

underlying the lumbodorsal fascia. As the muscle dissection continues anteriorly and superiorly, the latissimus is elevated from the ribs and from the external oblique muscle. The electrocautery is used to divide the bony origins of the muscle, and blunt dissection is used to separate the areolar tissue.

Continuation of the Latissimus Dorsi Flap Elevation (Figure 20-16)

As the serratus anterior muscle becomes visible, a fibrofatty bridge of tissue is encountered at that muscle's obliquely oriented inferior margin that connects the latissimus and the serratus anterior. This bridge of tissue must be divided to separate the two muscles so that the dissection does not progress beneath the serratus anterior. Once the fibrofatty connection is divided, the latissimus is elevated off the serratus anterior and reflected posteriorly. As the latissimus is elevated, the collateral branch of the thoracodorsal vessel to the serratus anterior muscle will be visible along its surface. If the main thoracordorsal pedicle has been ligated or injured by irradiation of the axilla, this collateral branch must be protected because it will provide circulation to the transposed flap.

The latissimus dorsi will now be attached only in the axilla. Extreme caution must be exercised to avoid inadvertent damage to the neurovascular structures while the muscle is being elevated in the axilla. Ten centimeters below the axillary vessels, the thoracordorsal neurovascular bundle separates from the muscle. As it approaches the axillary vessels, the many small branches connecting the thoracordorsal pedicle to adjacent structures must be ligated as they are encountered and before they are divided to avoid troublesome bleeding. If the dissection progresses close to the subscapular vessels, numerous venous branches with delicate, thin walls are encountered and can be easily injured. However, it is unnecessary to progress this far superiorly in the axilla unless the full length of the muscle is needed to recreate an anterior axillary fold.

Completion of Latissimus Dorsi Flap Mobilization (Figure 20-17)

As the branches from the thoracodorsal system are ligated and divided, the thoracodorsal pedicle is visualized and can be protected on the muscle's underside by superior reflection of the latissimus dorsi. Once the patency of the thoracodorsal vascular pedicle is confirmed, the collateral branch that runs to the serratus anterior muscle can be ligated and divided to maximize the arc of rotation of the flap.

Fibers intermingling and spiraling between the latissimus dorsi and the teres major make it difficult to distinguish the borders of the two muscles in the axilla, and the elevation of the latissimus in this region may be tedious. However, if the superior border of the latissimus is not completely detached from the teres major, the two interconnected muscles will bulge in the axilla when the flap is rotated into the chest.

After the dissection of the thoracodorsal vascular pedicle is completed and the latissimus is separated from the teres major, the flap is almost completely mobilized. At this point a decision is made regarding division of the muscle superiorly. Generally the muscle can be transposed without division superiorly. However, in an extremely thin patient, the muscle may be divided 2 or 3 cm superior to the point at which the thoracodorsal vascular pedicle enters it to avoid creating a bulge in the axilla when the muscle is transposed.

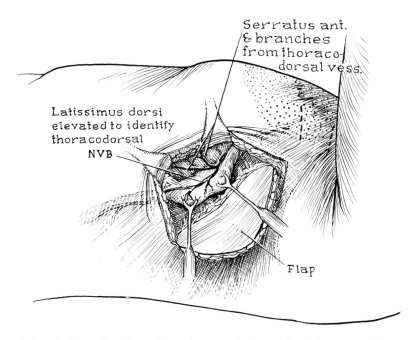

Fig 20-16. Continuation of the latissimus dorsi flap elevation.

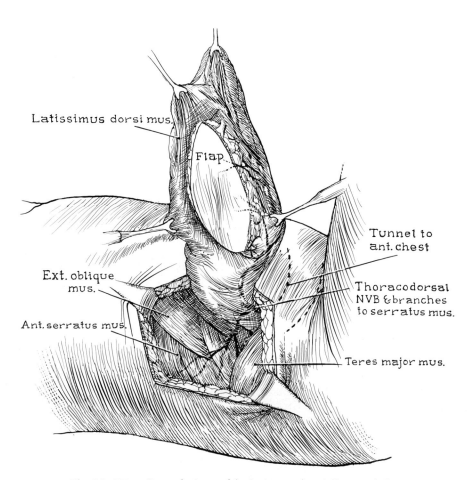

Fig 20-17. Completion of latissimus dorsi flap mobilization.

The latissimus tendon that inserts into the humerus is left intact, and the muscle is divided. If additional muscle length is needed to recreate an anterior axillary fold, the muscle is divided nearer the humerus through its tendinous insertion. With the latissimus now fully isolated on its tendinous attachment and neurovascular pedicle or on its neurovascular pedicle alone, it can be transposed to the chest through the tunnel.

Flap Transposition to the Anterior Chest Wall, and Closure of the Back Wound (Figure 20-18)

The elevated latissimus dorsi muscle is transposed to the chest wall pocket through a subcutaneous tunnel of sufficient size between the incisions on the chest and the back. After the flap has been transposed, the muscle and the vascular pedicle must lie free in the tunnel to avoid impairment of the circulation.

After the flap has been transposed to the breast pocket, the back wound is irrigated and hemostasis is achieved. Two 10-mm vacuum drains are placed under the skin flaps on the back and brought out through the skin near the axilla. The wound is then closed with interrupted absorbable sutures reinforced by a running subcuticular suture. Skin staples and cutaneous sutures are not used because the back wound will be tight, and the ensuing edema will cause unsightly crosshatching. After closure of the back wound, a sterile nonadherent gauze dressing is applied to the incision.

Insetting of the Flap on the Anterior Chest Wall (Figure 20-19)

After closure of the back wound the patient is moved to a supine or semisitting position with the ipsilateral arm abducted at a 90-degree angle. Although it is possible to inset the flap and insert an implant while the patient is in a lateral position, the best esthetic result is obtained if she is in a sitting or supine position. The skin is again prepared and draped so that the opposite breast is also in the sterile field.

For reconstruction following a radical mastectomy, part of the muscle is used to pad the chest wall from just below the clavicle to the inframammary crease. The appropriate position for the skin island is then determined. The flap is first secured with interrupted absorbable sutures along its superior and medial margins. Once the muscle is inset along the infraclavicular area and the medial border to the inframammary crease, the latissimus dorsi is sutured to the tendinous stump of the pectoralis major, creating an anterior axillary fold. The lateral margin is left open for implant insertion and breast mound contouring.

If additional volume is needed to achieve symmetry with the opposite breast, a sizing implant is placed beneath the flap to help determine the final contouring and placement of the skin island. Breast mound tailoring may require use of the entire skin island, excision of small skin segments, or deepithelialization and burial of the flap to provide additional axillary fill. The inferior margin of the skin island can be placed at the inframammary crease so the skin of the flap will lie low on the breast mound. Once the skin island is positioned as inferiorly as possible and all but the lateral margin of the flap has been inset, the final decision about implant size and positioning is made.

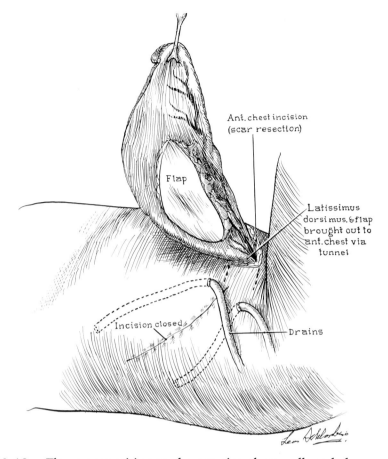

Fig 20-18. Flap transposition to the anterior chest wall, and closure of the back wound.

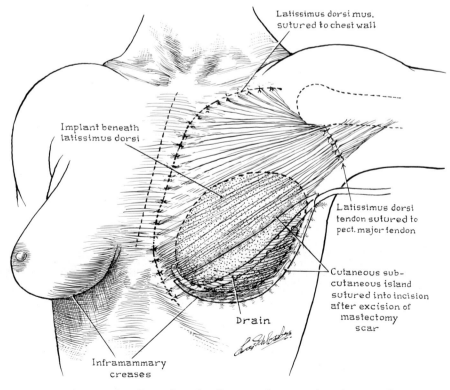

Fig 20-19. Insetting the flap on the anterior chest wall.

169

When the ideal breast mound size, contour, and position have been determined for symmetry with the contralateral breast and when the appropriate implant has been placed, a 10-mm constant vacuum drain is inserted beneath the flap and brought out in the axilla. Interrupted absorbable sutures are used to attach the lateral margin of the muscle to the chest wall. When the final breast mound contour is evaluated, the prosthesis is gently pushed laterally to ensure that the expander or implant will remain anterior to the midaxillary line. Because elevation of the latissimus leaves a large open space in the lateral portion of the chest, an implant can migrate into the back if the transposed latissimus dorsi muscle edge is not sutured to the chest wall.

When the flap and implant are finally positioned, skin staples are used to tailor the chest wall skin flaps to the skin island. Interrupted absorbable subcutaneous sutures then are placed between the staples, and the staples are removed. This layer of interrupted absorbable sutures is followed by a running subcuticular suture layer around the entire skin island margin. The chest wound incisions are dressed with an antibiotic ointment and with a nonadherent gauze dressing.

Modified Procedure for Latissimus Dorsi Flap Augmentation of an Atrophic Pectoralis Major Muscle Following Modified Radical Mastectomy
Insetting the Flap on the Chest Wall (Figure 20-20)

When the latissimus dorsi flap is used to augment an atrophic pectoralis major muscle, chest wall skin is generally sufficient to accommodate the muscle flap and implant. Therefore a skin island may not be needed, and only a strip of muscle is required. After the chest wall dissection has been completed, a single short incision in the back is made and the required amount of latissimus dorsi muscle and its vascular pedicle are elevated as previously described. The muscle can be harvested from its anterior border, where the primary vessels of the thoracodorsal system are located. The narrow flap is transposed through the subcutaneous tunnel and into the anterior chest wall pocket. A large portion of muscle should not be left in the axilla, or a bulge will appear when the arm is adducted. After the drains have been inserted and the back wound closed, the transposed section of the latissimus is attached with interrupted absorbable sutures to the lateral and inferior borders of the atrophic pectoralis major muscle; an opening is left for insertion of a tissue expander.

This entire process can usually be accomplished, if necessary, while the patient is in a lateral position. However, it is preferable to move the patient to a supine or semisitting position after the flap has been transposed to the chest and after the back incision is closed. This allows for additional chest wall dissection, completion of tailoring of the breast mound contour, and positioning of the prosthesis.

Positioning of the Implant Beneath the Augmented Pectoralis Major and Latissimus Dorsi Muscles (Figure 20-21)

The sling of muscle added to the inferior border of the atrophic pectoralis major produces sufficient coverage for an expander or implant and permits reconstruction of a properly contoured breast mound. The augmented pec-

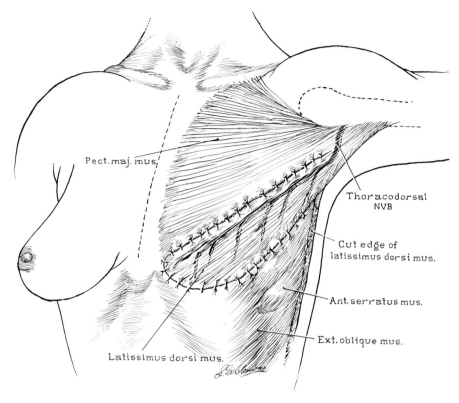

Fig 20-20.   Insetting the flap on the chest wall.

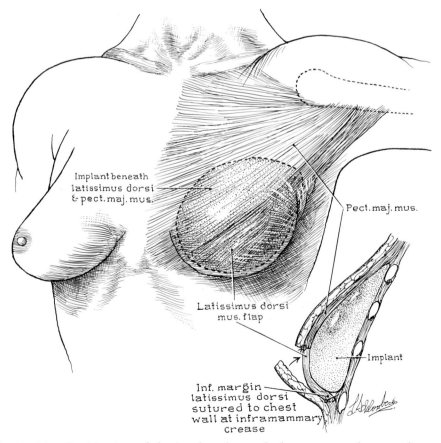

Fig 20-21.   Positioning of the implant beneath the augmented pectoralis major and latissimus dorsi muscles.

171

toralis major muscle is elevated from the chest wall to approximately 1 cm lateral to the midline of the sternum, starting inferiorly and proceeding superiorly to just beneath the clavicle. The implant or tissue expander then is placed beneath the joined muscles, and the latissimus portion is moved inferiorly to cover the implant (as shown in the inset). Interrupted absorbable sutures are used to attach the lower margin of the latissimus to the chest wall at the level of the inframammary crease and to affix its lateral edge to the chest wall just anterior to the midaxillary line.

The chest wall skin flaps are tailored to cover the joined muscles and the reconstructed breast mound. The wound is closed with a layer of interrupted absorbable sutures followed by a running subcuticular suture. A sterile dressing then is applied.

Postoperative Care

In the immediate postoperative period the patient is kept warm and well hydrated. Urine production and flap viability are closely monitored. If an initially well-perfused flap subsequently appears poorly perfused, prompt reexploration for evacuation of a wound hematoma may be required. Ambulation is started the day after surgery, and each drain is removed when its 24-hour accumulation is less than 30 ml. The patient may shower or bathe after the drains are removed, and usually she can be discharged from the hospital about 4 days postoperatively. Pressure under the arm on the side of flap transposition is avoided for 2 weeks. Normal daily activities and light physical activity may be resumed in 2 weeks. Excessive sun exposure and all strenuous activities, including sports and heavy lifting, must be avoided for 6 weeks. Smoking is prohibited for 8 weeks.

21

TRAM Flap

Introduction

The transverse rectus abdominis myocutaneous (TRAM) flap is the preferred technique for reconstructing the breast with distant autogenous tissue. It can be transposed to the chest on a superior epigastric vascular pedicle, or it can be transferred as a free flap, with microvascular anastomosis of the inferior epigastric vessels to appropriate vessels in the chest. The pedicled TRAM flap is discussed in this chapter. The free TRAM flap is discussed in Chapter 22.

Transposition of a standard TRAM flap involves elevation of a segment of the rectus abdominis muscle, with an overlying ellipse of subcutaneous tissue and skin based on a superior epigastric artery pedicle. The flap is rotated through a subcutaneous tunnel to the anterior chest wall.

A thorough knowledge of the anatomy of the anterior abdominal wall is essential to understanding the TRAM flap design and to understanding its use for breast reconstruction. Figure 21-1 shows the rectus abdominis muscle originating from the fifth, sixth, and seventh costochondral cartilages superiorly and attaching to the central crest of the pubic bone inferiorly. In the supraumbilical area three transverse tendinous inscriptions divide the muscle into neuromuscular units and connect it to the anterior fascial sheath. One or two incomplete tendinous bands also may be present below the umbilicus. The rectus abdominis muscle is broad and thin superiorly but narrow and thick inferiorly.

The rectus abdominis muscle supplements the functions of other abdominal wall muscles, particularly in flexion of the abdomen. No noticeable loss of function occurs when one rectus muscle is removed because the internal and external oblique muscles compensate for its absence. However, loss of both rectus muscles usually causes abdominal wall weakness, as well as difficulty in rising from a supine to a sitting position. Other functional changes are minimal if the strength and integrity of the rectus fascia are maintained. The location of the arcuate line partway between the umbilicus and the pubic symphysis is shown here. The arcuate line is a major anatomic landmark. Above the arcuate line (shown in Figure 21-2) the lateral anterior abdominal wall is composed of the external oblique muscle, the internal oblique muscle, and the transversus abdominis muscle. Each muscle is encased in a fascial compartment. Medial and lateral to the rectus abdominis

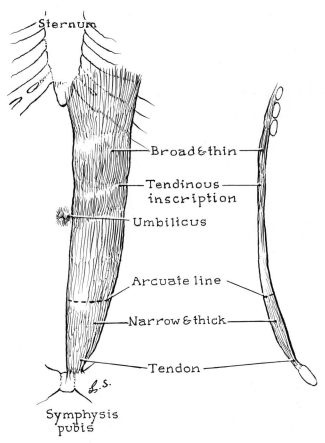

Fig 21-1. Anatomy of the rectus abdominis muscle.

muscle, aponeuroses are formed by the anterior and posterior layers of the fascia surrounding the external oblique and internal oblique muscles. The aponeurosis of the external oblique muscle passes medially and entirely anterior to the rectus abdominis muscle. The aponeurosis of the internal oblique muscle also passes medially and then splits, with the result that approximately half lies anterior and half lies posterior to the rectus abdominis muscle. The transversus abdominis muscle extends medially and posteriorly to the lateral border of the rectus muscle, where its anterior and posterior fascial layers, along with the posterior fascia of the internal oblique muscle, pass posterior to the rectus.

At the midline the external oblique aponeurosis and the anterior component of the internal oblique aponeurosis fuse with the posterior component of the internal oblique aponeurosis and with the entire aponeurosis of the transversus abdominis muscle to form the linea alba, a dense fascial sheath that lies between the two rectus muscles and extends from the xiphoid to the pubis. The linea semilunaris (not shown here), a sheath formed by fusion of the aponeuroses of the lateral abdominal muscles, extends from the ribs to the pubis along the lateral margin of each rectus muscle. The linea alba and linea semilunaris are important vertical supporting structures and always should be preserved when the rectus abdominis muscle is harvested.

The strong, thick posterior fascial layer, consisting of the posterior half of the internal oblique aponeurosis and the entire layer of the transversus

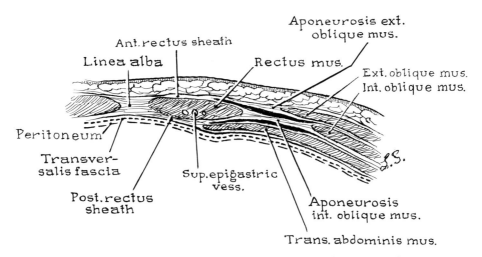

Fig 21-2. Abdominal wall anatomy above the arcuate line.

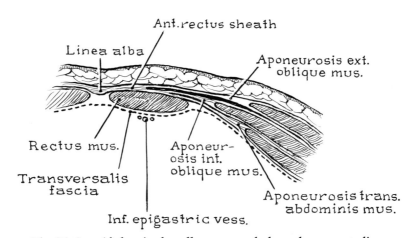

Fig 21-3. Abdominal wall anatomy below the arcuate line.

abdominis aponeurosis, provides strong posterior support for the rectus sheath. Even if a portion of the anterior rectus sheath is removed, a hernia is unlikely to develop in this area. At this level the superior epigastric artery runs near the center of the rectus abdominis muscle.

Below the arcuate line (shown in Figure 21-3), the transversus abdominis aponeurosis and the entire aponeurosis of the internal oblique muscle pass anterior to the rectus muscle. The transversus abdominis muscle ends laterally at the same level as the external oblique muscle. The transversalis fascia extends medially posterior to the rectus sheath. It is the only supporting structure at this level, and it makes the posterior rectus sheath much thinner below the arcuate line. At this level the inferior epigastric artery and vein are posterior to the rectus muscle. Few if any perforating branches course through the rectus abdominis muscle below the arcuate line. When a TRAM flap is elevated, all supporting structures inferior to the arcuate line should be left intact. Loss of the anterior rectus sheath below the arcuate line, particularly if the loss is combined with removal of the rectus abdominis muscle, weakens the anterior abdominal wall substantially and can result in a hernia unless the area is reinforced with fascia or synthetic material.

Figure 21-4 shows that the posterior sheath of the rectus abdominis muscle is thick and fibrous above the arcuate line. Below the arcuate line the sheath is thin and composed of the transversalis fascia and peritoneum only.

The rectus abdominis muscle receives its blood supply from the superior epigastric artery, the inferior epigastric artery, and branches of the intercostal arteries. The superior epigastric artery originates from the internal mammary artery and enters the abdomen approximately 3 cm lateral to the midline and beneath the costal margin. Almost immediately it enters the posterior rectus sheath and courses inferiorly for a variable distance before entering the muscle above the most superior tendinous inscription. Lying in the center of the midportion of the rectus muscle and traveling inferiorly to just above the umbilicus, the superior epigastric vessel then arborizes to anastomose with the ascending branches of the inferior epigastric artery.

The inferior epigastric artery originates from the external iliac artery and approaches the rectus muscle inferolaterally. A few centimeters below the arcuate line the inferior epigastric vessels enter the rectus sheath and ascend posterior to the muscle for a few centimeters. The vessels then enter the muscle and come to lie near the center of the muscle's midportion. The vessels then course superiorly to the umbilicus, where they arborize to connect with branches of the superior epigastric artery.

The inferior epigastric artery is the dominant blood supply to the rectus muscle, and it is a larger vessel than the superior epigastric artery. However, a TRAM flap will survive when it is based superiorly and transposed on the superior epigastric pedicle. The inferior epigastric pedicle serves as the primary blood supply when a TRAM flap is based inferiorly or transferred as a free flap. When anastomosed to vessels in the axilla or chest, the inferior epigastric artery can also be used to augment circulation to a pedicle TRAM flap based superiorly.

Several branches from the intercostal arteries enter the lateral aspect of the rectus sheath, accompanying the nerves in a segmental fashion throughout its length. These arterial branches communicate with the superior and inferior epigastric arteries. The intercostal arteries, particularly the musculophrenic artery (shown in Figure 21-4, *A*), can be important when the internal mammary artery has been damaged or when it is absent. Otherwise, these intercostal vessels are divided along with the motor nerves when the TRAM flap is elevated. Superior to the umbilicus, an arborization connects the superior and inferior epigastric systems. The venous drainage is cephalad in the superior epigastric veins and caudad in the inferior epigastric veins. This has practical importance because the inferior epigastric venous drainage must course cephalad through the arborized venous network when the pedicled TRAM flap, based on the superior epigastric system, is used.

The abominal skin and rectus muscle are innervated in a segmental fashion by intercostal nerves 8 through 12. These nerves enter the rectus sheath laterally alongside the intercostal vessels, pass behind the rectus muscle, and then enter the muscle posteriorly and just lateral to its midportion. Because flap elevation requires division of these nerves, a denervated rectus abdominis muscle results.

As shown in Figure 21-4, *B*, multiple vessels derive from the superior and inferior epigastric arteries, perforate through the rectus sheath, and

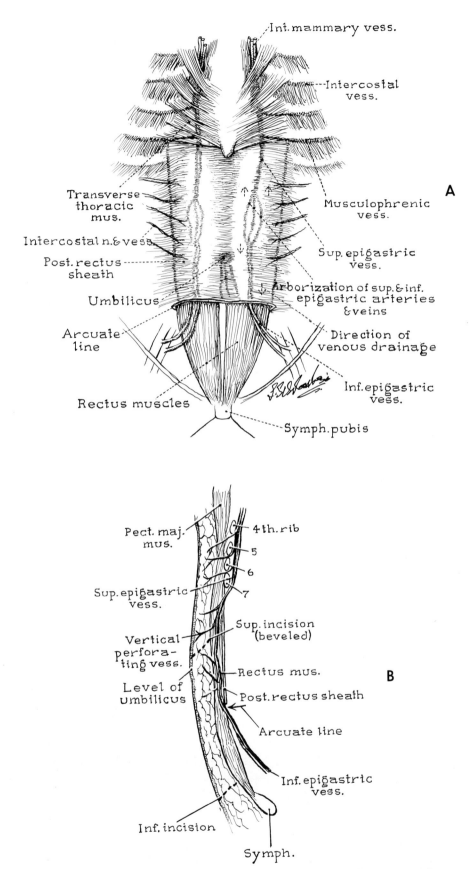

Fig 21-4. A, Posterior view of the anterior abdominal wall. B, Sagittal section of the anterior abdominal wall.

course into the level of the subdermal plexus, where they arborize laterally and medially to connect with similar vessels from the contralateral side. The density of this vascular network, which supplies the skin and subcutaneous tissue of the anterior abdominal wall, is greatest in the periumbilical area. Many perforating vessels are distributed between the umbilicus and the costal margin; however, they decrease in number in the region above the umbilicus. (This vascular network is best shown in Figures 21-6 and 21-7.) In the elevated TRAM flap these vertical perforating vessels form lateral and medial columns, coursing through each rectus sheath and spanning a 3- or 4-cm-wide area in the center of the muscle. This portion of the rectus sheath is harvested with the muscle, enabling these vertical perforators to be taken with the flap. The TRAM flap is designed with the beveled superior margin (shown in Figure 21-4, *B*) to take advantage of these perforating vessels that greatly enhance the flap's blood supply. The inferior epigastric artery enters the rectus muscle at the level of the arcuate line. No perforating vessels penetrate the subcutaneous tissues below this line. Therefore the inferior flap incision can be made vertically down to the rectus fascia because a bevelled incision benefits flap perfusion minimally.

Figure 21-5 shows the elevated skin island of a TRAM flap. The TRAM flap is divided into four circulatory zones defined in relation to the location of the muscle being transposed. Zone I (the myodermal portion directly perfused by the perforating vessels) is centered over the rectus muscle being transposed with the flap. Zone II (the portion perfused by axial vessels) is centered over the opposite rectus muscle. The medial portion of zone III, which is lateral to zone I, is also perfused by axial vessels. However, its lateral portion and all of zone IV, which is lateral to zone II, are randomly perfused by the subdermal plexus. After flap transposition the medial portion of zone III will usually survive; however, the whole of the lateral portion rarely survives. Zone IV is the least well-perfused area and rarely survives in its entirety. Frequently all of zone IV and the lateral portion of zone III will need to be resected. However, the perfusion of zones III and IV can be enhanced by using a delayed transposition procedure or by augmenting the circulation in the flap through microvascular anastomosis of the inferior epigastric artery and vein to vessels in the chest.

The TRAM flap, a well-vascularized, autogenous tissue block, produces an excellent tissue mound that closely matches the color and texture of the normal breast. The reconstructed breast tends to remain soft and well-contoured. Usually a breast prosthesis is not needed. The risks of capsular contracture and other implant-related problems are avoided. The patient does not have to be repositioned during the TRAM flap procedure because the chest and abdomen are in the same operative field. An additional advantage of the TRAM flap is that the abdominoplasty-type excision of tissue in the lower abdomen improves lower abdominal wall contour.

A major drawback of the TRAM flap involves the donor site. The fascia lying between the muscle and the skin in the abdomen is transposed with the flap. Therefore the abdominal wall can be weakened and is susceptible to hernia formation, particularly if both rectus abdominis muscles are transposed. A TRAM flap also leaves a large donor site scar that extends nearly the entire width of the abdomen. However, the scar usually is hidden with a swimsuit or underwear.

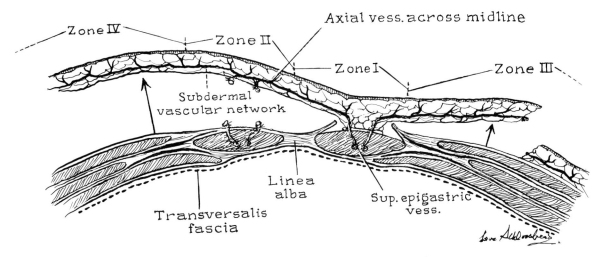

Fig 21-5. Elevated skin island of a TRAM flap.

Flap elevation requires division of the sensory innervation to the flap; therefore the resulting breast mound is insensate. After the TRAM flap has been transposed, the abdominal skin should regain some sensation during the first postoperative year.

Reconstruction with a TRAM flap is technically complex and may take twice as long as reconstruction with a latissimus dorsi flap and four times as long as a tissue expansion procedure. If microvascular anastomoses are necessary to ensure the vascular supply to the flap, the operative time is further increased. Once transposed the flap can be difficult to shape and set in place.

In planning for a TRAM flap preoperatively the surgeon must consider the amount of tissue that needs to be transposed to the chest, the type of mastectomy previously performed, the presence of radiation damage, the presence of an anterior axillary fold or an infraclavicular hollow, and the status of the pectoralis major muscle.

A radical mastectomy produces an extensive chest wall defect that necessitates a large TRAM flap. Because the entire flap will not survive on only one superior epigastric pedicle, modification may be necessary. Both rectus muscles may need to be transposed, a delayed flap may be transposed, or the blood flow may need to be augmented by microvascular anastomoses of the inferior epigastric vessels to vessels in the chest. Alternatively a flap centered higher in the abdomen will include a greater number of periumbilical perforating vessels and will enhance flap perfusion and survival. However, using such a flap results in a less satisfactory donor site scar. Reconstruction following bilateral radical mastectomies requires bilateral TRAM flaps taken from the low or the middle areas of the abdomen. However, if the chest wall defects are particularly extensive or if they include a marked infraclavicular hollow, a bipedicle or an augmented TRAM flap may be necessary to produce a single breast. Under these circumstances another pedicle flap or free flap can be used to reconstruct the other breast. Finally, the chest wall defect, resulting from the excision of radiation-damaged tissue, is usually quite extensive, and a TRAM flap is the best method for providing adequate coverage for breast reconstruction in this setting.

Transposition of a delayed TRAM flap can be used for women who have had previous abdominal surgery, for those who need flap reconstruction to cover an extensive area, or for those who are at increased risk for flap necrosis. This approach also may enhance survival of the standard pedicle TRAM flap when a bipedicle TRAM flap is contraindicated because of a previous division of a rectus muscle or when use of an augmented TRAM flap is not an option because of previous division of the inferior epigastric vessels.

Two methods for delaying the TRAM flap may be used to improve circulation to the flap. One involves elevating the flap and the muscle used for transposition until the flap is isolated on the perforating vessels through the rectus fascia, the rectus muscle, and the vascular pedicles. Then the flap is replaced in its abdominal bed, and the incision is closed. Usually within 1 week the flap can be reelevated and transposed for breast reconstruction.

An alternative, less extensive procedure for delay of the TRAM flap involves division of one or both inferior epigastric vessels through a small suprapubic incision. Division of these vessels increases the blood flow through the superior epigastric vessels. The flap then is transposed 1 or 2 weeks later. Delayed flap transposition with either method improves flap survival and decreases the incidence of fat and skin necrosis. Currently no studies have compared the two methods to determine if one is superior. Both delayed procedures require an additional operation.

Microvascular augmentation of the TRAM flap's circulation may be necessary when the tissue bulk of the flap is not adequately perfused by the superior epigastric pedicle alone. Several methods are available for augmenting the circulation to a pedicled TRAM flap. The most commonly used method is the microvascular anastomosis of the inferior epigastric vessels to vessels in the chest. This procedure is detailed in "Modification 2" in this chapter. This option should always be left available when a standard pedicled TRAM flap is elevated. If injury to the superior epigastric artery and vein occurs during flap mobilization or if the circulation through those vessels proves inadequate, the pedicled TRAM flap can be converted to a free flap by anastomosis of the inferior epigastric vessels to vessels in the chest. Anastomosis of the vein alone is most frequently performed because compromised venous drainage is relatively common and is a major cause of flap loss. Anastomosis of the inferior epigastric vein to a recipient vein, usually the thoracodorsal or thoracoacromial vein, will significantly improve venous drainage. This improves flap circulation and often results in complete survival of zones I, II, and III, and occasionally portions of zone IV. Theoretically it would be possible to anastomose only the inferior epigastric artery and not the vein; however, in practice this is rarely if ever done.

The other commonly used technique of augmentation (detailed as "Modification 4" in this chapter) is to raise the flap, not only as a pedicled flap in the classic sense of the TRAM flap but also to raise the side contralateral to the pedicled flap as a free flap. Under these circumstances the flap is converted from a pedicled flap, with zones I to IV of circulation, to hemiflaps, each with zone I and zone III territories. The inferior epigastric circulation is the dominant circulation to the TRAM flap, and anastomosis of these vessels to vessels in the chest significantly improves circulation to the entire flap. This technique is specifically indicated if a midline vertical incision has been made previously in the infraumbilical abdomen, which would limit the circulation from a contralateral pedicled flap or a contralateral pedicled flap with inferior epigastric augmentation. An additional indication for microvascular augmentation is a previously performed procedure involving the division of the ipsilateral superior rectus abdominis muscle (such as cholecystectomy). Such an operation precludes transposition of a bilateral pedicle flap. This alternate method of microvascular augmentation can also be used beneficially when the entire TRAM flap is needed for the high-risk patient with a substantial chest wall defect. A final method of augmentation is anastomosis of the free flap component vessels to the inferior epigastric vessels of the pedicled flap. This procedure is rarely done and is not illustrated in this chapter.

Indications

The TRAM flap is used primarily for reconstructing a breast mound. Additionally the TRAM flap can be used for simulation of the pectoralis major muscle, creation of an anterior axillary fold, and replacement of missing or inadequate skin following radical, modified radical, or subcutaneous mastectomy. The flap's large size permits correction of the foregoing defects and reconstruction of the breast mound at the same time.

The TRAM flap is useful for reconstruction of large chest wall defects, such as those that occur with radiation ulcers, and for correction of congenital deformities. The TRAM flap also can be used to reconstruct and to match a large or ptotic contralateral breast in an individual who is unwilling to undergo breast reduction or mastopexy. The TRAM flap may provide the only option for flap reconstruction when the latissimus dorsi muscle is atrophic, denervated, or absent. Finally, prior chest wall irradiation is another indication for breast reconstruction with autogenous vascularized tissue.

The TRAM flap alone, unlike the latissimus dorsi flap, can be used to reconstruct a breast mound. It therefore offers the best option for women who prefer totally autogenous tissue reconstruction or who have experienced serious implant-related problems, such as silicone mastopathy or severe capsular contractures.

Breast reconstruction in patients with denervation of the pectoralis muscle or those with thin, tight, or scarred chest wall skin and subcutaneous tissue requires the use of a vascularized skin island from a distant source. The latissimus dorsi or the TRAM flap may be used in breast reconstruction. However, the TRAM flap provides more skin with greater subcutaneous tissue bulk than the latissimus dorsi flap. The skin color and texture of the TRAM flap more closely simulate breast tissue, and the abdominal donor scar can be concealed more easily than can the back scar that accompanies a latissimus dorsi flap procedure.

Contraindications

Transposition of a TRAM flap is a lengthy operation, involving a dissection that spans from the pubis to the upper chest, and it creates two deep wounds. The postoperative period is stressful.

The best candidates for a TRAM flap have no major medical problems that might compromise flap survival. Older patients should undergo a thorough medical evaluation to ensure that they can safely tolerate a long operation. Obese women run a special risk of fat necrosis because the horizontal axial vessels preferentially supply the skin and not the subcutaneous fat. This is particularly true of individuals who are more than 25% above their ideal body weight. Conversely women who are very thin may be poor candidates because they generally lack sufficient tissue to reconstruct an adequate breast mound.

Safe transposition of a pedicle TRAM flap is usually precluded by previous subcostal, paramedian and transverse upper abdominal incisions, which typically divide the ipsilateral and perhaps both rectus abdominis muscles and consequently interrupt the superior epigastric artery and vein. Pflannenstiel incisions sometimes divide the vertical perforating vessels up to the level of the umbilicus, just as lower abdominal paramedian incisions may damage significant numbers of perforating vessels in the surrounding region. Midline abdominal incisions interrupt the horizontal axial vessels and limit the TRAM flap to the ipsilateral abdominal tissue, unless bipedicled flaps are used.

Complications

TRAM flap transposition may be associated with multiple systemic complications. Respiratory problems that may develop after the lengthy TRAM flap procedure include decreased ventilation, atelectasis, and pneumonia. Because the procedure is lengthy, patients are at risk for developing pulmonary emboli postoperatively. The development of a hematoma in the chest wall can produce excessive tension on the flap, or it can compress the vascular pedicle and result in partial or total loss of the flap. A hematoma in the abdomen can compromise circulation to the flap or to the remaining abdominal wall tissue. Infections in the TRAM flap or in the abdominal wall are uncommon and are often associated with fat necrosis. They usually respond to antibiotics and local wound care.

Fat and skin necrosis can be major problems with TRAM flap breast reconstruction and usually occur in the poorly perfused zones III and IV. Folding or kinking of the flap while shaping the breast mound also predisposes to subsequent tissue necrosis. Fat or skin necrosis in the abdominal wall is uncommon, unless some predisposing problem exists. When necrosis occurs, it develops in the infraumbilical area. Patients with fat necrosis typically have symptoms that include a low-grade fever, erythema, and wound induration, which is often followed by drainage of liquified fat. Fat or skin necrosis is treated conservatively, by local wound care, until the necrotic tissue becomes clearly demarcated. The nonviable tissue then should be debrided, and local wound care should be continued until the area of debridement heals by secondary intention. Often this treatment will not compromise the cosmetic result; however, a second-stage revision may be required.

A malpositioned or a misshapen breast mound can occur if the breast pocket is not correctly dissected or if the flap is not properly tailored and inset. If the pocket is dissected too far laterally, the breast may have too broad a base and project into the lateral portion of the chest. If the dissection is carried too far medially, the projection will appear abnormal in that direction. Both deformities will produce an asymmetric appearance that is difficult to correct. The breast mound also may be located too high because of an error in flap positioning (a rare occurrence). The inframammary crease also may be positioned too low. The inferior margin of the breast pocket should be placed higher than the contralateral inframammary crease because the inframammary crease will move inferiorly when the abdomen is closed.

Scars on the breast mound, at the periphery of the inset flap, or on the abdomen may become hypertrophic or wide and unsightly. Wide scars are more likely to form when the wound is closed under tension or if delayed healing has occurred secondary to skin or fat necrosis.

Seroma formation in the abdomen is an uncommon but difficult problem associated with the TRAM flap. The insertion of two constant vacuum drains will not prevent hematomas; however, the drains will remove small accumulations of blood and serum and can therefore reduce the risk of seroma. An abdominal wound with a large denuded surface occasionally will have prolonged serous drainage. If drainage continues for several weeks, a pseudobursa can form in the space between the abdominal skin flap and the abdominal wall. This condition usually resolves spontaneously over several months. Occasionally, reoperation with excision of the pseudobursa is required.

Hernias are rare when a single pedicle flap has been transposed. They are more common when both rectus muscles are either transposed with a bipedicle flap or transposed for a bilateral reconstruction. If both rectus muscles are used, the infraumbilical portion of the abdominal wall must be reinforced with synthetic mesh. If a hernia develops, it should be repaired with synthetic material. Abdominal laxity also can result from inadequate dynamic reinforcement of the abdominal wall after removal of the rectus muscle. The bulge is not a true hernia; however, it mimics a hernia and can be treated by reinforcing the lax area with synthetic material.

A malpositioned umbilicus is a relatively common complication associated with the TRAM flap. Most often the umbilicus will be horizontally malpositioned toward the side of the muscle used for transposition because of tightness resulting from removal of the anterior fascial strip. This complication is obviated by marking the midline before surgery so that the umbilicus can be centered during closure and by plication of the opposite anterior rectus sheath. A vertically malpositioned umbilicus most often occurs when it is positioned too high at closure. The umbilicus can be placed correctly by imagining a line drawn through the anterior superior iliac spines and by locating the umbilicus at or below the midpoint of that line. Necrosis of the umbilicus is extremely rare; however, it can be caused by excessive skeletonization when the umbilicus is cored from the TRAM flap.

Standing cones may form at the lateral ends of the abdominal closure and are best avoided by designing the flap so that its inferior and superior incision limbs are equal in length and by beginning closure of the abdomen laterally and advancing any excess tissue toward the midline.

Preoperative Evaluation

The patient's age, general medical condition, height and weight, prior abdominal or thoracic operations, and psychological disposition must be considered. Few candidates for this procedure are without potential risk factors. All risks and potential complications must be carefully explained to the patient before surgery to help establish realistic expectations in her mind. The surgeon must assess the amount of abdominal tissue available for use, as well as the quantity of tissue needed to fill the chest wall defect and to reconstruct a breast mound. The size and shape of the remaining breast also should be recorded. The patient should be asked if she prefers to have the reconstructed breast match the healthy breast or if the healthy breast should be modified to match the reconstructed breast.

Magnesium citrate and a cleansing enema usually are ordered the night before surgery to aid in subsequent abdominal closure. Patients should be well hydrated before surgery.

OPERATIVE PROCEDURE
Standard TRAM Flap Breast Reconstruction
Preoperative Marking (Figure 21-6)

While the patient is in a standing position, the skin is marked over the midline of the sternum, over the inframammary crease of the remaining breast (if present), and over the area of planned anterior chest dissection on the side of the previous mastectomy. The mastectomy side is marked to mirror the inframammary crease of the remaining breast. The proposed elliptically shaped TRAM flap then is outlined.

For a standard TRAM flap that is based on the contralateral rectus abdominis muscle (to the side of the mastectomy), the flap's superior margin is outlined approximately 2 cm above the umbilicus. The inferior margin is marked a few centimeters above the pubic hairline. The distance between these two points in the midline is usually 14 to 16 cm.

A line drawn between points *A* and *B* (the superior and inferior incision midpoints) determines the flap's width and serves as the short axis of its elliptical shape. The length of the flap *(CD)* should be three times its width; therefore the length is determined across the midpoint of the short axis. The lateral extent of the flap is in the area of the anterior superior iliac spine. If one half of the total long axis distance is on each side of the midpoint, the flap should be symmetrical. Both halves of the upper and lower incision limbs also should be the same length from the midpoint to avoid formation of standing cones when the abdomen is closed. The flap then is divided into zones I to IV and marked as shown. Two columns of perforating vessels penetrate each rectus muscle and provide the vascular supply to the skin and subcutaneous tissue of the flap.

After marking, the patient is placed on the operating table in a supine position, her hips are centered on the operating table, and both arms are abducted. After general anesthesia is induced, the patient's skin is prepped with an antibacterial solution from neck to pubic area, and the skin is draped, with the chest and abdomen included in the sterile field. Compression stockings are placed on the patient's legs. Her core temperature should be kept above 36° C during the operation.

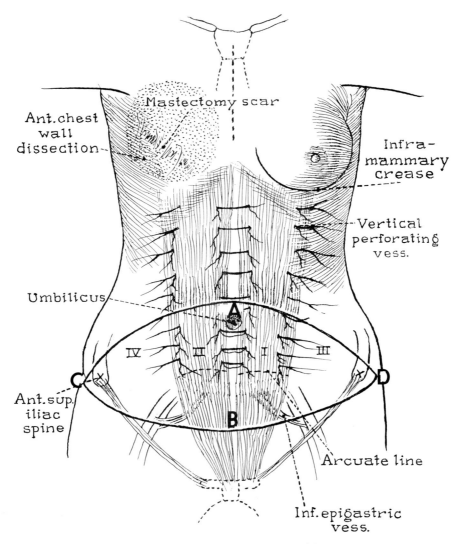

Fig 21-6. Preoperative marking.

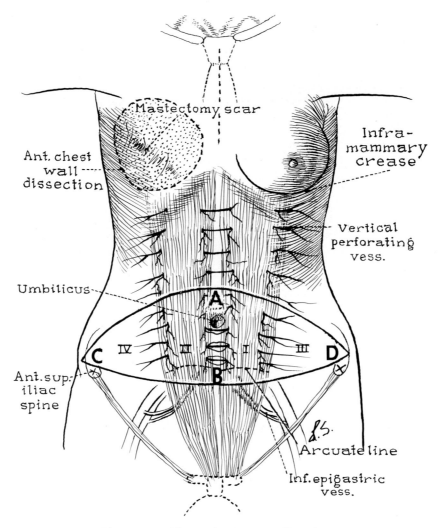

Fig 21-7. Alternative TRAM flap design.

Alternative TRAM Flap Design (Figure 21-7)

An alternative TRAM design centers the flap on the umbilicus so that it is located higher on the abdominal wall. This design places the inferior margin of the incision at the arcuate line. The superior limb is several centimeters above the umbilicus, and the lateral extent is immediately above the anterior superior iliac spine. The average width of this flap is between 12 and 15 cm. This design takes advantage of the rich concentration of vertical perforating vessels around the umbilicus. The flap is measured and is marked symmetrically according to the guidelines outlined for Figure 21-6.

Compared to the standard TRAM flap design this alternate produces a flap with a decreased arc of rotation and leaves a scar higher in the abdomen that is difficult to cover with a two-piece swimsuit or underwear. However, this upper or midabdominal TRAM flap is better vascularized because the superior epigastric vessels primarily supply the vascular territory of the upper abdomen, and the flap includes a greater number of periumbilical perforating vessels. This flap is useful in patients who have had previous surgery through a Pfannenstiel incision in which a lower portion of the abdominal wall skin is typically elevated off the anterior rectus sheath interrupting the perforating

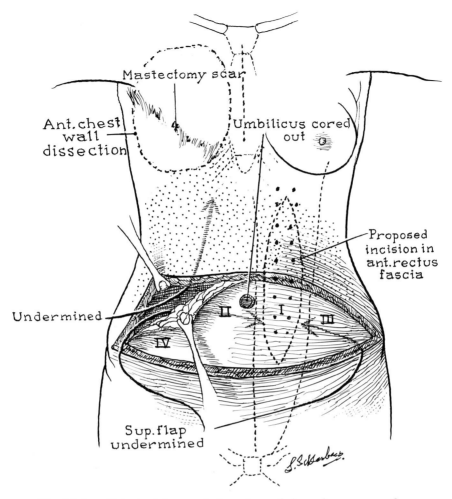

Fig 21-8. Skin incision and elevation of the subcutaneous flap.

vessels. This flap design also may be desirable in patients with chest wall radiation ulcers that require coverage with well-vascularized tissue, and in individuals who are at greater risk for abdominal wall weakness.

Skin Incision and Elevation of the Subcutaneous Flap (Figure 21-8)

Flap elevation begins on the side opposite the rectus abdominis muscle that is being transposed. The superior skin incision near the lateral margin is extended directly to the external oblique fascia. Medially and in the portion of the flap overlying the rectus sheath, however, the incision is beveled 45 degrees away from the flap and extended superiorly to include an additional 2 or 3 cm of subcutaneous fat, including the associated perforating vessels. The inferior limb of the incision is extended directly to the anterior abdominal wall fascia, without beveling, throughout its length.

The flap is raised toward the midline, beginning laterally at the level of the external oblique fascia on the ipsilateral side to the prior mastectomy and progressing toward the midline. Approximately 4 to 6 cm lateral to the midline the outermost column of vertical perforating vessels is identified exiting the rectus sheath and entering the subcutaneous fat. The inner column of perforators will be a few centimeters medial to this outer column. The rectus muscles are essentially symmetrical. Identification of the vertical per-forating vessels in the ipsilateral rectus sheath predicts their position in the contralateral muscle that will be used for transposition. A determination can now be made regarding how far dissection can continue past the midline on the contralateral side before encountering the perforating vessels that must be preserved with the flap.

The vast majority of perforating vessels pass through the anterior rectus sheath over a narrow area approximately 3 or 4 cm wide and near the center of the muscle. Only this strip of the fascia will need to be taken when the flap is mobilized.

As the flap elevation continues, the perforating vessels from the rectus muscle that is to remain in the abdomen are ligated and divided. After the linea alba is crossed, the umbilicus is cored out by cutting it free from the flap; however, it remains attached to the abdominal wall. Some subcutaneous fat is left around the base of the umbilicus to preserve circulation.

The TRAM flap now should be elevated 1 or 2 cm lateral to the midline on the contralateral side. Based on the location of the perforators on the ipsilateral side the most medial column of vertical perforating vessels is sought coming through the rectus sheath of the muscle that is to be used for transposition. Once these vessels are identified, medial dissection ceases. Then the inferior margin of the flap is elevated 3 or 4 cm below the arcuate line at the level of the rectus fascia.

The lateral margin of the flap on the side of the muscle being used for transposition is incised and elevated from lateral to medial in the same manner previously described. Once the TRAM flap has been elevated to the area where the most lateral column of vertical perforating vessels is seen coming through the rectus sheath, the dissection ceases and the subcutaneous tissue of the flap and the skin is placed in its original position. Next the upper abdominal skin and subcutaneous tissue should be undermined at the level of the fascia and elevated off the anterior abdominal wall to just above the costal margin and the xiphoid (shown by the stippling in this figure).

After the upper abdominal skin and subcutaneous tissue are elevated, the proposed fascial incision is drawn on the anterior rectus sheath. The elliptical outline (shown in the figure) extends from a few centimeters below the arcuate line to just above the most superior tendinous inscription. In-clusion of this superior portion of fascia facilitates muscle release with the tendinous bands attached. A TRAM flap designed to include this fascia contains the greatest number of perforating vessels in the portion of the anterior rectus sheath lying inside the ellipse. Thus the skin of the flap will be more richly perfused.

Fascial Incisions, and Mobilization of the Rectus Muscle (Figure 21-9)

After the skin and superior abdominal wall tissues have been elevated, the TRAM flap is isolated on a 3 to 4 cm band of anterior rectus sheath and centered over the portion of the rectus muscle that is most richly supplied by the vertical perforating vessels. At this point in the procedure the muscle is still attached to the xiphoid and pubis, and the flap is perfused by the

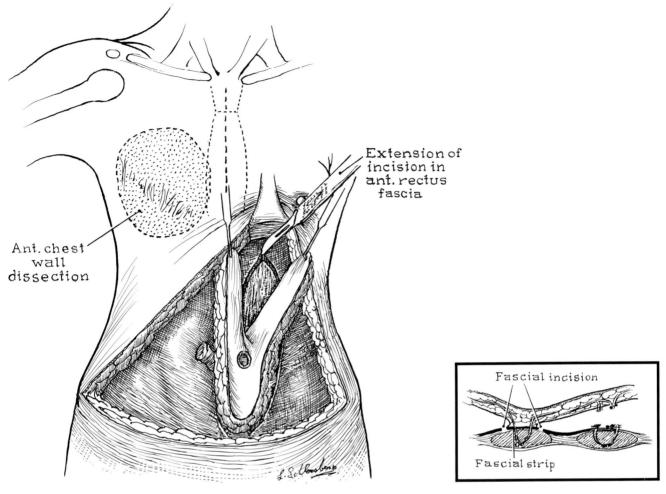

Fig 21-9. Fascial incisions, and mobilization of the rectus muscle.

inferior and superior epigastric pedicles. The flap should have normal circulation, with the possible exception being the most lateral part of zone IV.

The anterior rectus fascia is incised inferiorly to the lower margin of the flap just below the arcuate line. This elliptical fascial incision is designed to include the columns of perforating vessels that branch from the muscle into the subcutaneous tissue (see inset). The elliptical portion of the fascial incision is completed just beyond the most superior tendinous band and several centimeters above the superior edge of the flap. The incision then is continued upward in the middle of the anterior rectus sheath to 2 or 3 cm above the costal margin. Finally the portions of the rectus sheath lateral and medial to the elliptical strip of fascia are elevated off the anterior surface of the underlying rectus abdominis muscle.

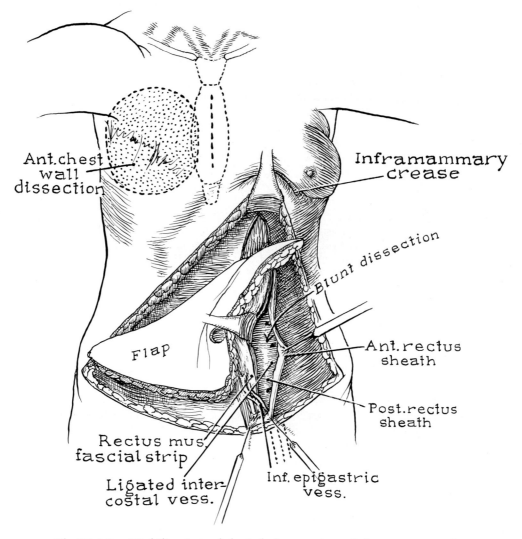

Fig 21-10. Mobilization of the inferior portion of the rectus muscle.

Mobilization of the Inferior Portion of the Rectus Muscle (Figure 21-10)

Mobilization begins in the midportion of the rectus muscle to minimize the risk of injury to the superior and inferior epigastric vessels. Blunt dissection is used to lift the rectus abdominis from its posterior fascia, and the muscle elevation proceeds toward its insertion inferiorly. As the lower half of the muscle is mobilized, the inferior epigastric artery and vein are identified and protected. The portion of the muscle superficial to the vascular pedicle is then freed.

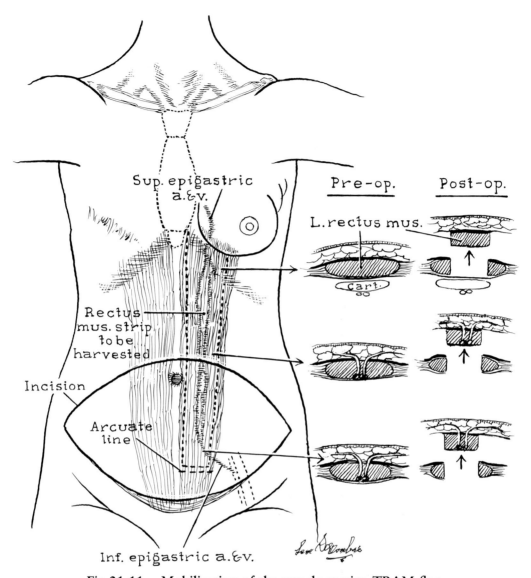

Fig 21-11. Mobilization of the muscle-sparing TRAM flap.

Mobilization of the Muscle-Sparing TRAM Flap (Figure 21-11)

It is not absolutely necessary to include the full width of the rectus muscle in the TRAM flap. A rectus muscle-sparing technique preserves the majority of the rectus muscle, which remains in the abdominal wall and possibly decreases the likelihood of abdominal wall weakness. A Doppler probe is used to identify the superior epigastric vessels within the muscle, and the path of the artery and vein is marked on the rectus sheath. A strip of the rectus muscle (usually 3 or 4 cm side) then is developed from just lateral to the vascular pedicle through the middle portion of the muscle surrounding the superior epigastric vessels. Only the strip containing the main vascular supply is mobilized. The lateral and medial edges of the rectus muscle remain in the abdomen and are sutured together before reapproximation of the anterior rectus sheath during abdominal wound closure. The inset depicts the sequential manner in which the muscle strip and its associated flap are harvested.

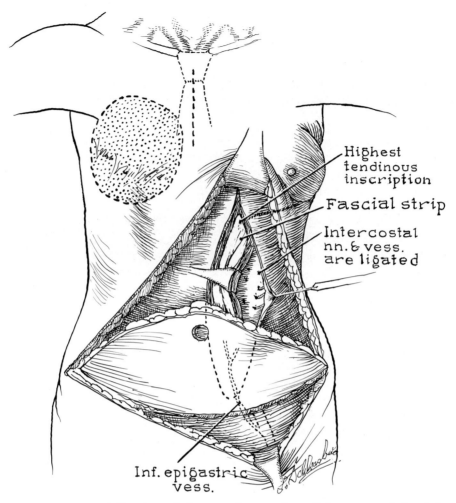

Highest tendinous inscription

Fascial strip

Intercostal nn. & vess. are ligated

Inf. epigastric vess.

Fig 21-12. Mobilization of the superior portion of the rectus abdominis muscle.

Mobilization of the Superior Portion of the Rectus Abdominis Muscle (Figure 21-12)

Elevation of the superior half of the rectus abdominis muscle proceeds from the midportion of the muscle toward the costal margin. As the dissection proceeds, the multiple intercostal nerve branches and associated small vessels that enter the lateral aspect of the muscle are ligated before that portion of the muscle is mobilized. Electrocautery is avoided to prevent muscle contraction. At the lateral edge of the muscle, near the costal margin, a large musculophrenic vascular branch usually enters the rectus abdominis. It is ligated and divided.

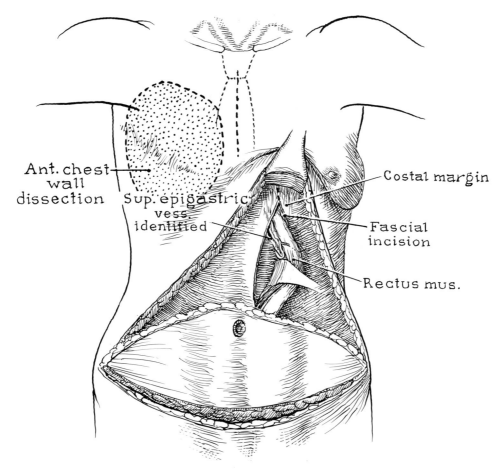

Ant. chest wall dissection

Sup. epigastric vess. identified

Costal margin

Fascial incision

Rectus mus.

Fig 21-13. Identification of the superior epigastric pedicle.

Identification of the Superior Epigastric Pedicle (Figure 21-13)

When the muscle is fully mobilized from the rectus sheath (except for its attachments near the arcuate line and the costal margin), the superior epigastric pedicle can be identified entering the posterior aspect of the rectus muscle. After the patency of the superior epigastric vessels is confirmed, the flap then is placed back in its bed to perfuse without restriction for 30 minutes. Time for perfusion is important because the flap has been folded upon itself during muscle mobilization, and circulation, especially venous drainage, may be impaired. During this time the anterior chest wall dissection is performed.

Anterior Chest Wall Dissection (Figure 21-14)

The anterior chest wall dissection begins by excision of the mastectomy scar. A transverse or oblique scar can be excised, and a chest wall pocket can be created beneath the scar. However, if the mastectomy scar is vertical or if it ends near the level of the opposite inframammary crease, a separate, obliquely oriented incision may be required.

Creation of the breast pocket begins with elevation of the skin and underlying subcutaneous fat off the chest wall. Superiorly the pocket is deepened to the pectoral muscle or to the fascia if present, so that the part of the TRAM flap used to pad the chest can be sutured to the muscle or to the fascia. The dissection margins are confined to the premastectomy breast pocket so that an envelope can be created to restrain the flap while tissue is tailored to a form that simulates the opposite breast. Such dissection also reduces the suturing required to inset the flap and to recreate the inframammary crease.

The final shape and position of the reconstructed breast depend largely on this dissection. If the pocket is too large, the breast will be flat and will lack projection. If the pocket is too small, circulation in the flap may be compromised or the reconstructed breast may be constricted. If the dissection is extended beyond the premastectomy envelope in any direction, the breast will appear misshapen.

The initial inferior dissection (except for the area of the tunnel) should be kept several centimeters above the opposite inframammary crease because the new inframammary crease will be several centimeters lower after the abdominal wall is closed following passage of the flap into the chest. The reconstructed breast mound will appear too low and asymmetric with the opposite breast if the inferior margin of the pocket is dissected to the level of the contralateral inframammary crease during the anterior chest wall dissection. However, if the dissection is carried too low, fat from the flap may migrate inferiorly, and the definition of the inframammary crease may be lost. It is difficult to elevate the inframammary crease if the dissection has extended too far inferiorly. However, if the inframammary crease seems too high, (after the abdominal wall has been closed), it can be easily lowered during insetting.

Generally the lateral dissection is carried only to the anterior axillary line unless a microvascular anastomosis is planned, in which case the dissection must be continued farther laterally to expose and mobilize the thoracodorsal vessels. However, if the dissection extends too far laterally, fat or skin from the flap can migrate into the area and make the breast appear malpositioned. Deformities that result from shaping and positioning errors destroy the symmetry of the breasts and are difficult to correct. Furthermore, insetting the flap into a pocket that is too large often necessitates using numerous deep sutures to mold the breast mound into an acceptable shape. Such excessive suturing can compromise the flap's circulation. It is preferable to create a smaller pocket that can be enlarged later if needed.

After the pocket has been fully dissected on the chest wall, a subcutaneous tunnel 7 to 10 cm wide is created by sharp and blunt dissection between the breast pocket and the abdominal wound at the fascial level. This tunnel must be wide enough to allow easy transposition of the flap to the pocket while protecting the muscle and the vascular pedicle.

194

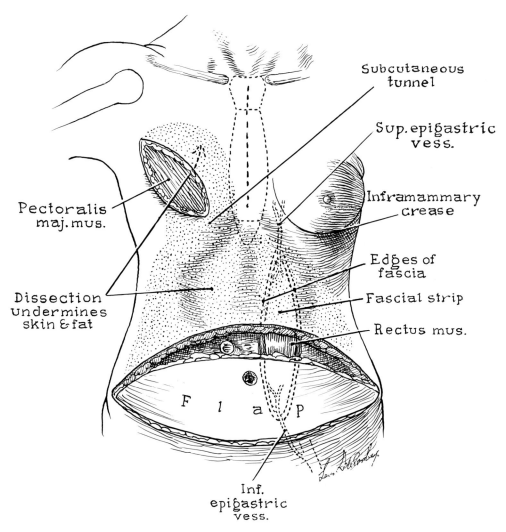

Subcutaneous
tunnel

Sup. epigastric
vess.

Inframammary
crease

Edges of
fascia

Fascial strip

Rectus mus.

Pectoralis
maj. mus.

Dissection
undermines
skin & fat

F l a P

Inf.
epigastric
vess.

Fig 21-14. Anterior chest wall dissection.

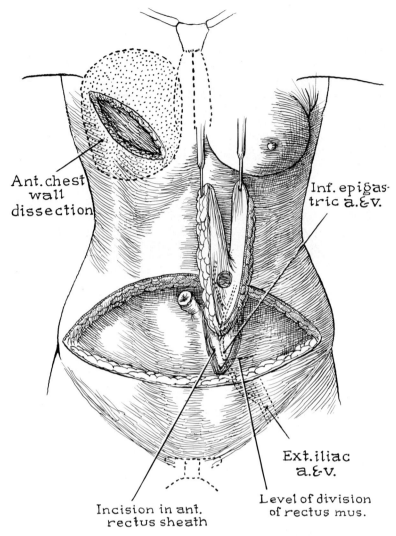

Ant. chest
wall
dissection

Inf. epigas-
tric a.&v.

Ext. iliac
a.&v.

Incision in ant.
rectus sheath

Level of division
of rectus mus.

Fig 21-15. Flap elevation for division of the rectus muscle.

Flap Elevation for Division of the Rectus Muscle (Figure 21-15)

After the surgeon ensures that the chest wall pocket has been dissected adequately, the flap is elevated superiorly to expose the underlying lower abdominal wall. The rectus muscle will be divided transversely at the lowest extent of the elliptical fascial incision. The inferior epigastric pedicle lies deep to the posterior rectus sheath at this level. Dividing the inferior epigastric artery and vein close to their origins from the iliac vessels will provide sufficient length for microvascular anastomoses if necessary.

Division of the Rectus Muscle and the Inferior Epigastric Pedicle (Figure 21-16)

The inferior epigastric vessels are identified as they enter the posterior side of the muscle slightly above the arcuate line. The muscle then is divided transversely just inferior to the point at which the inferior epigastric vessels enter the muscle. Then the vascular pedicle is isolated from the surrounding tissues.

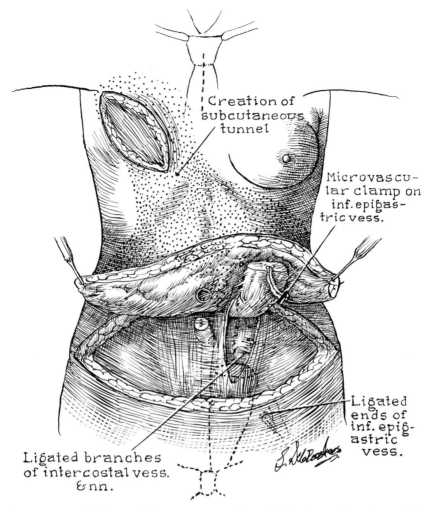

Fig 21-16.   Division of the rectus muscle and inferior epigastric pedicle.

Before the inferior epigastric pedicle is ligated and divided, the color and capillary refill of the flap are noted and any poorly perfused areas are identified. The origins of the inferior epigastric artery and vein from the external iliac vessels are identified, and a 5 cm vascular pedicle is dissected free from the surrounding tissues. The ends of the inferior epigastric artery and vein that will remain attached to the external iliac vessels are doubly ligated. Microvascular clamps are applied to the distal inferior epigastric pedicle to minimize trauma, and the vessels are divided.

After the rectus muscle and its inferior epigastric pedicle are divided inferiorly, the flap is isolated on the proximal rectus muscle and the superior epigastric vessels. At this point the superior portion of the rectus muscle and the vascular pedicle are evaluated to ensure that they are mobilized adequately for smooth transposition of the flap to the chest wall.

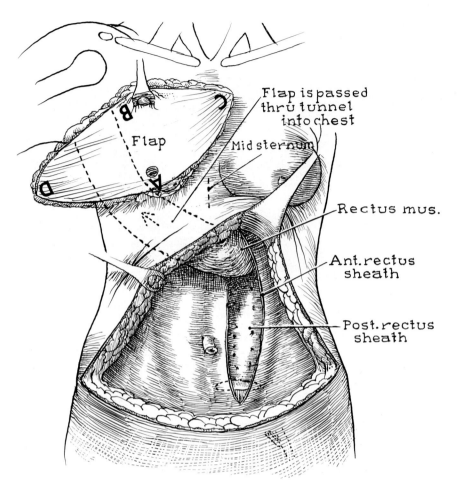

Fig 21-17. Transposition of the TRAM flap to the anterior chest wall.

Transposition of the TRAM Flap to the Anterior Chest Wall
(Figure 21-17)

Large retractors are used to elevate the upper abdominal skin and subcutaneous tissue. The flap is carefully rotated through the subcutaneous tunnel and into the chest wall pocket. After flap transposition the muscle and the vascular pedicle are inspected to ensure that they are not kinked, twisted, or compressed within the tunnel. If the tunnel is too small, it is enlarged.

The muscle must be separated adequately from its costal attachments and the superior portion of the rectus sheath, and it must lie flat to prevent vascular compromise. If the superior epigastric vascular pedicle seems too short, the muscle can be mobilized further, and additional length can be gained by resection of one or two of the costal cartilages. The internal mammary artery and vein lying beneath the cartilages must be identified and protected during this process.

If flap perfusion is satisfactory with the inferior epigastric vessels clamped, they are ligated. However, if the flap's circulation appears to be compromised, the pedicle is inspected again to ensure that it is not kinked or compressed within the tunnel. Occasionally, transient venous congestion develops following transposition of the flap to the chest wall. If this is not

198

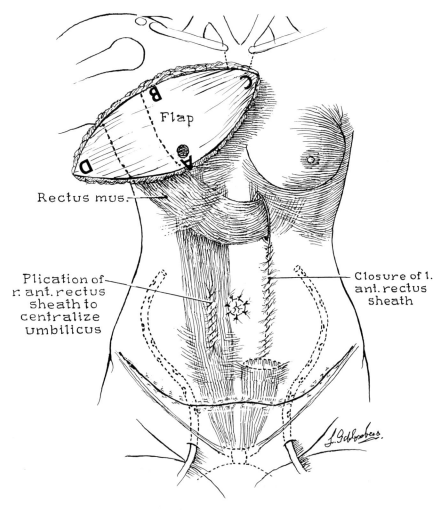

Fig 21-18. Closure of the anterior rectus sheath and the abdominal wound.

corrected quickly, the viability of the flap will be compromised. Venous congestion is relieved by releasing the microvascular clamp from the inferior epigastric vein to allow free venous drainage from the flap. The circulation often recovers promptly, and the vein can be ligated. Arterial insufficiency or persistent venous congestion is corrected by augmentation of the blood supply to the flap with anastomoses of the inferior epigastric vessels to appropriate vessels in the chest, most often the thoracodorsal vessels. This usually produces significant improvement in flap perfusion and venous drainage. A detailed discussion of the procedure for microvascular anastomosis appears later in this chapter.

The transposed TRAM flap is temporarily anchored to the anterior chest wall with sutures or skin staples to prevent tension on the flap, which may compromise the circulation when the abdomen is closed.

Closure of the Anterior Rectus Sheath and the Abdominal Wound (Figure 21-18)

After the TRAM flap has been passed into the chest and has been temporarily secured, the rectus fascia is closed. When a single muscle has been used in transposition, the anterior rectus sheath usually can be closed without the need for synthetic material to reinforce the fascia. The sheath

199

is closed with a monofilament suture from below upward. A running suture allows a gradual closure that distributes the tension evenly over the entire wound and prevents tearing of the fascia. At the point where the rectus muscle has been rotated, care is taken not to tighten the anterior fascia so much that the muscle or the vascular pedicle is compromised.

If the sheath closure is too tight, the umbilicus will be positioned abnormally on the abdominal wall and will be shifted toward the side of the muscle that is used for transposition. This horizontal shifting can be corrected by plication of the opposite rectus fascia in the same manner as done for the sheath closure previously described. The abdominal wound is irrigated following fascial closure with saline and povidone-iodine solutions, and hemostasis is achieved. Two 10-mm constant vacuum drains are inserted and brought out through separate stab incisions below the pubic hairline.

Before the abdominal wound is closed, the patient is placed in a semisitting position with thighs and knees flexed. A single interrupted absorbable suture is placed at the midpoint of the incision, and the location of the new umbilicus is marked with a needle and dye. The umbilicus is reconstructed at the level of a line drawn through the two anterior superior iliac spines. It is preferable to err on the low side in umbilicus placement because a location that is too high produces a more obvious deformity.

After the location of the umbilicus is marked, the abdominal wound is closed. Closure starts at the lateral margins and progresses medially to allow any excess tissue in the upper abdominal wall to be redistributed toward the midline. An initial closure is made with skin staples. Interrupted absorbable sutures then are placed in the superficial fascial layer between the staples, and the staples are removed. A layer of interrupted, absorbable sutures then is placed in the deep dermis and is followed by a running subcuticular suture.

To bring out the umbilicus at an appropriate midline location, a semicircular, convex, inferior incision is made. A core of fat underlying the incision is excised to allow a gentle indentation at the site of the new umbilicus. The umbilicus is anchored in each quadrant with through-and-through sutures to incorporate the abdominal wall skin, the anterior rectus sheath, and the umbilical skin. Finally a running absorbable suture is placed around the umbilicus. This produces a depressed umbilicus below the skin surface with a minimally visible scar. A dressing of nonadherent gauze and tape is placed on the closed abdominal wound.

Insetting of the TRAM Flap, and Closure of the Chest Wound (Figure 21-19)

Chest wound closure with creation of the breast mound is performed after the abdomen is closed. The patient is maintained in the same semisitting position as the proposed inframammary crease is marked to correspond with the opposite breast marking made preoperatively. Correct tailoring of the large, shapeless mass of skin and fat to create a natural-looking breast is probably the most esthetically demanding and time-consuming aspect of the TRAM procedure.

Insetting generally is started by positioning the flap so that its short axis (AB) lies parallel to the midline of the sternum. This placement improves blood flow to the flap and places most of the tissue bulk in the inferior half of the breast mound. A minimal amount of tissue bulk is required in the upper medial quadrant of the breast mound.

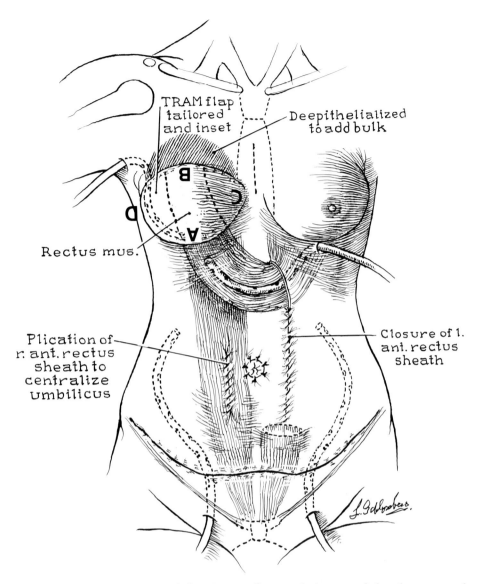

TRAM flap tailored and inset

Deepithelialized to add bulk

Rectus mus.

Plication of r. ant. rectus sheath to centralize umbilicus

Closure of l. ant. rectus sheath

Fig 21-19. Insetting of the TRAM flap, and closure of the chest wound.

Appropriate placement of the skin island is determined early in the tailoring process. If possible the inferior margin of the skin island is joined to the inferior border of the breast pocket at the inframammary crease to conceal one limb of the scar. However, this positioning may not be feasible if flap skin is needed to replace missing chest wall skin. Sometimes the skin island must be placed horizontally, vertically, or obliquely across the summit of the breast mound. The amount of skin needed for reconstruction will differ in each patient. Some patients may need a skin island only 6 cm wide, while others may require 10 cm or more of additional skin. Part of the challenge in tailoring the flap lies in finding the best position for the skin island.

The inferior half of the flap will provide the bulk of the breast mound, contribute to the new inframammary crease, and form much of the projection and natural ptosis of the breast mound. Trial tailoring typically begins by gently folding under the lower portion of the flap and by positioning it to rest on the inferior edge of the breast pocket. If it appears that the flap will

201

produce an excessively large breast mound, some tissue is excised in the lower area of the flap being turned under. If they are not needed, flap zones III and IV can be excised and removed, unless circulation is to be augmented by microvascular techniques.

The part of the flap that is to be included in the skin island and the part that will be folded under to add bulk can be determined by moving the flap around inside the pocket with the chest wall skin draped over it. The margin of overlap between the two areas is marked with dye, and the portion that is to be positioned beneath the chest wall skin is deepithelialized. The infra- mammary crease can be approximated by resting the tissue that is to become the inferior part of the breast mound on the inframammary shelf. The flap is stapled in place after the best position, contour, and symmetry are deter- mined.

The superior portion of the TRAM flap is tailored by first placing the upper part of the flap beneath the chest wall skin to determine the best position for correcting defects in the axillary and infraclavicular areas. If the pectoralis major muscle is absent, the cutaneous portion of the flap nearest the axilla is deepithelialized and attached to the pectoralis tendon stump to simulate an anterior axillary fold. After the chest wall skin is draped around the flap, the superior margin of overlap is marked with dye. Excess tissue is excised, and the portion of the flap to be buried for padding in the superior chest is deepithelialized. This deepithelialized portion of the flap then is tucked beneath the chest wall skin, and the upper part of the breast mound is secured temporarily with skin staples.

As the tailoring progresses, the flap may be trimmed and excess tissue may be discarded in any area. After each alteration the new breast mound is restapled, and its position, size, and contour are assessed until the optimal shape is formed. At this initial stage of reconstruction it is better to accept a less-than-ideal breast contour than it is to expend great effort to create an ideal breast mound and risk losing a large portion of the flap because of necrosis. The breast mound can be modified during subsequent stages of reconstruction when circulation has improved and the flap can withstand manipulation.

The buried superior portions of the flap are permanently sutured to the pectoralis major muscle when the best possible position and contour have been attained. The inferior portion of the flap must rest freely on the lower edge of the breast pocket to ensure the best appearance. Deep fixation sutures, which can constrict the vascular pedicle lying nearby, are not needed in the lower half of the breast mound. Before wound closure a constant vacuum drain is inserted beneath the flap and brought out through an axillary stab incision. A drain is also placed in the subcutaneous tunnel and brought out in the inframammary crease of the opposite breast. The tailoring of the chest wall skin to the margin of the skin island is completed using skin staples, and any excess tissue is excised. Interrupted dermal sutures are placed be- tween the staples. The staples are removed, and a layer of interrupted ab- sorbable sutures is placed around the entire skin island margin. The insetting is completed with a layer of running subcuticular sutures.

The following four modifications of the standard single-pedicled TRAM flap procedure are illustrated in detail:

1. Bilateral breast reconstruction using two TRAM flaps

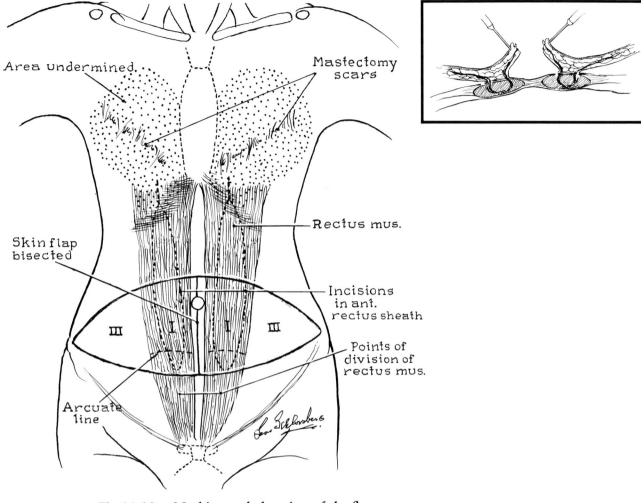

Fig 21-20. Marking and elevation of the flap.

2. Unilateral breast reconstruction: microvascular augmentation of standard, single-pedicled TRAM flap
3. Unilateral breast reconstruction: bipedicled TRAM flap
4. Unilateral breast reconstruction: microvascular augmentation of a modified bipedicled TRAM flap

The figures in this section are not drawn in the same detail as those provided for the standard TRAM flap procedure; rather the figures are designed to emphasize the unique aspects of the modifications illustrated.

Modification 1: Bilateral Breast Reconstruction Using Two TRAM Flaps
Marking and Elevation of the Flap (Figure 21-20)

Two pedicled TRAM flaps can be used for breast reconstruction following bilateral modified radical, total, or subcutaneous mastectomies. The standard TRAM flap is essentially split in two for reconstruction of bilateral defects so that one flap is transposed on one rectus muscle, and the other flap is transposed on the other rectus muscle. Use of a bisected TRAM flap for bilateral reconstruction permits two breast mounds, with matching skin color and texture, to be created from one donor site.

When a bisected TRAM flap is used for bilateral reconstruction, each flap will have a zone I and a zone III. In most instances the most lateral portion of each zone III will be poorly perfused and should not be used, unless a delayed TRAM procedure is performed or unless the blood supply to the flaps is augmented by anastomosis of the inferior epigastric vessels to vessels in the chest. After elevation and transposition of each flap the viability of zone III must be carefully assessed. Intravenous fluorescein is often used to assess flap circulation.

The procedure for marking and elevating the bisected TRAM flap is similar to that described for the standard TRAM flap (Figures 21-6 to 21-15). The superior incision is beveled 2 or 3 cm superiorly to include as many periumbilical vertical perforating vessels as possible. Flap elevation is begun at the level of the abdominal wall fascia. One half of the flap is elevated from lateral to medial, until the most lateral column of vertical perforating vessels is identified exiting the anterior rectus sheath. When these perforators are identified, a midline incision is made to the linea alba to bisect the flap. The umbilicus is cored out.

Then one half of the bisected flap is elevated from medial to lateral, until the most medial column of vertical perforators is encountered. This procedure is repeated on the opposite side of the abdomen to elevate the other half of the bisected flap. Once both flaps are isolated on the perforating vessels that run through the anterior rectus sheath and into the subcutaneous tissue (see inset), the upper abdominal skin and subcutaneous tissue are elevated to the level of the xiphoid process and the costal margin. The fascial incisions are made, and both rectus muscles are mobilized.

The anterior chest wall is prepared by dissection of two pockets conforming to the premastectomy breast envelopes. The chest wall incisions must be placed high enough to prevent inferior migration of the breast mounds when the abdominal wall is closed. Also, two subcutaneous tunnels, one between each breast pocket and the abdomen, are created. The two TRAM flaps can be rotated into ipsilateral or contralateral breast pockets. The best placement of each flap will be determined individually by the flap orientation that is dictated by the tissue needed to obtain an optimal breast mound.

After the anterior chest dissection is completed, the inferior portion of each rectus muscle is divided near the arcuate line below the point at which the inferior epigastric vessels enter the muscle. Microvascular clamps are applied to the flap side of the vessels. The inferior epigastric vessels then are ligated and divided.

Transposition of Bilateral TRAM Flaps, and Wound Closure (Figure 21-21)

After the rectus muscles and their pedicles have been divided inferiorly, each flap is rotated through its subcutaneous tunnel into a breast pocket. The muscles and vascular pedicles are carefully inspected in the tunnels to ensure that no compression or kinking has occurred. When a flap is rotated into an ipsilateral pocket, the muscle pedicle easily can become folded underneath the flap. This problem is corrected by straightening the pedicle at the point where it joins the flap and by adjusting the rotation. The flaps then are temporarily secured to the chest wall with sutures or with skin staples.

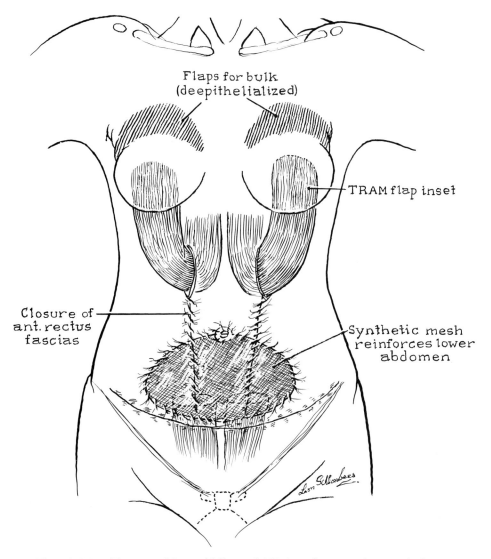

Fig 21-21. Transposition of bilateral TRAM flaps, and wound closure.

When both rectus muscles are used for reconstruction, the abdominal closure requires special attention. The fascia superior to the umbilicus can usually be closed with a running monofilament suture. When suturing near the most superior portion of the fascial incisions, care is taken to avoid a tight closure around the muscles and vascular pedicles. Below the umbilicus, primary closure of the anterior rectus sheath produces excessive tension around the wound, which may result in tears in the fascia and hernia formation. Therefore when both rectus muscles have been used to transpose two TRAM flaps, abdominal wall reinforcement with a synthetic material usually is required. After the fascial closure is complete and the lower abdominal wall is reinforced, the large abdominal wound is irrigated, drained, and closed as previously described. The umbilicus is brought out and inset at an appropriate location.

Both flaps are inspected again to ensure that the muscles and their vascular pedicles are not compressed or kinked in the subcutaneous tunnels. The flaps are examined for any evidence of venous or arterial insufficiency.

If circulation is compromised, the flap circulation must be augmented through anastomosis of the inferior epigastric pedicle to vessels in the chest.

Each flap is inset, and the anterior chest wounds are closed as illustrated in Figure 21-19. Each flap generally has a similar volume, so establishment of symmetry for size, contour, and placement is easier than it is when matching an in situ contralateral breast.

Two TRAM flaps are sometimes used for bilateral reconstruction following subcutaneous mastectomy or resection of extensive amounts of breast tissue for silicone mastopathy. In these situations adequate skin remains on the anterior chest for soft-tissue coverage so that the skin territory of both flaps is deepithelialized and the subcutaneous tissue is used as autologous implants. Flap elevation, abdominal wound closure, and flap transposition into the anterior chest wall pockets are performed as previously described.

Modification 2: Unilateral Breast Reconstruction: Microvascular Augmentation of Standard Single-Pedicled TRAM Flap

Preoperative Marking and Positioning of the Patient (Figure 21-22)

The preoperative marking and patient positioning for inferior epigastric augmentation of a pedicled TRAM flap are the same as those for the standard pedicled TRAM flap (described in Figure 21-6). The flap is drawn with the upper incision slightly above the umbilicus and the inferior incision slightly above the public hairline. The flap dimensions (previously described for the single pedicled TRAM flap) are the same. The endpoints of the short axis are marked *AB*, and the endpoints of the long axis are marked *CD*.

Elevation of the Flap on the Vertical Perforating Vessels, Division of the Inferior Rectus Abdominis Muscle with Dissection of the Inferior Epigastric Pedicle, and Elevation of the Anterior Abdominal Wall (Figure 21-23)

The previously marked skin incision is made in the area immediately over the anterior rectus sheath, and the superior incision is beveled 45 degrees. Flap elevation begins on the side contralateral to the pedicle muscle. The flap is elevated from lateral to medial at the level of the abdominal wall fascia. The vertical perforating vessels coming through the anterior rectus sheath on the contralateral side are identified, ligated, and divided. The perforating vessels will occupy a similar position on the side of the muscle that is to be transposed. The umbilicus is cored out in the midline, and the dissection is continued medially past the midline, until the most medial vertical perforating vessels are noted overlying the muscle that is to be transposed. The dissection on this side ends when these medial perforating vessels are encountered. The flap on the side of the muscle being transposed then is elevated in a similar manner from lateral to medial. This dissection stops when the most lateral perforating vessels are encountered over the anterior rectus sheath. The upper abdominal flap then is elevated at the level of the abdominal wall fascia to the costal margins and to the xiphoid process. When this dissection is completed, the flap is isolated on the vertical perforating vessels overlying the anterior rectus sheath from a few centimeters above the umbilicus to the level of the arcuate line. The fascial incision then

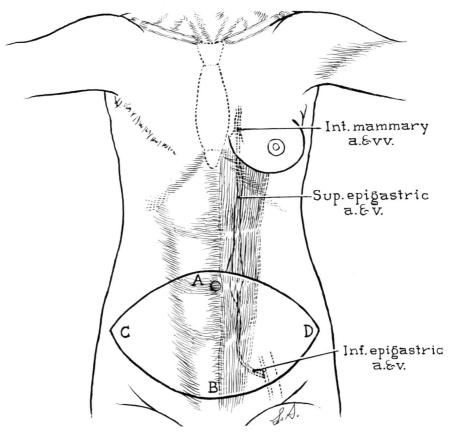

Fig 21-22.   Preoperative marking and positioning of the patient.

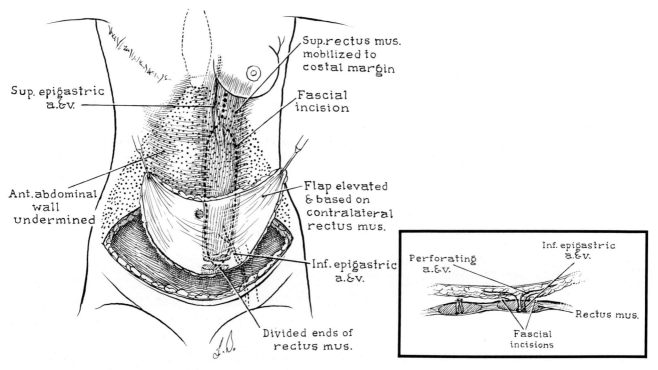

Fig 21-23.   Elevation of the flap on the vertical perforating vessels, division of the inferior rectus abdominis muscle with dissection of the inferior epigastric pedicle, and elevation of the anterior abdominal wall.

207

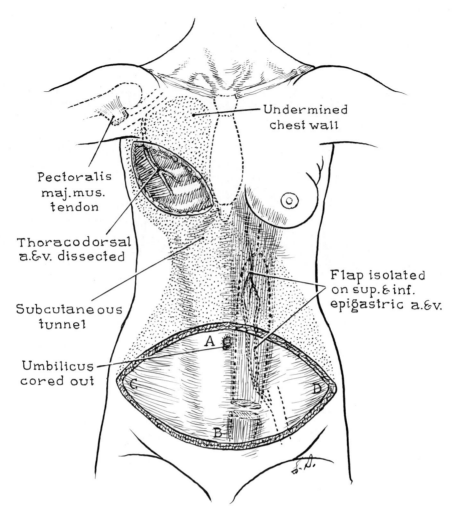

Fig 21-24. Chest wall dissection, and creation of a subcutaneous tunnel.

is marked as an ellipse around the vertical perforating vessels (see inset) and is extended superiorly to just past the most superior tendinous inscription and inferiorly to just below the arcuate line. A vertical extension of the incision is made superiorly to allow transposition of the flap after mobilization of the muscle. The outlined incision then is made through the fascia, and the rectus muscle is mobilized from its fascial sheath by beginning in the midpoint and moving inferiorly and then superiorly. The inferior epigastric pedicle will be identified during mobilization of the rectus. The epigastric pedicle is isolated, and the rectus muscle is divided inferiorly.

Chest Wall Dissection, and Creation of a Subcutaneous Tunnel (Figure 21-24)

After the mobilized TRAM flap is isolated on the superior epigastric vessels and the inferior epigastric vessels, the flap is returned to the abdominal bed. The chest wall dissection and the creation of the subcutaneous tunnel then are performed. The dissection to elevate the skin and subcutaneous tissue off the underlying muscle or chest wall extends to just below the clavicle superiorly, to 1 to 2 cm lateral to the midline of the sternum medially, to 1 to 2 cm above the inframammary crease inferiorly, and to the region of the

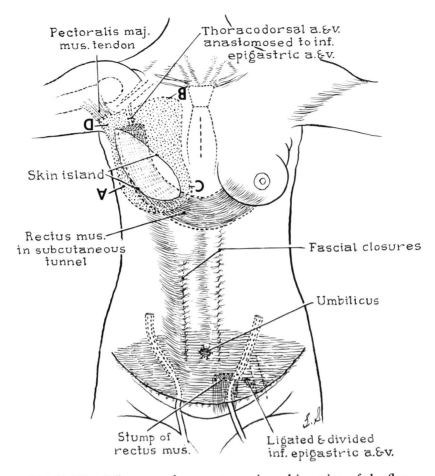

Fig 21-25. Microvascular anastomosis and insetting of the flap.

midaxillary line laterally. The dissection must be extended into the axilla far enough for the appropriate donor vessels to be identified and exposed sufficiently for the microvascular anastomoses. The thoracodorsal vessels are often used as donor vessels. The vessels must be prepared completely for microvascular anastomosis before division of the inferior epigastric pedicle to limit warm ischemia time. After completion of the chest wall dissection a subcutaneous tunnel is created between the chest wound and the abdominal wound to allow passage of the flap.

Microvascular Anastomosis, and Insetting of the Flap (Figure 21-25)

After completion of the chest wall pocket dissection and after preparation of the thoracodorsal vessels for microvascular anastomosis, the inferior epigastric pedicle is divided close to its origin. This division takes place after the vessels have been doubly ligated, and the vascular pedicle on the flap has been occluded with a microvascular clamp. The inferior epigastric artery and vein are irrigated with heparinized saline and prepared for the microvascular anastomoses. After the flap is passed through the subcutaneous tunnel into the chest wound and its satisfactory position is ensured, it is secured to the chest wall with skin staples. The operating microscope is used to facilitate anastomosis of the inferior epigastric artery and vein to the

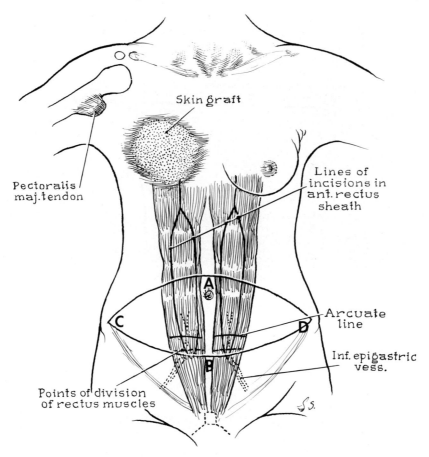

Fig 21-26.   Incision placement.

prepared artery and vein in the chest. After these anastomoses are completed, the vessels are evaluated for patency and the flap is inspected for capillary refill and dermal bleeding. The rectus muscle is sutured to the chest wall to stabilize the flap and to prevent tension or disruption of the microvascular anastomoses. Subsequently great care must be taken to ensure that the anastomoses are not compromised. The patient is converted to a semisitting position, and the fascial and abdominal wounds are closed in the same manner as described for a standard pedicled flap in Figure 21-18. The flap then is positioned, tailored, and inset as described in the standard pedicled flap in Figure 21-19. The anastomoses must be protected to avoid excessive tension, disruption, or kinking while the flap is being inset. If it is necessary to recreate the anterior axillary fold, a portion of the flap is deepithelialized and sutured to the pectoralis major muscle tendon.

Modification 3: Unilateral Breast Reconstruction: Bipedicled TRAM Flap
Incision Placement (Figure 21-26)

A TRAM flap based on both rectus abdominis muscles has sufficient blood flow to ensure viability of the entire tissue bloc. A bipedicled TRAM flap contains a dual vascular supply with both superior epigastric pedicles

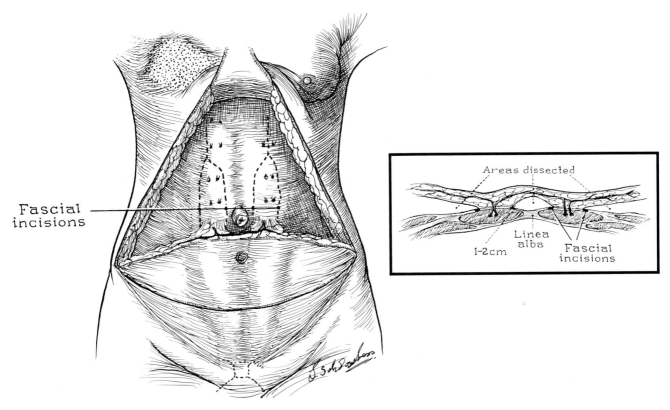

Fig 21-27. Elevation of a bipedicled TRAM flap.

and therefore has an enhanced capacity for arterial inflow and venous drainage. This flap is sufficient to fill a large chest wall defect and to create a single breast mound when it is needed in reconstruction following radical mastectomy.

The bipedicled TRAM flap also may be used for patients who are at high risk for developing flap complications, even when the entire TRAM flap is not needed to reconstruct extensive defects. A bipedicled TRAM flap is typically based low in the abdomen to maximize its arc of rotation. The flap is marked as previously described in Figure 21-6 for the standard TRAM flap. Points *AB* and *CD* indicate the short axis and the long axis, respectively.

Elevation of a Bipedicled TRAM Flap (Figure 21-27)

The incisions are beveled to develop a bipedicled TRAM flap as described for the standard TRAM flap. One side of the flap at a time is elevated by incising from lateral to medial at the level of the abdominal wall fascia, until the lateral column of vertical perforating vessels is identified emerging through the anterior rectus sheath. After both sides of the flap are elevated to this point, the upper abdominal skin and subcutaneous tissue are elevated to the level of the xiphoid and costal margins bilaterally to enhance exposure for the midline dissection and flap transposition. The umbilicus is cored out before dissection of the flap.

A relatively narrow space exists between the two medial columns of perforating vessels for freeing the flap from the linea alba and rectus sheath. The large skin island overlying this area cannot be bisected as it can with bilateral TRAM flaps. However, a headlight, long retractors, facelift scissors, or an electrocautery with an extended insulated tip will aid in the dissection. The dissection can be performed from the superior and inferior margins of the flap, with the skin island reflected in front of the field as the dissection progresses to the center of the flap. The skin island is freed first over the midline; then it is freed for an additional 1 or 2 cm laterally on each side of the linea alba as shown in the inset. The dissection ends where the most medial vertical perforators exit the anterior rectus sheaths. When the midline dissection is completed, the fascial incisions overlying each rectus muscle are marked so that a 3- to 4-cm-wide strip of fascia will be harvested with the vessels. The inferior margin of each of the elliptical fascial incisions extends to just below the arcuate line, and the superior margin ends above the most superior tendinous inscription. The vertical incision on each side continues up the middle of the anterior rectus sheath and ends slightly above the costal margin.

Mobilization of the Rectus Muscles from the Fascial Sheath (Figure 21-28)

The medial portion of the rectus sheath underlies the large skin island, which cannot be moved entirely out of the way. It may be impossible to complete the medial limbs of the elliptical fascial incisions until the inferior margin of the flap is developed and the flap is elevated superiorly. Blunt dissection is used to lift the inferior portions of the rectus muscles from the posterior fascia. As the inferior epigastric vessels are identified, they are protected while the portion of the muscle that is superficial to the vascular pedicle is freed.

Division of the Rectus Muscles and Inferior Epigastric Pedicles (Figure 21-29)

The muscles and vessels are divided inferiorly. The inferior epigastric vessels are left as long as possible. The medial limbs of the fascial incisions then can be completed, while the rectus muscles are mobilized from below. As the muscles are elevated superiorly, branches of the intercostal nerves and vessels from the arcuate line to the costal margin are divided as they enter the muscles laterally.

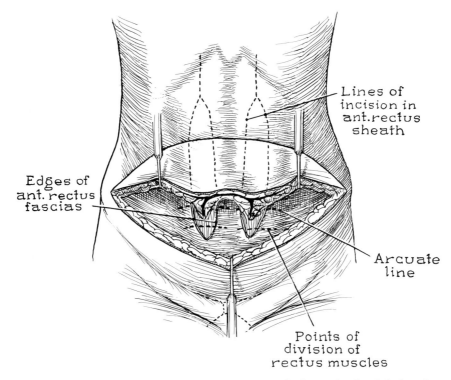

Fig 21-28.   Mobilization of the rectus muscle from the fascial sheath.

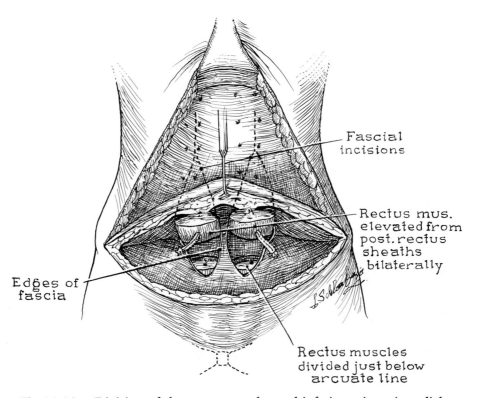

Fig 21-29.   Division of the rectus muscles and inferior epigastric pedicles.

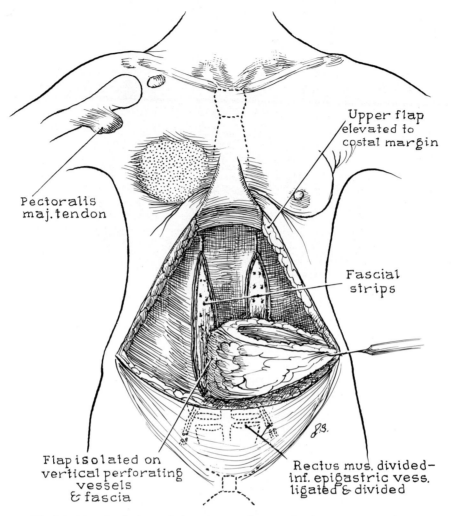

Pectoralis
maj. tendon

Upper flap
elevated to
costal margin

Fascial
strips

Flap isolated on
vertical perforating
vessels
& fascia

Rectus mus. divided-
inf. epigastric vess.
ligated & divided

Fig 21-30. Isolation of the TRAM flap on both rectus muscles.

Isolation of the TRAM Flap on Both Rectus Muscles (Figure 21-30)

After the muscles are completely mobilized, the TRAM flap is isolated on the vertical perforating vessels that connect the skin island to the rectus abdominis muscles through the strips of anterior rectus sheath lying within the ellipses of the incised fascia. The flap is attached superiorly to both rectus muscles and their associated superior epigastric pedicles. At this point the flap is replaced in its original bed and is perfused for 30 minutes before it is transposed to the anterior chest. The anterior chest wall dissection can be performed during this interval.

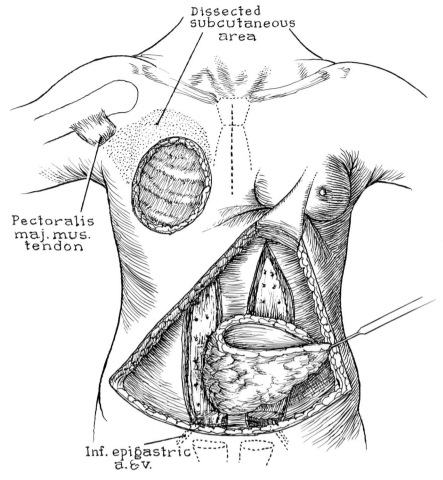

Fig 21-31. Anterior chest wall dissection for transposition of a bipedicled TRAM flap.

Anterior Chest Wall Dissection for Transposition of a Bipedicled TRAM Flap (Figure 21-31)

The breast pocket dissection is performed as previously described for the standard TRAM flap transposition. Because the bipedicled flap is often used to cover an extensive chest wall defect, a large segment of tissue may need to be excised. If the anterior axillary fold is to be recreated, the dissection is continued to expose the tendon stump of the previously resected pectoralis major muscle.

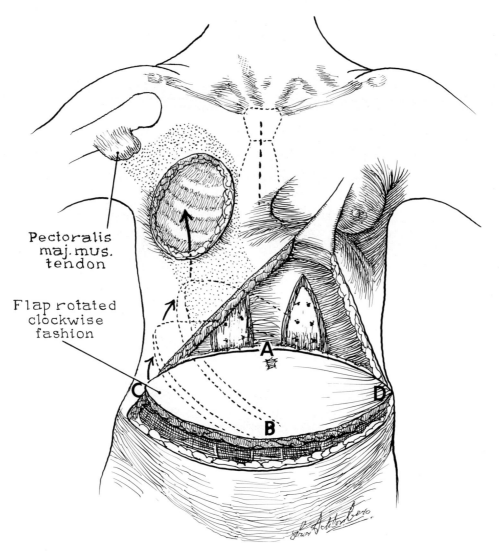

Pectoralis
maj. mus.
tendon

Flap rotated
clockwise
fashion

Fig 21-32. Creation of a subcutaneous tunnel, and transposition of the TRAM flap to the anterior chest wall.

Creation of a Subcutaneous Tunnel, and Transposition of the TRAM Flap to the Anterior Chest Wall (Figure 21-32)

A wide subcutaneous tunnel is created between the chest and the abdominal wound by blunt dissection at the level of the chest wall and the anterior rectus sheath. This tunnel must accommodate easy passage of the skin island and both rectus muscles and their vascular pedicles into the chest. Clearly nonviable or otherwise excess portions of the flap can be excised and discarded before transposition to facilitate flap passage through the subcutaneous tunnel.

The flap is transposed gently into the anterior chest to avoid avulsion of the perforating vessels from the muscle. Typically the flap is rotated clockwise, placing the lateral tip *(C)* of the ipsilateral-based portion in a medial chest location. The contralateral tip *(D)* of the flap is relocated near the lateral edge of the chest.

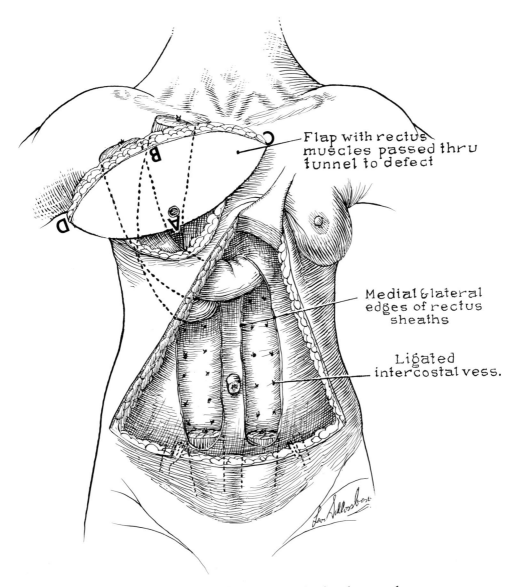

Fig 21-33. TRAM flap position in the chest pocket.

TRAM Flap Position in the Chest Pocket (Figure 21-33)

The muscles and their pedicles then are closely inspected to ensure that they are reposing smoothly and are under no tension within the tunnel. The muscles can be mobilized further if necessary by detaching the lateral portion of the contralateral muscle from the costochondral cartilages or by further releasing the medial portion of the ipsilateral muscle. Once the muscles and the vascular pedicles are in a satisfactory position, the flap is temporarily attached to the chest wall with sutures or staples before the abdominal wound closure is started.

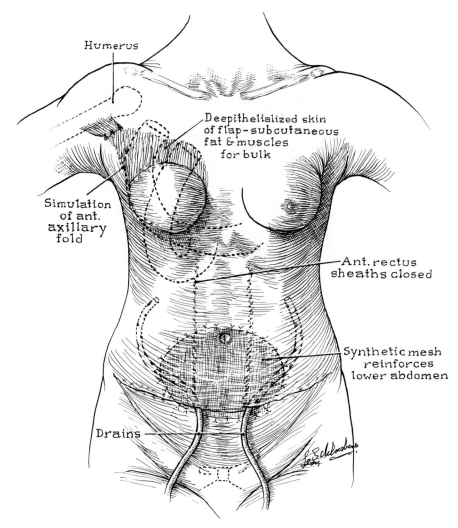

Fig 21-34. Closure of the anterior rectus sheath, reinforcement of the abdominal wall, and insetting of the flap.

Closure of the Anterior Rectus Sheath, Reinforcement of the Abdominal Wall, and Insetting of the Flap (Figure 21-34)

A running monofilament absorbable suture is used to close the anterior rectus sheaths superior to the umbilicus. The fascial closures below the umbilical level are reinforced with synthetic mesh. The abdominal wound then is irrigated with copious amounts of saline solution, and two 10-mm constant vacuum drains are inserted and brought out in the pubic region. Once more, before the final abdominal closure, the muscles and the vascular pedicles are inspected to ensure that they are lying smoothly and are not compressed or under tension within the tunnel. The patient then is placed in a semisitting position with her thighs and knees flexed, and the abdomen is closed as previously described.

The flap then is tailored and inset as described in Figure 21-19. If an anterior axillary fold needs to be created (as shown here), a portion of the flap is deepithelialized and attached to the pectoralis major tendon or to the periosteum of the humerus. Finally, vacuum drains are inserted into the chest wall wound (not shown here), and the wound is closed and dressed.

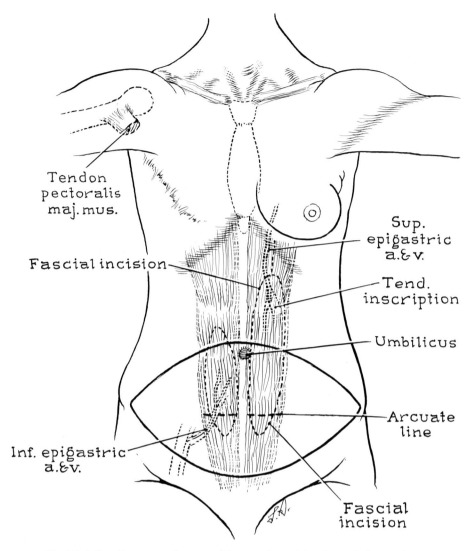

Fig 21-35. Preoperative marking and positioning of the patient.

Modification 4: Unilateral Breast Reconstruction: Microvascular Augmentation of a Modified Bipedicled TRAM Flap

Preoperative Marking and Positioning of the Patient (Figure 21-35)

A TRAM flap based on the contralateral rectus abdominis muscle and on its superior epigastric pedicle can also carry the inferior portion of the ipsilateral rectus muscle and its inferior epigastric pedicle. The vascular supply of the flap then can be augmented by anastomosing the ipsilateral inferior epigastric vessels to vessels in the chest. The patient is marked preoperatively in the standing position and in the same manner as for a unilateral pedicled TRAM flap (illustrated in Figure 21-6).

The superior epigastric-based hemiflap (shown contralateral to the mastectomy side in these figures) is similar to the standard pedicled TRAM flap. The inferior epigastric-based hemiflap (shown ipsilateral to the mastectomy side in these figures) essentially is a free flap component.

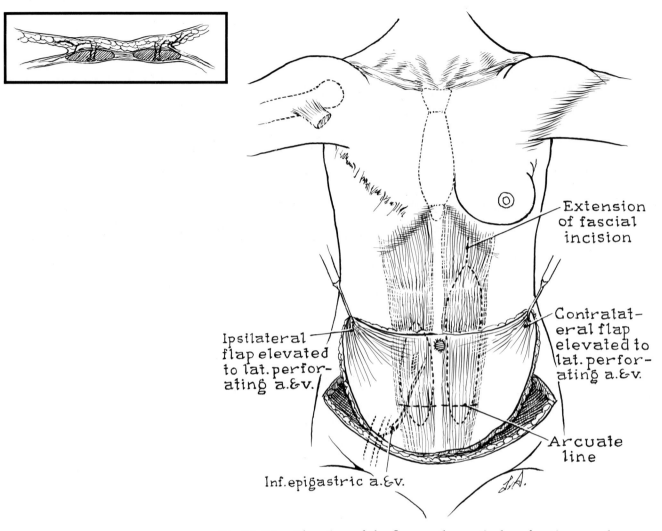

Fig 21-36. Elevation of the flap on the vertical perforating vessels.

Elevation of the Flap on the Vertical Perforating Vessels
(Figure 21-36)

Elevation of a flap based on the contralateral rectus muscle and on the inferior portion of the ipsilateral muscle is similar to elevation of the bipedicled flap described in Figure 21-20. Flap dissection can begin laterally on either side by deepening the superior and inferior incisions to the fascial margins. Superiorly over the anterior rectus sheath the incision should be beveled as previously described. Flap elevation then begins from lateral to medial at the level of the abdominal wall fascia, and the flap is elevated to the most lateral perforating vessels, as shown on the inset. When both flaps have been elevated, the lateral to medial dissection is stopped.

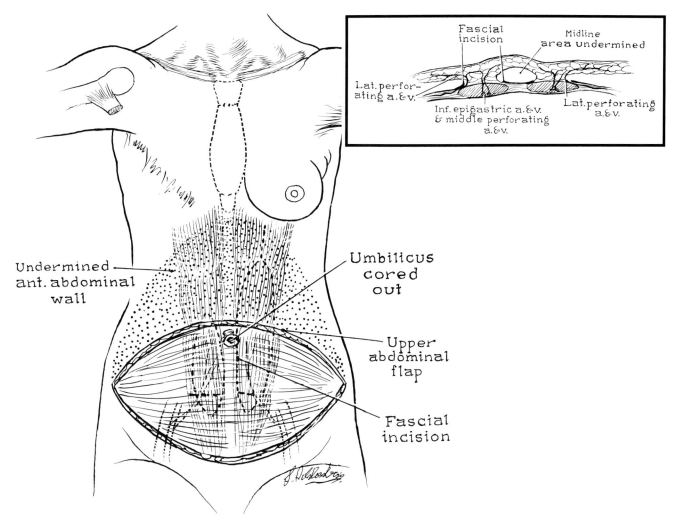

Fig 21-37. Completion of flap elevation, elevation of the anterior abdominal wall, and marking of fascial incisions.

Completion of Flap Elevation; Elevation of the Anterior Abdominal Wall; Marking of Fascial Incisions (Figure 21-37)

The umbilicus is cored out, and the flap is separated in the midline by sharp and blunt dissection. Work progresses from medial to lateral on each hemiflap until the medial vertical perforating vessels are exposed (see inset). The dissection usually proceeds superiorly and inferiorly to the midportion of the flap. At this point the flap will be isolated on the vertical perforating vessels from both rectus muscles.

The upper abdominal wall is undermined to the costal margins, and the xiphoid process, at the level of the abdominal wall fascia. The fascial incisions are then marked for mobilization of the muscles. On the pedicled side the elliptical incision extends to just superior to the most superior tendinous inscription and then is extended as a straight line above the costal margin. The elliptical outline encloses the vertical perforating vessels medially and laterally and ends just below the arcuate line. On the opposite side the elliptical incision extends to just above the superior margin of the flap and inferiorly to just beneath the arcuate line, without a superior straight line extension.

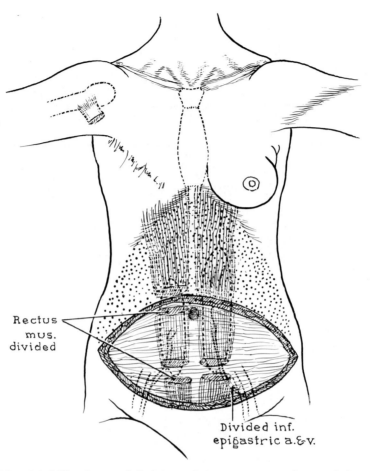

Rectus
mus.
divided

Divided inf.
epigastric a.&v.

Fig 21-38. Mobilization and division of the rectus muscles, and dissection of the ipsilateral inferior epigastric pedicle.

Mobilization and Division of the Rectus Muscles, and Dissection of the Ipsilateral Inferior Epigastric Pedicle (Figure 21-38)

Although dissection can begin by mobilizing either rectus muscle, the ipsilateral hemiflap component usually is dissected first by making the fascial incision outlined and then mobilizing the lateral portion of that muscle to expose the inferior epigastric pedicle. The pedicle is protected, and the flap is dissected to the point where the vessels separate from the muscle, and then the muscle is divided just inferior to the arcuate line. The muscle then is dissected superiorly and mobilized from the rectus sheath. The muscle is divided again just superior to the fascial strip and the anterior fascial incision. It is usually impossible to complete the medial fascial incisions until both rectus muscles have been fully mobilized. The inferior epigastric artery and vein are dissected close to their origin from the external iliac artery and vein. The inferior epigastric vessels are then doubly ligated close to their origin and divided. The inferior epigastric pedicle attached to the muscle is irrigated with heparinized saline solution and is occluded with a microvascular clamp. The fascial incisions then are made over the superior epigastric hemiflap muscle, and the muscle is mobilized superiorly, laterally, and inferiorly. The inferior epigastric vessels can be divided and ligated on this side without attempting to gain length because the rectus muscle and flap will be supplied by the superior epigastric pedicle. At this point the medial fascial incisions

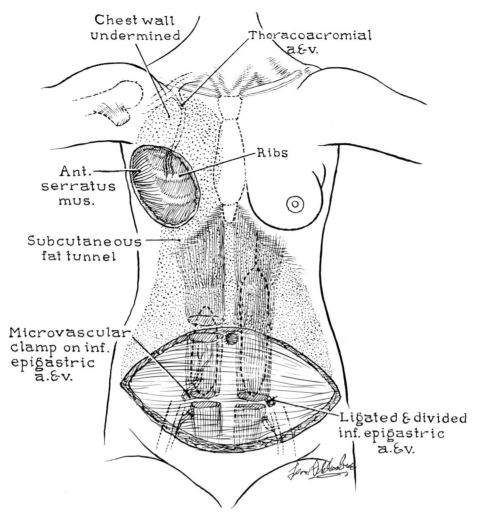

Fig 21-39. Chest wall dissection.

can be completed, and the superior epigastric hemiflap muscle can be elevated and fully mobilized to expose the superior epigastric vessels. The inset flap will be perfused on the contralateral side by the superior epigastric vessel pedicle and on the ipsilateral side by the inferior epigastric vessels, which will be anastomosed to recipient vessels in the chest.

Chest Wall Dissection (Figure 21-39)

After muscle mobilization and flap isolation on the contralateral superior epigastric vessels the flap is placed back in its bed and is allowed to perfuse during the chest wall dissection. The chest wall dissection for this procedure is identical to that described in Figure 21-24. The locations of the potential recipient vessels and the orientation of the flap in the chest determine which chest vessels will be used for anastomosis. The tissue requirements in the chest dictate the flap orientation and determine accordingly which vessels are the best recipient vessels. Usually the thoracodorsal vessels or the thoraco-acromial vessels are used, and the extent of the chest wall dissection will vary, depending on which vessels are chosen. The vessels must be mobilized and prepared for microvascular anastomosis before transposition of the flap to the chest.

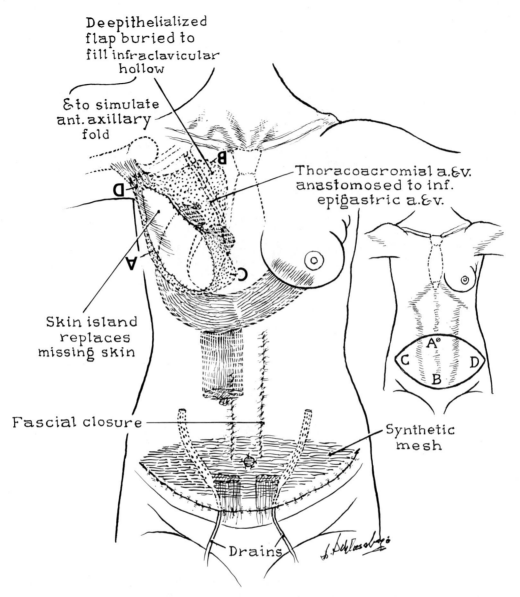

Deepithelialized flap buried to fill infraclavicular hollow

& to simulate ant. axillary fold

Thoracoacromial a.&v. anastomosed to inf. epigastric a.&v.

Skin island replaces missing skin

Fascial closure

Synthetic mesh

Drains

Fig 21-40. Flap transposition to the chest, microvascular anastomosis, insetting of the flap, and closure of the abdominal wound.

Flap Transposition to the Chest, Microvascular Anastomosis, Insetting of the Flap, and Closure of the Abdominal Wound (Figure 21-40)

After the inferior epigastric pedicle is divided, the flap is transposed through the subcutaneous tunnel into the chest wound and secured with skin staples. The pedicle is inspected to ensure that the rectus muscle has been mobilized adequately, that it lies smoothly in the subcutaneous tunnel, and that the superior epigastric vessels are not kinked or compressed. The orientation of the flap on the chest wall after transposition can be compared with the original flap orientation shown on the inset. The flap is inspected for capillary refill, dermal bleeding, and venous congestion. The operating microscope is used while the thoracoacromial vessels (shown in this illustration) are anastomosed to the inferior epigastric artery and vein. After the anastomoses are completed, the microvascular clamps are removed. Once

224

the patency of the anastomoses is confirmed, the muscle of the flap is sutured to the chest wall to stabilize the flap and to prevent disruption of the anastomoses during manipulation. The patient then is placed in a semisitting position, and the anterior rectus fascia is reapproximated and reinforced with synthetic mesh, as described for the bipedicled TRAM flap in Figure 21-34. The abdominal wound is closed in the standard manner for a TRAM flap (described in Figure 21-18). The flap then is positioned, tailored, and inset to produce an esthetic breast mound (described in Figure 21-19) without compromising flap circulation or disrupting the microvascular anastomoses. The chest wall wounds are also drained with vacuum drains (not shown).

Postoperative Care

When surgery is completed, the chest incisions are dressed with a nonadherent gauze or an antibiotic ointment and a loose light dressing. A portion of the skin island is left exposed to permit regular monitoring of flap circulation for 4 or 5 days. The patient is transferred from the operating table to a hospital bed with an Egg-Crate mattress, while she is maintained in a semisitting position to enhance venous drainage and to reduce abdominal tension.

In the recovery room the patient is given humidified oxygen and is kept warm. The flap circulation is closely monitored. Initially the flap appears pale and feels cool; however, its temperature and color should gradually improve. If a flap that seemed adequately perfused in the operating room becomes mottled later, the patient's shoulders are elevated further to assist venous drainage, her blood volume is expanded, and room temperature is increased. If these simple steps do not improve circulation to the flap, the patient is returned to the operating room for reexploration. Whenever an initially well-perfused flap develops signs of vascular compromise, the reason for the change must be promptly identified and corrected.

The patient is kept warm and well hydrated. She should remain in a semisitting position for approximately 1 week to enhance venous drainage of the flap. Oral intake of fluids is started on the first postoperative day. The bladder drainage catheter is removed, and ambulation is begun on the first or second postoperative day. The intravenous fluids are discontinued when the patient is taking sufficient fluids by mouth. Chest and abdominal drains usually are removed by the fifth or sixth day, or they are removed when the drainage is less than 30 ml per 24 hours. The patient may shower after the drains are removed, and she must gently pat dry the reconstructed breast. Usually the patient can be discharged from the hospital by the seventh to tenth day.

Upon discharge the patient must be clearly informed of restrictions. Smoking is forbidden for 8 weeks. Heating pads, hot water bottles, or ice packs near the reconstructed mound are not used; however, a warmed towel may be used to relieve discomfort. Significant patient discomfort postoperatively is not unusual because of the required sitting position. Abdominal pain, tenderness, and tightness will be bothersome and especially pronounced in patients undergoing a bipedicled flap procedure.

22

Free Flap

Introduction

A free flap procedure involves isolation of a block of tissue on a single dominant vascular pedicle, division of the artery and vein, and transfer of the flap to a distant site with reconstitution of the vascular supply by anastomosis to in situ vessels. At present the transverse rectus abdominis myocutaneous (TRAM) is the free flap most often used for breast reconstruction.

The internal mammary, the thoracoacromial, the thoracodorsal, and the subclavian vessels (shown in Figure 22-1) can be used for microvascular anastomoses. Selection of the appropriate vessels to be used depends primarily on the vessels' availability, length, and location and on the orientation of the flap on the chest wall. The vessels for anastomoses should closely match the size of the inferior epigastric or the superior gluteal vessels because the anastomosed arteries and veins must provide flow to and drainage from the free flap. The thoracodorsal pedicle is used most commonly in the transfer of a free TRAM flap because the size, length, and location of the artery and vein are best suited for anastomoses with the inferior epigastric pedicle and for positioning the flap. However, use of the thoracodorsal pedicle for the chest wall anastomoses can preclude later transposition of the ipsilateral latissimus dorsi muscle if extensive tissue loss occurs with the free tissue transfer. By contrast use of the thoracoacromial vessels does not preclude future employment of any of the standard flaps used in breast reconstruction. Although the thoracoacromial vessels are less accessible than the thoracodorsal vessels, the size and location of the vessels make them an acceptable choice for anastomoses with the inferior epigastric system if the thoracodorsal artery and vein are unavailable. The internal mammary artery is best suited for use with the superior gluteal flap because the transferred pedicle typically is positioned toward the medial aspect of the chest. The internal mammary artery provides robust and reliable flow because its 1.5- to 3-mm diameter is similar to that of the superior gluteal artery. Exposure of the internal mammary artery requires resection of the medial portion of the third or fourth costal cartilage. However, it is still the recipient vessel of choice when a superior gluteal free flap is transferred. Whenever the internal mammary vessels are used for free tissue transfer, the surgeon should have a contingency plan for alternate venous drainage because the venae comitantes associated with the internal mammary artery are small, thin walled, and difficult to handle. A vein graft will often be required. The subclavian artery also provides excellent flow; however, a vein graft will be required to bridge

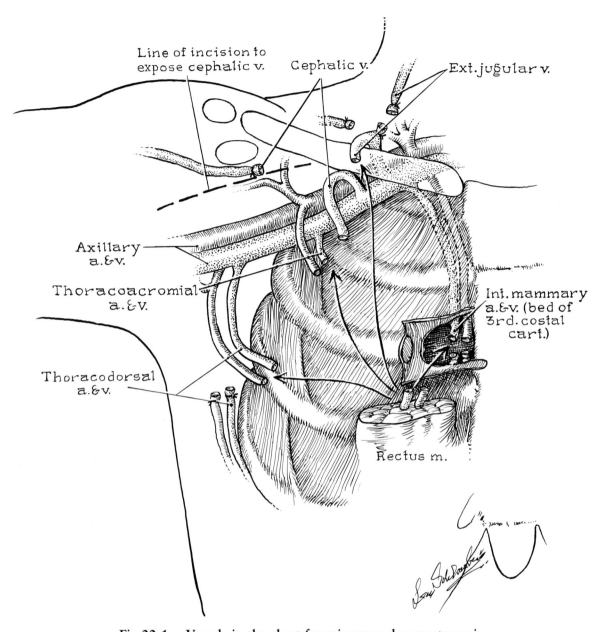

Fig 22-1. Vessels in the chest for microvascular anastomosis.

it to the flap's artery in the breast pocket. Use of the subclavian artery also necessitates an infraclavicular incision for adequate exposure.

The internal mammary, thoracodorsal, thoracoacromial, cephalic, subclavian, or external jugular veins can be used for venous drainage of a free flap. Choice of a vein should be based on its availability, the flap's orientation, and cosmetic considerations. Use of the subclavian vein, like the artery, also requires a bridging vein graft to connect the transferred and recipient vessels. Furthermore, a separate incision in the infraclavicular area is required. The cephalic vein, which provides an excellent source for venous drainage, can be transferred to the anterior chest by making a small transverse incision in the upper arm, and the external jugular vein can be exposed through several transverse, stair-stepped incisions in the neck. Because good venous drainage is so critical, a vein graft from a lower extremity can also be used to obtain adequate drainage if necessary. A minor drawback to using a vein graft is the resultant scar at the site of the harvested vein.

Free flaps offer several important advantages. Because free tissue transfer with the superior gluteal or TRAM flap provides a large amount of autologous tissue, an implant is generally not needed. The color and texture of the transferred tissue generally closely match the contralateral breast. With either flap the donor site is easily concealed, and removal of tissue from the lower abdomen or buttock causes minimal functional disability or surgical morbidity. The abdominal wall is disrupted less with the free TRAM flap than it is with the pedicle TRAM flap because the dissection extends only slightly above the umbilicus for the free TRAM flap and leaves a large portion of the muscle intact within the rectus sheath. The free TRAM flap also allows greater versatility in positioning, tailoring, and contouring of the breast mound compared with the pedicle TRAM flap. When the pedicle TRAM flap is transposed to the chest, a bulge may appear, along with some associated discomfort, in the upper abdomen caused by the bulk of the muscle. The bulge can be avoided with a free TRAM flap. The free TRAM flap, based on a single rectus muscle, can be used for reconstruction following total, modified radical, or radical mastectomy and is illustrated in detail in this chapter. When bilateral reconstruction is performed, bilateral free TRAM flaps may be used. The use of bilateral free TRAM flaps (also illustrated in this chapter) avoids the need for implants and disrupts the abdominal wall less than does the use of bilateral pedicle flaps. The free flap procedure also permits reconstruction of two breast mounds, with matching skin color and texture, from one donor site. However, weakening of the abdominal wall occurs with bilateral free TRAM flaps because portions of both rectus muscles are transferred.

The superior gluteal free flap (also illustrated in detail), unlike the TRAM flap, does not disrupt the abdominal wall and produces the least noticeable donor site scar of all flap procedures for breast reconstruction. However, for several reasons the free TRAM flap is currently favored over the superior gluteal free flap. The vascular pedicle of the rectus abdominis muscle is long, the dissection is straightforward, and the entire operation can be done while the patient is in the supine position. With the superior gluteal flap, dissection of its short vascular pedicle can be tedious, and the patient must be repositioned during the operation. Following the free TRAM flap procedure, the patient can comfortably maintain a semisitting position because the surgical procedure only involves the anterior surface of the body. Posterior and anterior wounds follow the superior gluteal free flap procedure, and it is difficult for the patient to find a comfortable position for the first week postoperatively because she must remain semiupright. Bilateral free TRAM flap procedures can also be performed in a single operation. Bilateral breast reconstruction with superior gluteal flaps must be staged and is associated with an increased risk and morbidity. Therefore the gluteal free flap generally is used only when other myocutaneous flaps, including the free TRAM flap, the pedicle TRAM flap, or the latissimus dorsi flap, are unavailable or when their use is contraindicated.

A thorough understanding of the anatomy and vascular supply of the tissue involved in free flap transfer is essential to successful breast reconstruction. The anatomy and vascular supply of the TRAM flap, currently

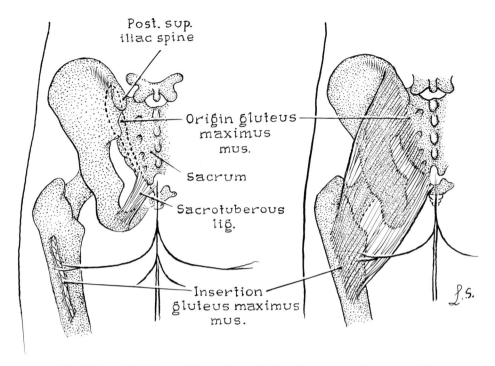

Fig 22-2.   Origin and insertion of the gluteus maximus muscle.

used more frequently than the gluteus maximus flap, are illustrated in Chapter 21. The anatomy of the gluteus maximus muscle is illustrated in Figure 22-2. The gluteus maximus muscle originates from the lateral margin of the sacrum and from the posterior superior iliac spine and has additional, small attachments to the coccyx and the sacrotuberous ligament. The muscle fibers extend obliquely and insert into the greater trochanter of the femur and the iliotibial tract. The gluteus maximus muscle is the strongest external rotator and extender of the hip and forms the bulk of the buttock. It also contributes to abduction of the thigh and stabilization of the hip in rising from a stooped position and in the motions associated with stair climbing and jogging. Transfer of the portion of the gluteus maximus muscle superior to the piriformis muscle does not produce a limp; however, it detracts from performance of these specific activities.

The vascular supply and innervation of the gluteus maximus muscle is shown in Figure 22-3. The arterial supply is derived from the superior gluteal and the inferior gluteal branches of the internal iliac artery. The two branches are separated by the piriformis muscle. The superior portion of the gluteus maximus muscle is supplied by the superior gluteal artery, which is usually 2 or 3 mm in diameter, and has slightly larger venae comitantes than the inferior gluteal artery. Its 4- or 5-cm-long vascular pedicle is located approximately 5 cm below the posterior superior iliac spine and 3 cm lateral to the border of the sacrum. The superior gluteal artery emerges superior to the piriformis muscle through a space between the piriformis and the gluteus medius muscles. The gluteus medius and gluteus minimus muscles lie deep to the anterior and superior portion of the gluteus maximus. The inferior portion of the gluteus maximus muscle is supplied by the inferior gluteal artery. With this double vascular supply the muscle can be split. For breast reconstruction, the superior half generally is used as a free flap and the inferior half is preserved to maintain function. However, a flap can be based on either half, and the main difference is the location of the resultant scar and cosmetic deformity. The gluteus maximus muscle is innervated by the inferior gluteal nerve, which originates from the L5, S1, and S2 spinal segments.

Indications

The superior gluteal flap and the free TRAM flap, rather than the standard TRAM pedicled flap, can be used for reconstruction in patients who are at high risk for flap failure or when previous surgery precludes the use of a pedicled TRAM flap. Bilateral free TRAM flaps can be used for reconstruction following bilateral mastectomy. The vascular supply of the free flap is superior to that of the standard single-pedicled TRAM flap. A free bilateral TRAM flap yields sufficient bulk to fill the large chest wall defect that results from radical mastectomy. A superior gluteal flap generally is not used for reconstruction following radical mastectomy; however, this flap provides sufficient volume to create a breast mound after modified radical or total mastectomy. In addition, the superior gluteal free flap may be the optimal flap to use in women who have a thin body habitus, with minimal subcutaneous fat in the lower abdomen.

Contraindications

The microvascular anastomosis for free flap reconstruction is technically demanding and time consuming; therefore a free flap procedure should not be used when a suitable, simpler alternative method of reconstruction could produce a comparable result. Also, it should not be used in patients with cardiovascular, pulmonary, or renal disease in whom safe administration of general anesthesia and successful completion of the flap cannot be ensured. A previous injury or surgical procedure that has compromised the dominant vascular supply to the gluteus maximus muscle or to the rectus abdominis muscle and its perforating vessels precludes use of that muscle in a free flap.

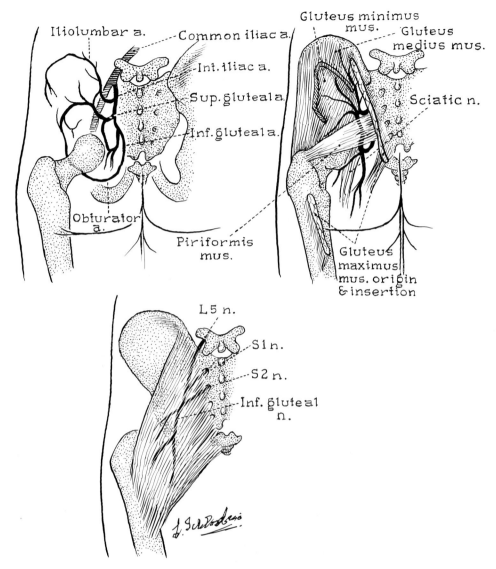

Fig 22-3. Vascular supply and innervation of gluteus maximus muscle.

Complications

The rectus abdominis and gluteus maximus free flap procedures are associated with significant complications. Respiratory problems, such as decreased ventilation, atelectasis, and pneumonia, may develop because of the length of the procedure. Thrombophlebitis and pulmonary emboli are risks of the surgery. The length of the surgery and the extensive dissection involved may bring about hypothermia and hypovolemia.

The most significant complication related to the free flap is vascular thrombosis. Free flaps should have a failure rate of less than 5% because of the excellent perfusion provided by the sizable inferior epigastric artery or by the superior gluteal artery. However, flap circulation must be monitored continuously, and immediate reexploration of the anastomoses must be performed if the patency of the artery or the vein is questionable. Vascular thrombosis, if it is not promptly detected and corrected, can result in complete loss of the flap. Other flap-related and chest wound complications include hematoma, infection, delayed healing, and an unsatisfactory appearance of the breast mound. A hematoma at the recipient site must be promptly evacuated to avoid compromise of the circulation to the flap or to the chest wall skin. Hematoma evacuation should be performed in the operating room to minimize the risk of disruption of the anastomoses and to have access to the microscope should revision of the anastomoses be required. If the anastomoses are properly performed and if the flap is not excessively manipulated during insetting, fat necrosis is unlikely to occur. Wound infection is infrequent and generally resolves with local wound care and systemic antibiotics. Fat necrosis and wound infection increase the likelihood of delayed wound healing. A malpositioned or misshapen breast mound can result if the breast pocket is not correctly dissected and if the flap is not properly tailored and inset.

Donor site complications for both types of free flaps include seromas and hematomas. Proper attention to hemostasis during transfer will minimize the risk of hematoma. However, if a hematoma develops, it must be promptly evacuated in the operating room. Insertion of constant vacuum drains into the donor sites to remove accumulated blood and serum usually will prevent formation of seromas. The free TRAM flap procedure may result in hernia formation, a lax abdominal wall, a malpositioned umbilicus, or formation of a standing cone at the lateral ends of the abdominal incision. These complications are more likely to occur when the abdominal closure is improperly performed. Finally, with a superior gluteal free flap, the contour of the buttocks can become distorted after flap transfer.

Preoperative Preparation

Breast reconstruction with a free flap usually requires replacement of 2 to 3 units of blood; therefore autologous blood should be donated at least 2 weeks before surgery. Cigarette smoking and aspirin ingestion are discontinued 2 weeks before surgery.

Antiembolism stockings and sequential compression devices should be placed preoperatively to help prevent thrombophlebitis and pulmonary emboli. The operating room must be kept warm, the patient should be placed on a warming blanket, and warm intravenous fluids should be administered to maintain a core temperature above 36° C. A bladder drainage catheter should be inserted to monitor urinary output. Prophylactic intravenous antibiotics and humidified oxygen are routinely administered, and blood replacement should begin early in the procedure. Preoperative steroid administration, although a controversial treatment, is frequently used because, postoperatively, it may diminish edema in the flap.

OPERATIVE PROCEDURE
Transverse Rectus Abdominis Free Flap
Preoperative Marking; Patient Positioning (Figure 22-4)

A free TRAM flap from the lower abdomen can be based on the ipsilateral or on the contralateral rectus abdominis muscle. The standard free

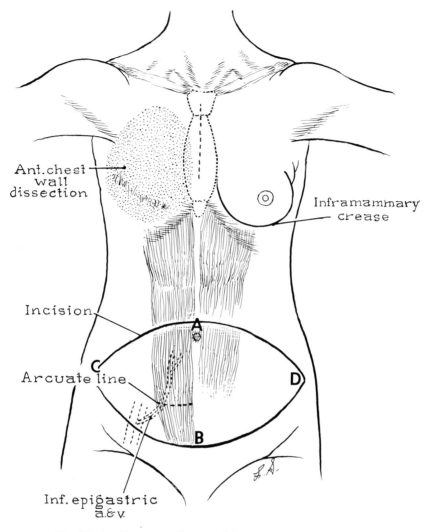

Fig 22-4. Preoperative marking; patient positioning.

TRAM flap design, shown here, produces a scar that is easily covered with underwear or with a two-piece swimsuit. The chest wall is marked while the patient is sitting in an upright position. The midline of the sternum, the inframammary crease on the opposite breast, and the proposed dissection pocket are marked. The elliptical outline of the flap is marked while the patient is standing. The flap's superior margin is outlined approximately 2 cm above the umbilicus, and the inferior margin is marked a few centimeters above the pubic hairline. The distance between these two margins in the midline is usually 14 to 16 cm.

A line drawn between the superior incision midpoint *(A)* and the inferior incision midpoint *(B)* determines the flap's width and serves as the short axis of the ellipse. The flap should be designed so that its width will approximately equal the width of the chest wall defect. The width distance is multiplied by 3 to determine the long axis of the ellipse, which extends from *C* to *D* just below the anterior superior iliac spine. Both halves of the upper and lower incision limbs should be the same length from the midpoint to avoid standing cones when the abdomen is closed. The flap then is divided into zones I through IV as described for the standard TRAM flap in Figure 21-5.

After marking, the patient is placed in the supine position, with the hips centered on the operating room table and with both arms flexed. After general anesthesia has been induced, the skin is prepared from the neck to the pubic area with an antibacterial solution and is draped, with the chest and abdomen in the operative field.

Elevation of the Contralateral Side of a Free TRAM Flap Based on a Single Muscle (Figure 22-5)

Flap elevation will begin on the side opposite the rectus abdominis muscle that is being used for transfer. The lateral portion of the superior skin incision can be extended directly down to the external oblique fascia. However, medially and in the portion of the flap overlying the rectus sheaths the incision should be beveled 45 degrees and extended superiorly to include an additional 2 or 3 cm of periumbilical subcutaneous tissue with its perforating vessels. The inferior limb of the incision is extended directly down to the anterior abdominal wall fascia throughout its length.

The flap is elevated, starting laterally, at the level of the external oblique fascia on the side from which only the skin and subcutaneous tissue will be harvested. The dissection proceeds medially, to the area 2 or 3 cm medial to the linea semilunaris, at which point the lateral-most column of vertical perforating vessels is identified as it exits the rectus sheath and enters the subcutaneous fat. The medial-most column of perforators is only a few centimeters medial to the lateral row. Because the rectus muscles are essentially symmetrical in an individual, the location of the vertical perforators coming through the rectus sheath on this side will mirror their location in the rectus sheath overlying the muscle on the side to be used for transfer, as shown in cross section in the inset. The extent to which the dissection is continued across the midline to the other side before encountering the perforating vessels, which must be preserved with the flap, can be determined.

The vast majority of perforating vessels pass through the anterior rectus sheath over a narrow area, approximately 3 or 4 cm wide, located near the muscle's center, and only this strip of the fascia will be included when the muscle is mobilized. The remaining 2 or 3 cm of the anterior rectus sheath laterally and 1 or 2 cm of the sheath medially will be preserved and repaired to reinforce the posterior rectus sheath and facilitate closure of the anterior abdominal wall after the flap is transferred.

As the flap is elevated, the perforating vessels that will remain in the abdomen are ligated as they emerge through the anterior rectus sheath and before they are divided. Otherwise, they retract beneath the rectus sheath after division and are difficult to control. As the elevation of the flap extends across the linea alba, the umbilicus is cored out and left attached to the abdominal wall, with some subcutaneous fat around its stalk to preserve circulation.

The TRAM flap will now be elevated 1 or 2 cm beyond the midline on the side from which part of the rectus muscle will be elevated. When the medial-most column of vertical perforating vessels coming through the rectus sheath that overlies the muscle used for transfer is identified exiting the fascia, (shown on cross section), the medial dissection is stopped. The flap's inferior margin then is elevated to 3 or 4 cm below the arcuate line at the level of the rectus fascia.

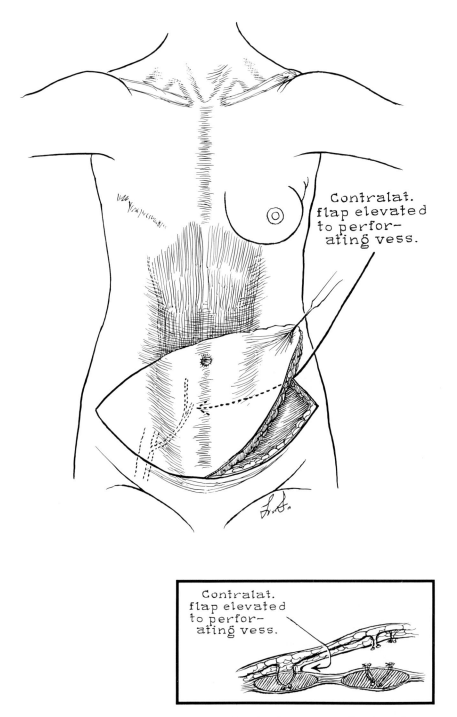

Fig 22-5. Elevation of the contralateral side of a free TRAM flap based on a single muscle.

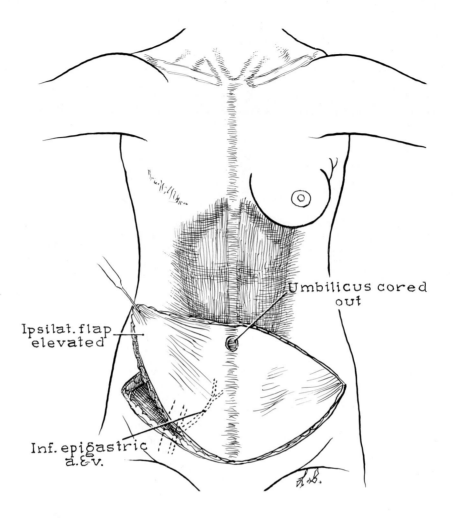

Ipsilat. flap elevated

Umbilicus cored out

Inf. epigastric a.&v.

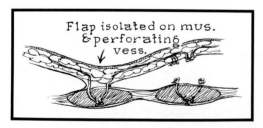

Flap isolated on mus. & perforating vess.

Fig 22-6. Elevation of ipsilateral side of a free TRAM flap based on a single muscle.

Elevation of the Ipsilateral Side of a Free TRAM Flap Based on a Single Muscle (Figure 22-6)

The flap's lateral margin on the side of muscle transfer is elevated, starting laterally and in the same manner as described for the flap elevation on the contralateral side. The dissection continues to the point at which the lateral-most vertical perforating vessels are seen coming through the rectus sheath (shown on cross section). The dissection is stopped at this point, and the flap is replaced on the abdominal wall.

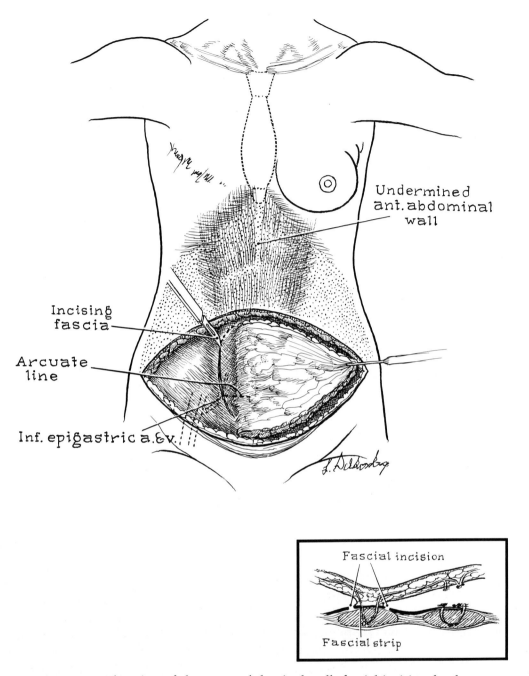

Fig 22-7. Elevation of the upper abdominal wall; fascial incision for free TRAM flap.

Elevation of the Upper Abdominal Wall; Fascial Incision for Free TRAM Flap (Figure 22-7)

The upper abdominal wall is elevated at the level of the muscular fascia to the costal margin and to the xiphoid. The TRAM free flap then is isolated on the 3- or 4-cm-wide strip of anterior rectus sheath that is richly supplied with the periumbilical perforating vessels. At this point the muscle is still lying intact within the rectus sheath and is perfused by the inferior and superior epigastric vessels. Most of the flap should appear to have normal circulation except, possibly, the most lateral part of zone IV.

237

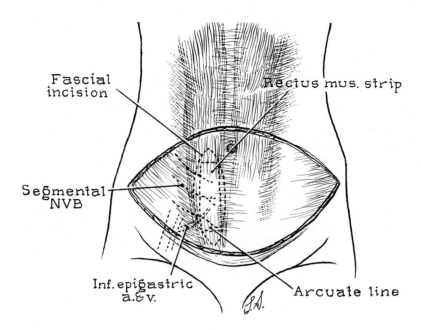

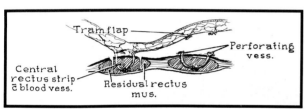

Fig 22-8. Muscle-sparing procedure for rectus abdominis muscle mobilization.

Thus far the steps for the dissection and elevation of the TRAM free flap have been the same as for the TRAM pedicle flap. The procedures diverge when the fascial incision is made. For the free TRAM flap the fascial incision is started at the flap's lower margin just inferior to the arcuate line, and it is continued superiorly as an ellipse that extends around the columns of vertical perforating vessels exiting the muscle. The fascial incision ends slightly above the superior margin of the flap, a few centimeters above the umbilicus. The strip of fascia lying within the borders of the incised ellipse incorporates a large number of perforating vessels (cross section in the inset). When the fascial incision is complete, the portions of the anterior rectus sheath lateral and medial to the elliptically shaped strip of fascia are elevated off the surface of the rectus muscle by blunt dissection.

Muscle-Sparing Procedure for Rectus Abdominis Muscle Mobilization (Figure 22-8)

The risk of injury to the inferior epigastric pedicle, which enters the muscle's posterior surface near the arcuate line, is minimized by starting the mobilization of the rectus abdominis muscle at the lateral edge of the flap's superior margin. A TRAM free flap can be developed by using a thin strip of the muscle or, more commonly, the entire width of the muscle. To elevate a thin strip of muscle, a Doppler probe is used to identify the path of the inferior epigastric vessels as they flow through the muscle. The lateral and medial portions of the muscle outside the vascular pathway are left intact in the abdomen to preserve abdominal wall strength. Approximately the

238

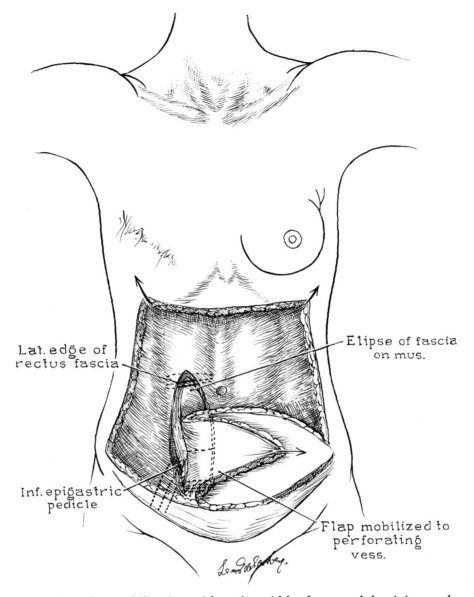

Fig 22-9. Flap mobilization with entire width of rectus abdominis muscle.

middle third of the muscle, which contains the inferior epigastric artery and vein, as well as the perforating vessels, is harvested. The free flap will include only a small strip of muscle with the inferior epigastric vessels as shown in the inset. The defect from this muscle strip harvest should be closed before closure of the anterior rectus sheath. The pedicle is then prepared as described in the next figure.

Flap Mobilization with Entire Width of Rectus Abdominis Muscle
(Figure 22-9)

The free TRAM flap also can be developed using the entire width of the rectus muscle. To elevate the entire width of the muscle, the rectangular segment of the rectus abdominis muscle underlying the flap is mobilized by blunt dissection, beginning near the flap's superior margin. As the muscle is elevated, the multiple intercostal nerves and associated small vessels that enter the lateral aspect of the rectus muscle are ligated as they are encountered. Electrocautery, which causes muscle contraction, is avoided.

The vascular pedicle should be readily identified and protected as it enters the posterior aspect of the muscle slightly above the arcuate line. Once the pedicle's point of entry into the rectus abdominis is identified, the portion of the muscle superficial to the pedicle is elevated and divided inferior to this point. The vascular pedicle then is freed from the surrounding tissues and carefully inspected to confirm that the vessels are suitable for planned anastomoses in the chest. The inferior epigastric artery and vein must be traced as far toward the external iliac vessels as practical in order that 4- or 5-cm lengths of artery and vein can be isolated.

The superior margin of the muscle is divided at this time so that all of the flap dissection and manipulation will be completed except for division of the inferior epigastric pedicle. The flap is then allowed to perfuse for 30 minutes after it has been isolated only on the inferior epigastric pedicle. During dissection of the anterior rectus sheath and muscle mobilization, the flap is folded upon itself and is poorly perfused. It should be well perfused before it is transferred to the chest. Although zone IV may be visibly congested, the remainder of the flap should appear viable, and as the perfusion of the flap improves, the congestion in zone IV may diminish.

Dissection of the Anterior Chest Wall (Figure 22-10)

A transverse or an oblique mastectomy scar can be excised as the initial incision for creation of the breast pocket. However, if the scar is oriented vertically, or if it ends near the opposite inframammary crease, a new oblique incision is made instead.

The breast pocket is created by elevation of the skin and underlying subdermal fat from the chest wall. Because part of the free flap will be used to pad the chest, the superior portion of the pocket is deepened to the pectoral muscle so that the flap can be sutured to the chest wall. The dissection should be confined to the margins of the premastectomy breast pocket as much as possible. Confining the dissection will create an envelope that will naturally restrain the flap during tailoring and therefore assist with the shaping of flap tissue. Also limiting the pocket to its premastectomy margins can reduce the amount of suturing required for insetting the flap and recreating the inframammary crease.

The initial inferior dissection ends several centimeters above the opposite inframammary crease because closure of the abdominal wall following transfer of the flap will pull the incision 2 or 3 cm inferiorly. The crease easily can be further lowered during insetting if it seems too high. The extent of the dissection laterally is determined by the vessels that are to be used for the anastomoses. The thoracodorsal vessels are the most commonly used vessels for the anastomoses when a free TRAM flap is used for breast reconstruction. When the thoracodorsal vessels are used for anastomosis, the lateral dissection has to be continued further laterally than the premastectomy pocket to gain access to these vessels and to provide sufficient exposure to safely perform the microvascular anastomoses. Medially the dissection extends to 1 to 2 cm lateral to the midline.

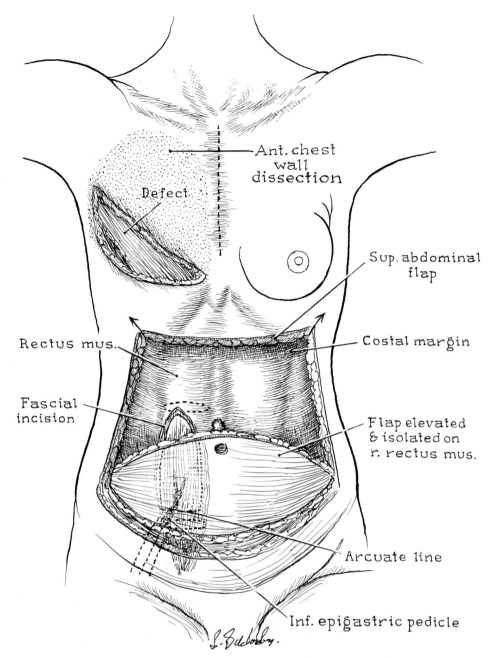

Fig 22-10. Dissection of the anterior chest wall.

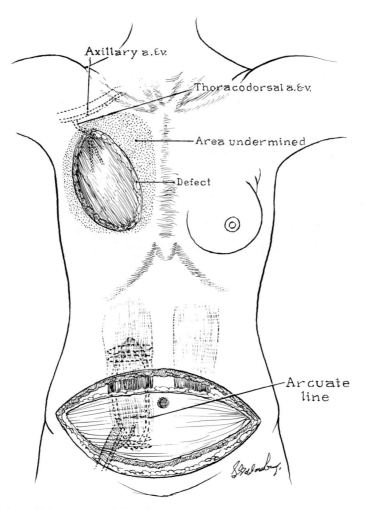

Fig 22-11. Dissection of the thoracodorsal pedicle; completion of lateral chest wall dissection.

Dissection of the Thoracodorsal Pedicle; Completion of Lateral Chest Wall Dissection (Figure 22-11)

It is essential to gain as much length as possible on the recipient vessels to facilitate the microvascular anastomosis and to allow for movement while the flap is positioned and inset into the breast pocket.

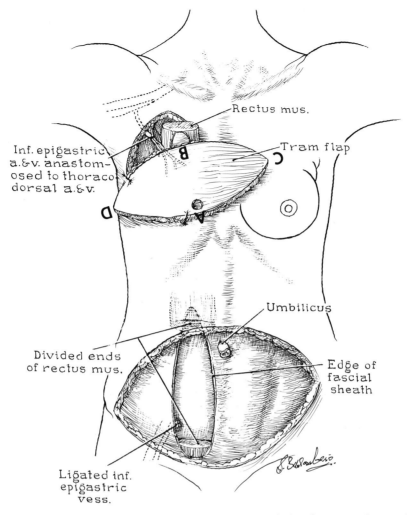

Fig 22-12. Division of the inferior epigastric pedicle; flap transfer to chest; microvascular anastomoses.

Division of the Inferior Epigastric Pedicle; Flap Transfer to Chest; Microvascular Anastomoses (Figure 22-12)

After the flap is perfused in situ and the recipient artery and vein are prepared for anastomoses, the inferior epigastric pedicle is clamped as close to the external iliac vessels as possible. The stump of the pedicle on the external iliac vessels is doubly ligated. The inferior epigastric artery and vein are irrigated with heparinized saline solution and are prepared for the microvascular anastomoses.

The completely detached flap then is positioned on the chest wall and is stabilized with skin staples or with sutures before the microvascular anastomoses are begun. The patient then is positioned so that the donor and recipient vessels lie in the same focal plane.

With the aid of the operating microscope the vessels are anastomosed with fine, interrupted nylon sutures. After the circulation has been restored, the anastomosed vessels are carefully checked for patency. The muscle of the flap then is secured to the chest wall so that the anastomoses will not be disrupted or be under tension as the flap is tailored and inset. The flap is allowed to perfuse undisturbed while the abdominal wound is closed.

Abdominal Closure; Insetting of the Flap (Figure 22-13)

Because the TRAM flap donor site covers nearly the entire width of the abdomen, abdominal closure must be performed carefully to prevent postoperative complications and unsightly scarring. The anterior rectus sheath can be closed primarily with a monofilament suture. Use of a running suture allows a gradual closure that distributes the tension evenly over the entire wound. If the fascial closure is too tight, the umbilicus will shift toward the side of the muscle used for transfer and will be abnormally positioned on the abdominal wall. This horizontal shifting can be corrected by plication of the opposite rectus fascia. After fascial closure and plication the abdominal wound is irrigated with saline and povidone-iodine solutions, and hemostasis is obtained. Two 10-mm constant vacuum drains are inserted and brought out through separate stab incisions in the pubic hair region.

For closure of the abdominal wall the patient is placed in a semisitting position with the thighs and knees flexed. A single, interrupted absorbable suture is placed at the midpoint of the incision, and the new umbilicus location is marked with a needle and brilliant green. The umbilicus is repositioned at or slightly below the level of a line drawn through the two anterior superior iliac spines. It is better to err on the low side when placing the umbilicus because placement at a site that is too high produces a more obvious deformity.

After the location of the umbilicus is determined, the abdominal wound is closed in three layers, starting at the lateral margins and progressing medially, so that any excess tissue in the upper abdominal wall can be redistributed to a medial position. An initial closure is made with skin staples. Then sutures are placed between the staples in the superficial fascial system, and the staples are removed. A layer of interrupted absorbable sutures then is placed in the deep dermis and followed by a running subcuticular suture. The umbilicus is brought out at an appropriate midline location through a semicircular convex inferior (or smile) incision. A core of fat underlying this incision is excised to form a gentle indentation at the new umbilical location. The umbilicus is sutured with four quadrant sutures that go through the abdominal wall skin, the anterior rectus sheath, and the umbilical skin. Finally a layer of running absorbable sutures is placed around the umbilicus. This produces a depressed umbilicus and a minimally visible scar below the skin surface. The closed wound is dressed with nonadherent gauze and tape.

After the abdomen is closed, the breast mound is created. While not technically difficult, correct tailoring of the flap is probably the most esthetically demanding and time consuming part of a free flap procedure. The formation of a natural-looking breast from a large shapeless mass of skin and fat requires patience and creativity. The flap is gently rotated until the best positions for the skin island and for the tissue bulk are determined. Usually a free TRAM flap is inset with its width lying perpendicular to the midline of the sternum. Such placement maximizes the flap's blood flow and adds tissue bulk in the inferior half of the breast mound where it is usually most needed. In general the least amount of tissue is required in the upper medial quadrant of the breast mound.

The most appropriate placement of the skin island is determined early in the tailoring process. If possible the inferior margin of the skin island should be joined to the inferior border of the breast pocket to ensure that

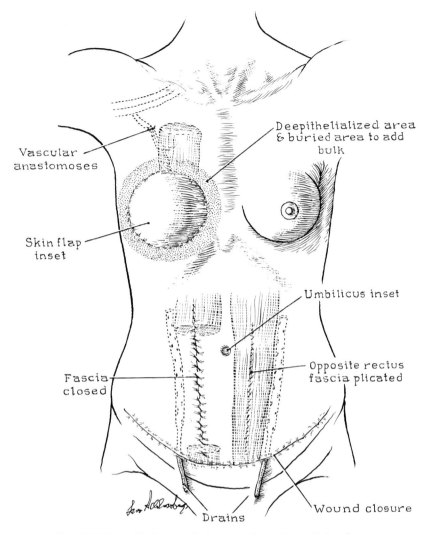

Vascular anastomoses

Deepithelialized area & buried area to add bulk

Skin flap inset

Umbilicus inset

Fascia closed

Opposite rectus fascia plicated

Drains

Wound closure

Fig 22-13.   Abdominal closure; insetting of the flap.

one limb of the scar will be concealed. However, the fitting of the flap to the defect does not always permit this positioning. Sometimes the skin island must be placed across the summit of the breast mound horizontally, vertically, obliquely, or even in the superior portion of the breast. Some patients may need a skin island only 4 cm wide, while others require 8 cm or more of additional skin. The following general guidelines must be individualized because the location and the amount of skin needed for reconstruction will differ in each patient. Part of the challenge of tailoring the flap lies in finding the best position for the skin island.

To start the actual insetting process the proposed inframammary crease is marked to correspond with the opposite breast marking made preoperatively. The inferior half of the flap will provide the bulk of the breast mound, contribute to the new inframammary fold, and form much of the breast mound's projection and ptosis. Trial tailoring is begun by gently folding under the flap's lower portion and positioning it to rest on the inferior edge of the breast pocket. If the trial placement indicates that the flap will produce a breast mound that is too large, some of the tissue in the lower area of the flap is excised. In addition, when insetting a TRAM free flap that is based on a single rectus muscle, zone IV tissue and as much of the zone III tissue as possible are discarded because these areas are the least well perfused.

The flap is moved around the pocket and the chest wall skin is draped over it to determine the part of the flap that will be included in the skin island and the part that will be folded under to add bulk. The margin of overlap between those two areas is marked with brilliant green, and the portion that will be positioned beneath the flap or chest skin is deepithelialized. The inframammary crease is approximated by resting the tissue that is to become the inferior part of the breast mound on the inframammary shelf. The trial tailoring thus far completed should be stapled in place until the best position, contour, and symmetry are finalized.

The superior portion of the flap is tailored next. The upper part of the flap is placed beneath the chest wall skin to determine the best use of tissue components for filling defects in the axillary and infraclavicular areas. If the pectoralis major muscle is absent, the portion of the flap nearest the axilla should be deepithelialized and attached to the pectoralis tendon stump to simulate an anterior axillary fold. After draping the chest wall skin around the flap, brilliant green is used to outline the superior margin of overlap of the skin island. Any excess tissue is excised, and the portion of the flap to be buried for padding in the superior chest is deepithelialized. Once the deepithelialized edge of the flap is tucked beneath the chest wall skin, the upper part of the breast mound is temporarily secured in position with skin staples.

As the tailoring progresses, the flap may be trimmed and any excess tissue may be discarded. Every new alteration requires restapling of the new breast mound and reassessment of its position, size, and contour until the best shape is found. Caution must be exercised while tailoring to avoid compromising the circulation by folding or kinking the flap.

Creation of a perfect breast mound does not have to be achieved at the initial operation. It is better to accept a less-than-ideal breast contour at this stage than to risk losing a large portion of the flap because of necrosis caused by excessive manipulation. The breast mound can be modified and improved at later revisions when circulation has improved and when the flap can withstand additional manipulation.

When a satisfactory position and contour have been attained, the buried superior portions of the flap are permanently sutured to the pectoral muscle or chest wall. The inferior portion of the flap must rest freely on the lower edge of the premastectomy breast pocket to produce a natural-appearing inframammary fold. If the pocket has been correctly dissected, deep fixation sutures should not be needed in the lower half of the breast mound.

Before final wound closure a constant vacuum drain is inserted beneath the flap and is brought out through an axillary or a lateral incision (not shown here). The tailoring of the chest wall skin to the margin of the skin island is finalized, using skin staples, and any excess tissue is excised. Interrupted dermal sutures are placed between the staples, the staples are removed, and a layer of interrupted absorbable sutures is placed around the entire skin island margin. The insetting is completed with a layer of running subcuticular sutures. The location of the vascular pedicles should be marked on the patient's skin to prepare for an examination with a Doppler probe postoperatively.

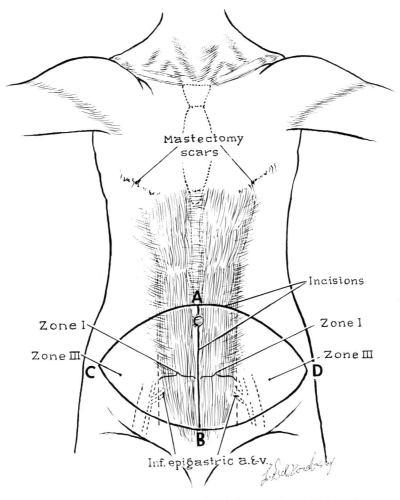

Fig 22-14. Patient marking for bilateral free TRAM flaps.

OPERATIVE PROCEDURE

Bilateral Free TRAM Flaps for Bilateral Breast Reconstruction

Patient Marking for Bilateral Free TRAM Flaps (Figure 22-14)

The bilateral free TRAM flaps are marked in the same manner as the standard pedicled TRAM flap described in Figure 21-6. The superior incisions are outlined by marking a point (*A*) approximately 2 cm above the umbilicus in the midline and by marking another point (*B*) approximately 2 cm above the pubic hairline. The line *AB* connecting these points represents the short axis of the flap. The distance *AB* is typically 14 to 16 cm. The long axis of the flap can then be determined by measuring a distance (*CD*) that is three times the length of *AB* to cross the midpoint of the line *AB*. Points *C* and *D* are marked just superior to the anterior superior iliac spines bilaterally. A horizontal ellipse is drawn around these points as shown. In comparing the marking for the bilateral free TRAM flaps with the marking for the standard pedicled flap the primary difference is the additional line

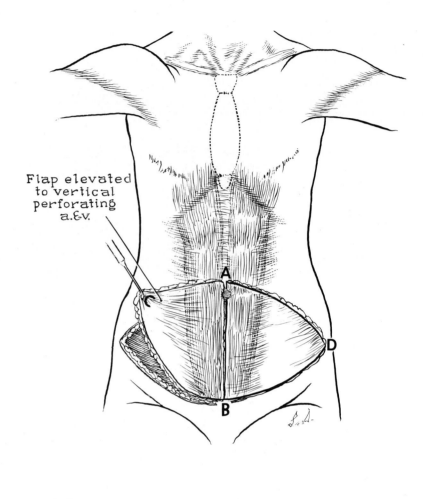

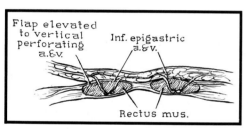

Fig 22-15. Lateral elevation of one hemiflap.

AB that is drawn through the midline of the flap to delineate two separate halves of the abdominal flap. With this design each hemiflap has a zone I and a zone III. If tissue requirements are different on the two sides of the chest, the line *AB* can be shifted approximately 1 to 2 cm from the midline depending on the location of the medial column of vertical perforating vessels. After the patient is marked, she is placed on the operating table in a supine position and general anesthesia is induced.

Lateral Elevation of One Hemiflap (Figure 22-15)

Elevating the flaps begins by making the incisions down to the fascia. Over the anterior rectus sheaths and medially the incision through *CAD* is beveled superiorly to leave some additional fat on the anterior rectus fascia. Laterally the incision is extended directly to the fascia. Inferiorly the incision is extended directly to the fascia throughout its full length. The flap elevation then begins laterally at point *C*. The flap is elevated at the level of the abdominal wall fascia until the lateral-most vertical perforating vessels are encountered exiting the anterior rectus sheath, as illustrated in cross section on the inset. The lateral to medial dissection is stopped when these vertical perforating vessels are encountered.

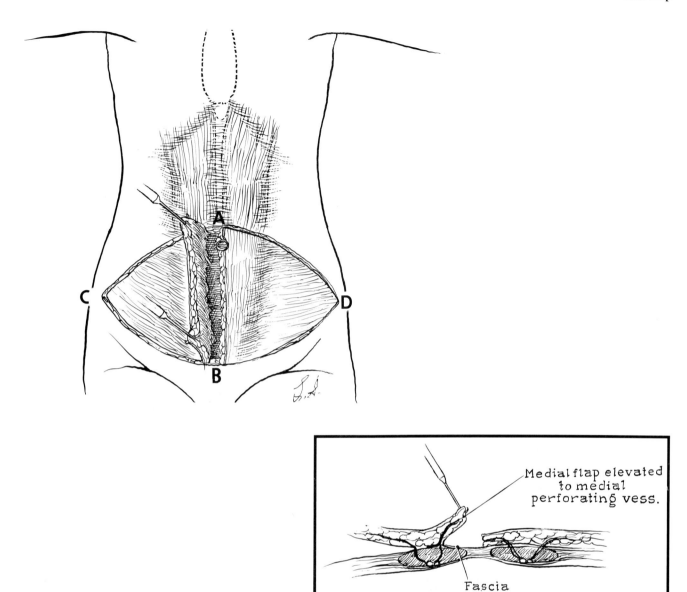

Fig 22-16. Medial elevation of hemiflap.

Medial Elevation of One Hemiflap (Figure 22-16)

After completing the lateral elevation of one hemiflap the medial dissection begins by coring out the umbilicus and by making the midline incision along line *AB*. Dissection then proceeds laterally from this incision toward *C* at the level of the abdominal wall fascia for 2 to 3 cm from the midline of the abdomen until the medial column of vertical perforating vessels is encountered, as shown in cross section on the inset.

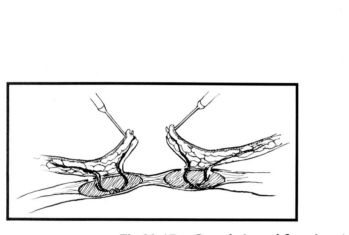

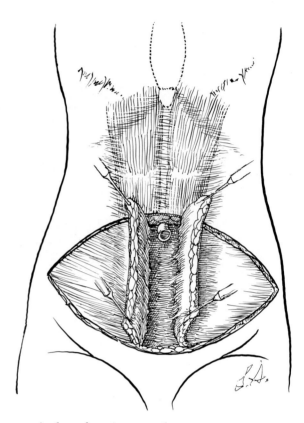

Fig 22-17. Completion of flap elevation to vertical perforating vessels.

Completion of Flap Elevation to Vertical Perforating Vessels (Figure 22-17)

After one hemiflap is completely elevated to the level of the vertical perforating vessels, this process is repeated on the contralateral side so that each hemiflap is isolated on its two columns of vertical perforating vessels coming through the anterior rectus sheath, as shown in cross section on the inset.

Undermining of the Upper Abdominal Wall; Fascial Incisions; Mobilization of the Rectus Muscles (Figure 22-18)

The upper abdominal flap then is elevated at the level of the abdominal wall fascia to the costal margin and xiphoid process. The area of undermining is shown here as stippling. After the mobilization of the upper abdominal wall is completed, the fascial incisions are marked about the vertical perforating vessels. These elliptical incisions extend from a few centimeters above the umbilicus to just below the arcuate line. After the incisions are marked, one fascial ellipse is incised. A strip of fascia is left on the anterior surface of the rectus muscle. Mobilization of the rectus muscle from its fascial sheath by blunt dissection then is begun at approximately the midportion of the hemiflap and sufficiently superior to the arcuate line to allow retraction of the muscle and exposure of the inferior epigastric vessels with minimal risk. After the inferior epigastric vessels are identified, the muscle is mobilized from its fascial sheath within the area of the ellipse. Below the arcuate line the inferior epigastric vessels emerge posteriorly from the muscle. Segmental

250

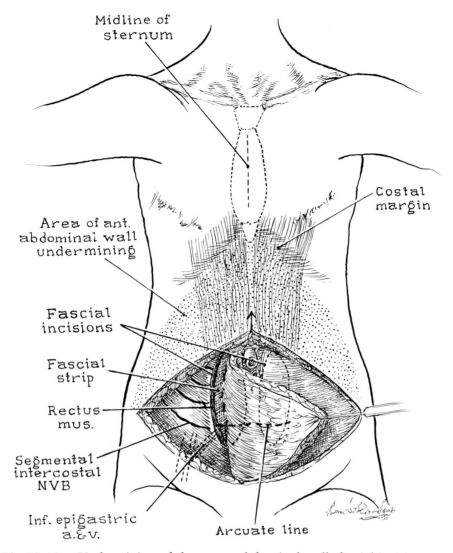

Fig 22-18. Undermining of the upper abdominal wall; fascial incisions; mobilization of rectus muscles.

intercostal neurovascular bundles are ligated as the muscle is mobilized from its fascial sheath. The inferior epigastric pedicle then is dissected as close to its origin at the external iliac artery and vein as possible to gain sufficient length for anastomoses to recipient vessels in the chest. Occasionally it may be beneficial to divide the rectus muscle inferiorly (not shown here) to gain additional exposure for dissection of the inferior epigastric pedicles. However, division of the rectus muscle superiorly at this point is premature because it will preclude performance of a pedicle transposition of the flap if an injury should occur to the inferior epigastric vessels which would prevent their use for the microvascular anastomoses. Both hemiflaps are dissected in the same manner.

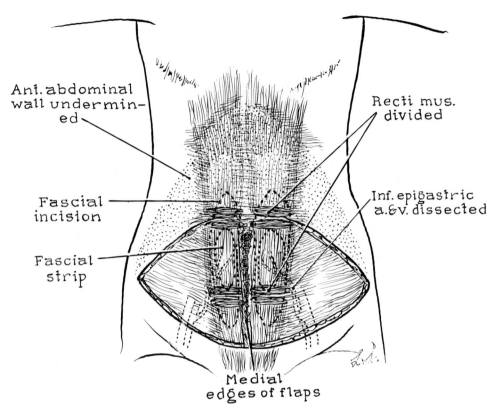

Ant. abdominal
wall undermin-
ed

Recti mus.
divided

Fascial
incision

Inf. epigastric
a.&v. dissected

Fascial
strip

Medial
edges of flaps

Fig 22-19. Division of rectus muscles; isolation of free TRAM hemiflaps on inferior epigastric vessels.

Division of Rectus Muscles; Isolation of Free TRAM Hemiflaps on Inferior Epigastric Vessels (Figure 22-19)

After completing the dissection of the inferior epigastric pedicles, the rectus muscles are divided inferior (if not already done) and superior to the fascial ellipses. The dissection should be done with a scalpel to avoid the risk of damage to the inferior epigastric vessels which could occur if electrocautery is used. The use of electrocautery could be particularly hazardous at this point because the only remaining ground through which the electrical current can pass from the hemiflap tissue, including the rectus muscle, is the inferior epigastric pedicle. After division of the muscles both hemiflaps are perfused only by the inferior epigastric vessels. At this point the hemiflaps are replaced in the abdomen and are allowed to perfuse while the chest wall dissection is performed.

Chest Wall Dissection for Bilateral Free TRAM Flaps
(Figure 22-20)

Each side of the chest wall dissection for bilateral free TRAM flaps is similar to that for a unilateral free TRAM flap. The dissection should extend superiorly to just below the clavicle, medially to 1 to 2 cm lateral to the midline of the sternum, inferiorly to the sixth rib, and laterally to approximately the midaxillary line. The primary difference between the chest dissection for a free TRAM flap and the dissection for a standard pedicle TRAM flap is that the dissection for the free TRAM flap extends farther laterally—

252

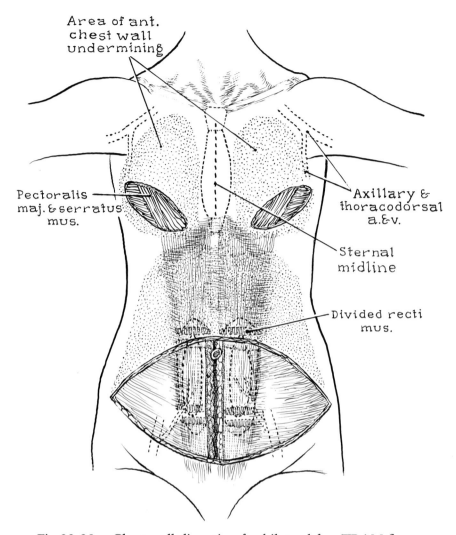

Fig 22-20. Chest wall dissection for bilateral free TRAM flaps.

to the midaxillary line and into the axilla sufficiently to mobilize the thoracodorsal or thoracoacromial vessels for the anastomoses. The incision in the chest should use a preexisting scar if the scar is oriented transversely or obliquely and will provide adequate exposure for the microvascular anastomoses. However, if the previous scar location is unsuitable, a new incision is made. If the chest incision is made too low, the breast mound may be placed too far inferiorly. The inframammary crease should ultimately be located at the level of about the seventh rib. The chest incision should be made above that. Additional tissue can be excised later, if necessary, to allow insetting of the flap at the level of the desired inframammary crease. The dissection is performed at the level of the pectoralis fascia or at the level of the chest wall if a radical mastectomy has been performed. When the flaps have been elevated and the vessels dissected and prepared for the microvascular anastomoses on one side, the corresponding dissection is performed on the opposite side. The chest wall dissection must be finished, with the vessels completely dissected, inspected for suitability, and prepared for the microvascular anastomoses before the flaps are detached from the abdomen by dividing the inferior epigastric pedicles.

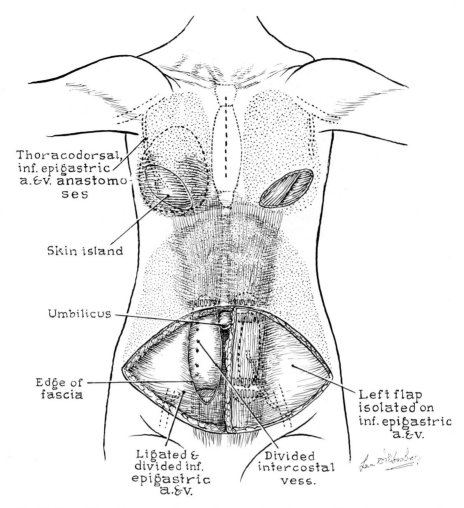

Thoracodorsal, inf. epigastric a.&v. anastomoses

Skin island

Umbilicus

Edge of fascia

Left flap isolated on inf. epigastric a.&v.

Ligated & divided inf. epigastric a.&v.

Divided intercostal vess.

Fig 22-21. Hemiflap transfer to the anterior chest wall and microvascular anastomoses.

Hemiflap Transfer to the Anterior Chest Wall and Microvascular Anastomoses (Figure 22-21)

After the preparation of the chest wall recipient sites for transfer of the TRAM hemiflaps is completed, one hemiflap (in this case the right) is detached by division of its inferior epigastric vessels and by double ligation of the vessel stumps on the external iliac artery and vein. The inferior epigastric artery and vein are irrigated with heparinized saline solution and prepared for the microvascular anastomoses. The flap then is transferred to the chest wall and stabilized with skin staples. If necessary the patient's position is modified to facilitate performance of the microvascular anastomoses, with the vessels in a single focal plane. The artery and vein are anastomosed, and circulation is restored to the transferred hemiflap, while the other hemiflap remains perfused in the abdomen (as shown here). Once the hemiflap is adequately revascularized and the patency of the artery and vein confirmed, the hemiflap is allowed to perfuse on the chest. After one hemiflap is completely revascularized, the muscle should be secured to the chest wall to prevent inadvertent kinking or disruption of the anastomoses during insetting. The other hemiflap then is similarly detached, and the microvascular anastomoses are performed on the opposite side.

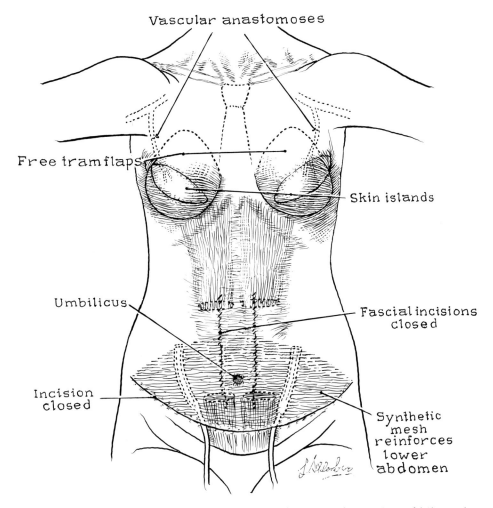

Fig 22-22. Abdominal wound closure; tailoring and insetting of bilateral free TRAM flaps.

Abdominal Wound Closure; Tailoring and Insetting of Bilateral Free TRAM Flaps (Figure 22-22)

After both flaps are vascularized and while the abdomen is being closed, the flaps are allowed to perfuse in the chest in a manner similar to that described in detail in Figure 22-13. Each anterior rectus sheath is closed with a running monofilament absorbable suture to distribute tension equally between the two sides. The abdominal wall then is strengthened by reinforcement with synthetic mesh. The abdomen is drained with two constant vacuum drains brought out through stab wounds in the pubic hair region. The remainder of the closure is performed with the patient in a flexed position. The abdominal wound is closed in three layers with absorbable sutures. Skin staples initially are used to close the wound. Excess tissue is distributed toward the midline. The skin staples then are removed and are replaced with a layer of sutures in the superficial fascia. A second layer of interrupted sutures is placed in the deep dermis, and finally a running subcuticular layer is used to complete the closure. The umbilicus is brought out and inset in the midline.

The TRAM flaps then are positioned in the predissected pockets and are tailored for final insetting. The flaps are manipulated until the best position is achieved to provide the optimal use of the subcutaneous fat and the skin components, as described in Figure 22-13 for the unilateral free TRAM flap. The areas to be buried are deepithelialized and if necessary sutured in place. The skin island is inset with a two-layer closure of interrupted and running absorbable sutures. Constant vacuum drains (not shown here) are placed in the chest beneath the flaps at sites remote to the vascular pedicles. The location of the vascular pedicles should be marked on the patient's skin to permit an examination with a Doppler probe postoperatively.

OPERATIVE PROCEDURE

Gluteus Maximus Free Flap Breast Reconstruction

Preoperative Marking (Figure 22-23)

The midline of the sternum and the opposite inframammary crease are marked while the patient is in an upright or sitting position. The proposed chest wall dissection is outlined and the paths of the external jugular vein, the cephalic vein, and a lower extremity vein suitable for grafting are marked because a vein graft may be needed for the microvascular anastomoses.

The patient may be standing or lying with the donor hip in a lateral position for marking the superior gluteal flap. The ipsilateral side (with respect to the mastectomy) is most often used as the flap donor site so the surgeon can gain access to the chest and to the donor hip without repositioning the patient. As illustrated here the elliptically shaped skin island is marked in the area overlying the superior gluteal artery. The flap's long axis should run essentially parallel to this artery, whose pedicle is typically located 5 cm below the posterior superior iliac spine and 3 cm lateral to the border of the sacrum. The superior gluteal artery usually can be mapped with a Doppler probe. Once this artery is identified, the medial and superior margins of the flap can be determined.

The maximum flap width that allows primary wound closure is about 12 or 13 cm, and the flap length is typically designed to be approximately three times the width. Usually the tissue on the flap's long axis provides the breadth of the reconstructed breast, and the tissue on the short axis contributes to breast projection and ptosis. However, if necessary, the flap's length can be extended when extra bulk is needed to fill larger defects. The lateral tip then would be deepithelialized and buried to fill the anterior axillary fold. The depth of the flap, which is defined as the distance between the skin surface and the vascular pedicle, is usually 13 to 15 cm.

As the flap is dissected, only a relatively short and narrow strip of muscle is harvested beginning near the sacrum medial to the superior gluteal pedicle and ending at the lateral border of the muscle. In general the muscle should comprise approximately 15% of the flap's total volume. Transfer of a larger strip of muscle increases the risk of functional impairment, makes the anastomoses more difficult to perform, and may cause the superior portion of the breast mound to change in size and contour as the muscle subsequently atrophies.

After marking, the patient is placed on the operating table with the donor hip elevated in a lateral position. If two surgical teams are available,

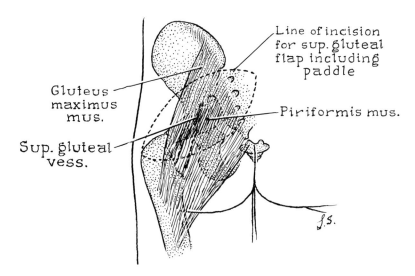

Fig 22-23. Preoperative marking.

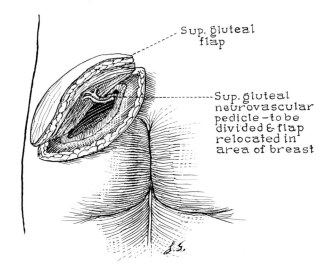

Fig 22-24. Superior gluteal flap dissection.

the patient usually can be positioned so that the chest wall dissection and the flap elevation can be performed simultaneously. If one team performs the procedure, the flap is elevated first and then the anterior chest wall dissection is done. Once the flap is removed and the buttock wound is closed, the patient will be moved to a supine position for the microvascular anastomoses.

Superior Gluteal Flap Dissection (Figure 22-24)

The superior skin margin is incised and deepened to the gluteus maximus fascia. The upper border of the muscle is identified and followed to its lateral margin. The deep fascia that covers the gluteus maximus is incised so that the muscle fibers at the lateral edge of the strip being transferred can be divided with the electrocautery. When the lateral margin is freed and elevated from the underlying gluteus medius muscle, the superior gluteal vessels are identified emerging superior to the piriformis muscle when the gluteus maximus muscle is reflected toward the midline. The inferior margin incision then is made and is extended to the fascial layer.

The superior and inferior fascial incisions are extended circumferentially to elevate the elliptical tissue flap except for the medial attachments of the muscle. By sharp dissection the muscle is detached from its origins at the sacrum and posterior superior iliac spine. The portion of the gluteus maximus muscle to be transferred then is separated from the inferior part of the muscle that will remain by proceeding obliquely with the dissection from the lateral border toward the iliac spine to carefully split the muscle parallel to its fibers.

The superior gluteal pedicle is freed from the surrounding soft tissue. Good exposure of the superior gluteal pedicle is obtained by using a retractor to widen the space between the gluteus medius and the piriformis muscles. Many smaller venous and arterial branches coming off the pedicle will be encountered at the level of the piriformis muscle. These vessels must be cauterized or ligated before the pedicle is divided. The pedicle will be divided at the level of the piriformis because the large network of branching vessels makes dissection beyond the piriformis difficult because the superior gluteal vein is fragile and easily injured. The dissected vascular pedicle will be 4 or 5 cm long and sufficient for anastomoses to vessels in the chest. The reliability of the flap's circulation is evaluated to ensure that the tissue can be transferred safely. The superior gluteal flap now is isolated only on the superior gluteal vessels, and the underlying gluteus medius and piriformis muscles are exposed. At this point the flap should be allowed to perfuse on its vascular pedicle for at least 30 minutes while the chest wall dissection is completed.

Chest Wall Dissection; Microvascular Anastomoses (Figure 22-25)

Because the patient is in a lateral position for the gluteus maximus free flap procedure, the anterior chest dissection can be more tedious than it is when the patient is in a supine position. The internal mammary artery and vein usually fit best with the flap's orientation; therefore the medial portion of the third costal cartilage overlying these vessels is resected to gain exposure. The internal mammary artery is constant in its size and suitability for microvascular anastomoses. However, the vein is delicate and friable, and often multiple small veins, rather than a single large vein, are present. If the vein is inadequate, a vein graft should be harvested at this point for the venous anastomosis and a suitable recipient vein should be exposed. If the chest wall dissection is particularly difficult (a rare occurrence), it may be necessary to reposition the patient to complete the chest wall dissection. If necessary the vascular pedicle to the flap can be divided, the flap vessels can be irrigated with heparinized saline solution, and the flap can be cooled on sterile ice slush. The buttock wound then is closed, and the patient is repositioned, prepared, and draped in the supine position to facilitate completion of the chest wall dissection. However, despite the awkwardness of the dissection, the flap's vascular pedicle generally should not be divided before the vessels in the chest are ready for anastomoses to the artery and the vein of the transferred flap. Premature pedicle division can result in prolonged flap ischemia and in an increased risk of flap failure.

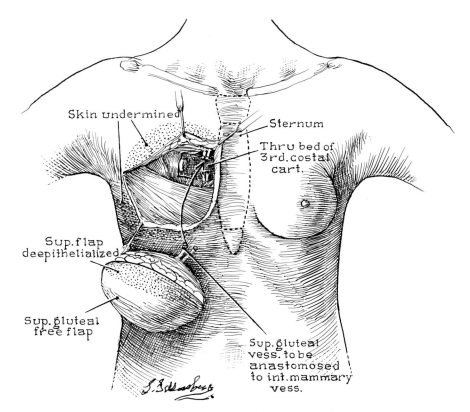

Labels in figure: Skin undermined; Sternum; Thru bed of 3rd. costal cart.; Sup. flap deepithelialized; Sup. gluteal free flap; Sup. gluteal vess. to be anastomosed to int. mammary vess.

Fig 22-25. Chest wall dissection; microvascular anastomoses.

After the chest wall vessels have been prepared for anastomosis, the superior gluteal vascular pedicle is divided as a unit to avoid injury to the vessels, and then the artery and vein are separated, flushed with heparinized saline solution, and prepared for anastomoses just before flap transfer. The flap is kept cool on crushed ice while the donor site wound is closed.

Before repositioning the patient for the microvascular anastomoses and flap tailoring, hemostasis is obtained at the donor site. A constant vacuum drain is inserted deep to the donor site and is brought out through a separate stab wound. The donor site is closed with a layer of interrupted absorbable sutures and followed by a layer of running subcuticular sutures. Some of the surrounding buttock skin may be undermined and mobilized as necessary to prevent formation of a depression in the contour. Finally the suture line is reinforced with sterile strips, and the donor site incision is dressed with nonadherent gauze and tape.

After the donor site has been closed, the patient is placed in a supine position. The microvascular anastomoses now can be performed with the vessels in a single focal plane. The anastomoses are performed most easily with the superior gluteal flap positioned so that the vascular pedicle lies superiorly to the harvested muscle and the skin island lies inferiorly. Before the anastomoses are begun, the flap is stabilized temporarily on the chest wall with skin staples or sutures.

With the aid of the operating microscope the arterial and venous anastomoses are performed with interrupted sutures of fine nylon. When the

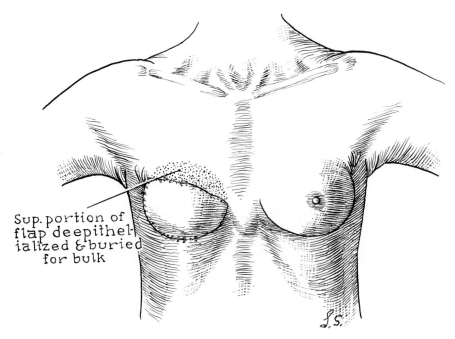

Sup. portion of
flap deepithel-
ialized & buried
for bulk

Fig 22-26. Flap insetting and tailoring.

anastomoses are completed and circulation is restored to the flap, the vessels and their anastomoses are carefully evaluated for patency and satisfactory blood flow. The portion of the muscle transferred with the flap is sutured to the chest wall so the anastomoses will not be disrupted while the flap is inset. The flap then should be allowed to perfuse undisturbed in its new chest wall location for approximately 30 minutes before insetting.

Flap Insetting and Tailoring (Figure 22-26)

After the flap has perfused for 30 minutes on the chest, the patency of the anastomoses should be confirmed and the patient should be moved to a semisitting position for tailoring and insetting. With the anastomotic sites secured the flap can be rotated gently until the best position for the skin island is found. In most patients a transverse or oblique orientation produces the best breast mound contour. The flap's position in the breast pocket is determined to some extent by the location of the recipient vessels. The inferior portion of the skin island can be used to form the lower half of the breast mound and inframammary crease. Part of the superior portion of the skin island can be deepithelialized and buried beneath the chest wall skin to provide bulk for the superior portion of the breast mound and padding for the chest. Detailed guidelines for insetting the flap are provided in the text accompanying Figure 22-13. At the end of the procedure the location of the vascular pedicles should be marked on the patient's skin so that they can be examined with a Doppler probe postoperatively.

Postoperative Care

Following reconstruction with the free TRAM flap or with the gluteus maximus flap the anterior chest wound is dressed with a nonadherent gauze (or antibiotic ointment) and light dressing. A portion of the skin island remains exposed to enable regular monitoring of the flap circulation for the first few days postoperatively. The patient is transferred from the operating table to a hospital bed with an Egg-Crate mattress while she is maintained in a semisitting position for gravity-assisted venous drainage. In the recovery room, warmed intravenous fluids and humidified oxygen are administered and the patient is kept warm.

Close monitoring of the flap's circulation begins in the recovery room. During the first few postoperative hours the flap will appear pale and will feel cool. Its temperature and color should improve gradually. If a flap that seemed adequately perfused in the operating room later becomes mottled, the patient's shoulders should be elevated further to assist venous drainage. The blood volume and the room temperature also can be increased. If these steps do not improve the flap's circulation, the patient is returned to the operating room for reexploration. When a flap that was initially well perfused subsequently develops signs of vascular compromise, the cause of the problem must be identified and corrected promptly.

Perfusion of a free flap can be monitored in several ways, including taking the patient's temperature, Doppler probe assessment, intravenous administration of fluorescein, and evaluation of capillary refill in the skin island. Loss of capillary refill or increasing venous congestion indicates vascular compromise. If vascular thrombosis develops, it must be detected within 2 or 3 hours, and corrective action must be taken, or the flap may be lost.

The patient is kept warm and well hydrated and is maintained in a semisitting position for approximately 1 week except when ambulating. Arm movement on the side of the anastomoses is restricted, and any pressure on the anastomosed vessels is avoided for 7 to 10 days. The patient should not lie on the side of the reconstruction, and care givers should not attempt to lift the patient by her arm.

Although heparin and dextran are not routinely used, one or two aspirins a day may prevent vascular thrombosis. The bladder drainage catheter can be removed and ambulation can begin on the first or second postoperative day. The antiembolism stockings can be removed at this time also. Oral intake is resumed on the first postoperative day, and intravenous fluids are discontinued. Chest and donor site drains are removed by the fifth or sixth day as the fluid accumulation from each drain decreases to 30 ml per 24 hours. The patient may shower once the drains are removed and gently pat dry the reconstructed breast. Usually between the seventh and tenth day the patient can be discharged from the hospital.

Upon discharge the patient must be clearly informed of restrictions. Smoking and exposure to passive smoke are forbidden for 8 weeks. Heating pads, hot water bottles, or ice packs near the new breast mound should not be used; however, a warmed towel is permitted if it relieves discomfort. Driving and the performance of light household duties are not allowed for 3 weeks. Any breast manipulation or constriction is prohibited for 6 weeks.

23

Nipple-Areolar Reconstruction

Introduction

As techniques for breast reconstruction have improved, procedures that render excellent cosmetic results for nipple-areolar reconstruction have been introduced. The reconstructed nipple-areolar complex converts the flesh mound into a natural-appearing breast and creates symmetry with the contralateral nipple-areolar complex. This symmetry is achieved by duplicating the size, color, and position of the areola and by the equal projection of the nipple with that of the existing structures in the opposite breast. Generally the nipple is reconstructed first, and the areolar reconstruction follows as a single staged operation.

The most difficult problem in nipple reconstruction is maintenance of long-term projection. An adequate nipple reconstruction often loses projection during the first postoperative year. A number of techniques, including free composite grafts or local flaps, have been developed to maintain long-term nipple projection. Free composite grafts are harvested most often from the opposite nipple-areolar complex and have variable rates of success. The major disadvantages of these grafts are scarring and the loss of projection of the donor nipple. However, several alternate harvest sites have been used, such as an earlobe, a toe, or the labia minora. The earlobe has often been used to reconstruct the nipple in individuals who do not have a donor nipple or who do not wish to have the remaining nipple used. The donor site in the earlobe usually heals imperceptibly. However, the skin color of this composite graft generally is lighter than the surrounding areola, and projection is often inadequate after the graft heals.

The skate flap offers the most uniformly reliable outcome for maintenance of long-term nipple projection. The flap's name comes from its design on the reconstructed breast mound, which resembles the skate (stingray) fish.

The three methods used for areolar reconstruction are nipple-areolar complex banking, free skin grafting, and tattooing. Nipple-areolar complex banking in the groin at the time of mastectomy is no longer practiced for several reasons. Most important, tumor spread to the groin lymph nodes from the transplanted nipple-areolar complex has been reported even though frozen section of the undersurface of the graft had been negative for malignant cells at the time of mastectomy. In addition, during the double transfer of the nipple-areolar complex from the breast to the groin and back to the breast, loss of pigmentation and nipple projection often occurred. Finally, improvements in other reconstructive techniques now provide more uniform and reproducible results than nipple-areolar complex banking.

Creation of the areola by free skin grafting is the procedure of choice for most surgeons. With present techniques a graft can be obtained from any convenient location, including the upper inner thigh, the opposite areola, or the postauricular region. Most surgeons prefer to take the graft from the lower abdomen or the upper inner thigh just beneath the pubic hairline. A skin graft from either of these areas typically develops a natural-appearing pigmentation as it matures, and the easily concealed donor site heals inconspicuously. The graft's pigmentation can be enhanced with ultraviolet light in the first several months postoperatively or with tattooing at a later date if desired. In selected cases a contralateral areola of sufficient size (at least 5 cm in diameter) can provide ideally pigmented skin for the new areola. This techniqe generally is used only for patients undergoing mastopexy or reduction mammoplasty of the contralateral breast to establish symmetry after reconstruction. The advantage to areolar sharing is that it produces a graft with perfect color and texture match. With this technique an areolar graft is harvested from the peripheral edge of the contralateral areola. It is important to harvest the areola graft in a concentric ring because a spiral donor site produces a conspicuous scar. From an areola 5 cm in diameter a 3- to 5-cm areola can be harvested leaving a donor areola of the same size. This sharing procedure has a minor drawback; it produces a radial scar at the seam where the graft is sutured after being wrapped concentrically around the reconstructed nipple. Fortunately any conspicuous scarring on the areola can be camouflaged by tattooing. Occasionally the use of postauricular tissue can produce an excellent color match for light-skinned or red-headed individuals who have light pink areolae. Bilateral donor sites are needed to obtain enough tissue; however, the bilateral harvesting ensures that both ears will be set back symmetrically. An elliptical incision is made around the crease of the ear to harvest the tissue, and the resultant scar is inconspicuous. Also the labia minora has been used for areolar reconstruction; however, the tissue generally is too deeply pigmented after it heals to provide a satisfactory match for the contralateral areola. Tattooing has an established place in nipple-areolar reconstruction, particularly to increase the pigmentation of a nipple reconstructed with a local flap. Usually it is performed as an outpatient procedure under local anesthesia 2 to 3 months after nipple-areolar reconstruction with a full-thickness skin graft. Tattooing can be used to create an entire areola at the time of nipple reconstruction if the reconstruction has not included an areolar graft. However, the uniform coloration that typically is produced by tattooing alone can give an unnatural appearance.

Immediate nipple-areolar reconstruction at the time of breast mound creation occasionally may be indicated; however, a multistage approach generally is preferred. After a breast mound is created, the second stage of reconstruction typically involves minor adjustments on the reconstructed breast and if necessary modifications to the contralateral breast to establish symmetry. The nipple-areolar reconstruction is the third and final stage.

To achieve symmetry the reconstruction of the nipple-areolar complex should be delayed until the breast mound has settled into a stable shape. This stability usually occurs within 4 months of surgery. Also if a modification, such as mastopexy, augmentation, or reduction, has been performed on the opposite breast as a second-stage procedure, a similar length of time should elapse to allow the contralateral breast to obtain its final position before the nipple-areolar complex is reconstructed. If the nipple-areolar complex is created prematurely or is created before the opposite breast has been balanced, it may be malpositioned and lack symmetry.

Indications

Nipple-areolar reconstruction is indicated in women who are undergoing breast reconstruction and want to have a complete and natural-appearing result. Nipple-areolar reconstruction is also useful in women who have lost all or part of the nipple-areolar complex following partial mastectomy because of a complication of reduction mammoplasty or because of a congenital breast deformity, such as Poland's syndrome. In addition, when the nipple-areolar complex is distorted following a biopsy or a subcutaneous mastectomy, excision of the distorted nipple-areolar complex and reconstruction often produce an improved cosmetic result.

Contraindications

Prior radiation to the native breast or the reconstructed breast produces a relative ischemia and decreased tissue elasticity, which increase the risk of flap necrosis and graft failure after nipple-areolar reconstruction. Tobacco smoking is a relative contraindication, and patients with this risk factor must be approached with caution if surgery is to be undertaken.

Complications

Esthetic complications associated with nipple-areolar reconstruction include a malpositioned complex, incorrect areolar size, inadequate nipple projection, and a poor color match of the nipple to the areola or to the contralateral nipple-areolar complex. Malpositioning of the nipple-areolar complex is the most serious complication and generally requires surgical revision, with the attendant additional scarring, for correction. An areola that is too small can be treated with overgrafting or tattooing. In contrast revision of an overly large areola is more problematic and usually requires excision of the excess areolar tissue around the periphery with the creation of a new margin. To a large extent this complication can be avoided by anticipation of residual spreading of the areola, which frequently occurs postoperatively. Inadequate projection of the nipple must be corrected surgically. Other minor complications relate primarily to the donor site scar and include pain and hypertrophic scarring.

Preoperative Preparation

Nipple-areolar reconstruction often can be done with the patient under local anesthesia as an outpatient procedure. Local anesthesia suffices when this reconstruction is combined with other minor procedures, such as scar revision or removal of a tissue expander fill port. General anesthesia is used if the patient prefers it or if the nipple-areolar reconstruction is performed simultaneously with a more extensive procedure.

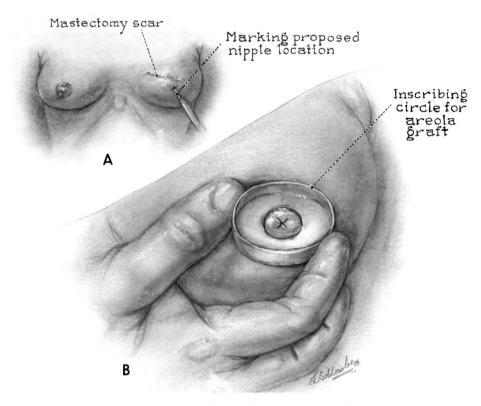

Mastectomy scar

Marking proposed nipple location

Inscribing circle for areola graft

A

B

Fig 23-1. Nipple-areolar position marking.

OPERATIVE PROCEDURE
Nipple-Areolar Position Marking (Figure 23-1)

The location of the nipple-areolar complex is designed with the patient awake and sitting in an upright position (Figure 23-1, *A*). Ideally the complex is constructed on the summit of the breast mound; however, positional similarity with the contralateral nipple-areolar complex is so essential that it takes precedence over other considerations. The best esthetic position is determined by the examiner's eye rather than by direct measurements. The surgeon first should locate the nipple-areolar complex in a freehand manner. Several direct measurements then can be made bilaterally to check distances from the nipple to the suprasternal notch, to the midline of the sternum, and to the midclavicular line. Final nipple-areolar positioning is estimated best with the surgeon standing several steps from the sitting patient to assess the symmetry. The patient may look in a mirror to see if the location appears appropriate. The marked position should be viewed from above because this is how the patient will most often view the complex. Slight deviation of the nipple-areolar complex laterally, inferiorly, or both is more acceptable than deviation medially or superiorly.

As shown in Figure 23-1, *B*, a cookie cutter can be used to inscribe a circle around the nipple to demarcate the planned areola.

Following marking of the nipple-areolar position the patient is placed in a supine position. The skin is cleansed and draped to fully expose the natural breast and the reconstructed mound. Planned donor sites for tissue grafts are similarly prepared.
(Four different techniques for nipple reconstruction are presented and labeled 1 to 4)

Nipple Reconstruction 1
Nipple-Sharing by Donor Nipple Transection (Figure 23-2)

When the nipple height is greater than its diameter, the terminal one half of the nipple can be transected transversely and transferred as a free composite graft to the reconstructed breast. As shown in Figure 23-2, *A*, the distal one half of the nipple is amputated through a transverse incision. The height of the amputated part should not exceed 5 mm; if the height is greater, the graft should be thinned. The graft then is sutured in place at the de-epithelialized recipient site. Hemostasis at the recipient site must be meticulous. The graft is secured with interrupted absorbable sutures. The donor site can be allowed to heal by secondary intention, as shown in Figure 23-2, *B*. Alternatively it can be closed primarily with a running absorbable suture. The donor site is dressed with a light, nonadherent gauze dressing. The reconstructed nipple is covered appropriately after areolar reconstruction has been completed.

Nipple Reconstruction 2
Nipple-Sharing by Donor Nipple Bisection (Figure 23-3)

When the nipple diameter is greater than its height, a graft is obtained by bisection of the nipple. As shown in Figure 23-3, *A* and *B*, an initial incision bisects the nipple through its center. A second incision connects the ends of the first incision across the inferior base of the nipple. Half of the nipple is excised, as shown in Figure 23-3, *C*. After hemostasis is achieved, the donor site is closed primarily with a running absorbable suture, as shown in Figure 23-3, *D*. The harvested graft is thinned if necessary to a maximal height of 5 mm. The graft then is transferred to the reconstructed breast mound after the recipient site is deepithelialized. The graft is sutured in place with interrupted absorbable sutures. The donor site is dressed with a light, nonadherent gauze dressing. The reconstructed nipple is covered appropriately after areolar reconstruction has been completed.

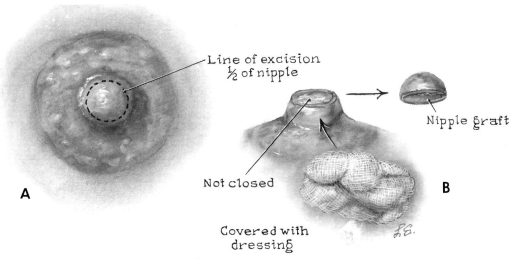

Fig 23-2.   Nipple sharing by donor nipple transection.

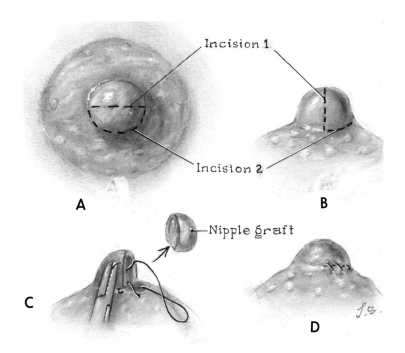

Fig 23-3.   Nipple sharing by donor nipple bisection.

Nipple Reconstruction 3
Graft Harvest from the Earlobe for Nipple Reconstruction
(Figure 23-4)

Figure 23-4 shows the technique for harvesting a composite graft from the earlobe. The graft can be harvested from any portion of the earlobe. The exact location is determined by identification of an area that will give a rounded graft corresponding closely in size and projection to the existing nipple. As illustrated in Figure 23-4, *A*, the graft is outlined as a wedge on the earlobe. The graft is harvested through full-thickness incisions as illustrated. After the graft has been excised, it can be recontoured by excision of the apex of the wedge, as shown by the dotted line in Figure 23-4, *B*. The maximum thickness of the graft after recontouring should not exceed 5 mm. As shown in Figure 23-4, *C*, the defect in the ear is closed with a single layer of interrupted sutures. The incisions should be designed to ensure that the two sides are equal in length to prevent the development of standing cones. The nipple graft is sutured in place on the breast mound with interrupted absorbable sutures after the recipient site has been deepithelialized. A light, nonadherent gauze dressing is placed around the donor site. The reconstructed nipple is covered appropriately after areolar reconstruction has been completed.

Nipple Reconstruction 4
Nipple Reconstruction with a Skate Flap (Figure 23-5)

The skate flap is marked as illustrated in Figure 23-5, *A*, after a circle to demarcate the areola has been inscribed around the planned nipple location. In this figure the body of the flap is stippled, and the wings are crosshatched. The circle *a* is centered 1 to 2 mm higher than the center of the demarcated areola because the nipple position will shift during closure. This will ensure that the reconstructed nipple will be appropriately centered in the areola. A tear-shaped ellipse, *b*, is extended from the lateral margins of the circle *a* to a point at the base of the areolar circle. This tear-shaped ellipse subsequently will be elevated as part of the body of the skate flap, incorporating dermis and subcutaneous fat to add bulk and to ensure projection of the nipple. Next, a transverse superior line, marked *c*, is drawn tangent to the upper border of the circle *a*, and a transverse inferior line, marked *d*, is drawn tangent to the lower border of the circle *a* to establish the upper and lower borders of the wings of the skate flap. The skate flap marking, as oriented in these illustrations, presumes that no scar traverses the flap site. Should a scar cross the site, the orientation of the flap would need to be rotated to ensure that the blood supply to the reconstructed nipple is not compromised. The direction in which the blood supply will enter the final reconstructed nipple is indicated by the vertical arrow in Figure 23-5, *B*.

As shown in Figure 23-5, *B*, the crescent-shaped superior and inferior portions of the areolar circle are deepithelialized and the excised tissue is discarded. The wings of the skate flap, lying between the two transverse lines and lateral to circle *a*, are elevated as full-thickness skin grafts; the wings begin peripherally and end at the lateral border of the body of the skate, as

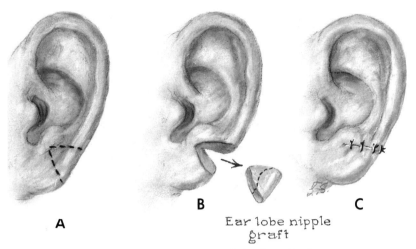

Ear lobe nipple
graft

Fig 23-4.   Graft harvest from the earlobe for nipple reconstruction.

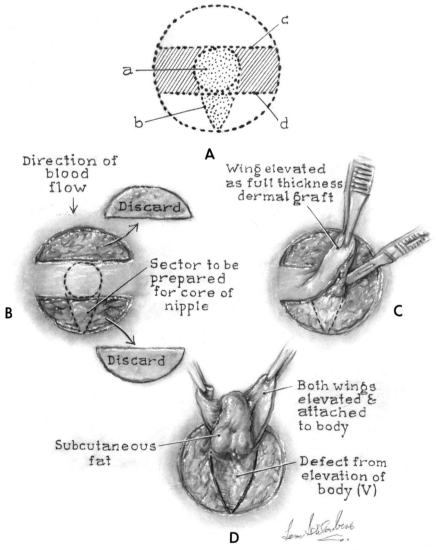

Fig 23-5.   Nipple reconstruction with a skate flap.

shown in Figure 23-5, *C*. The body of the skate includes the skin and subcutaneous tissue in circle *a* and the adipose tissue within the teardrop outline.

After both wings have been elevated, as shown in Figure 23-5, *D*, the body of the skate flap is raised. Incisions are made through the subcutaneous fat corresponding to the outlined V. These incisions must be made carefully if a prosthesis is in a subcutaneous location because the prosthesis can be perforated inadvertently. The subcutaneous tissue underlying the circle *a* is elevated in continuity with the subcutaneous tissue in the teardrop *b*. Sufficient subcutaneous fat is included with the body of the skate to provide a nipple of appropriate size. Extra tissue initially raised can be excised if the resultant nipple is too bulky. After the skin and subcutaneous fat that constitute the body of the skate flap are fully elevated, a defect will be left in the dermis at the site of the teardrop *b*.

Completion of Skate Flap Reconstruction (Figure 23-6)

As illustrated in Figure 23-6, *A*, the defect in the dermis is closed with interrupted absorbable sutures placed at the base of the new nipple. As shown in Figure 23-6, *B*, as the apex of the teardrop *b* is elevated by a forceps, the wings of the skate flap then are brought around the body of the skate inferiorly. The wings are anchored together at the base of the nipple to the areola. A running absorbable suture is used to join the edges of the wings together around the body of the nipple.

Closure of the defect resulting from elevation of the skate flap distorts the original circle that inscribed the areola. A new circle is marked by centering a cookie cutter on the reconstructed nipple, as illustrated in Figure 23-6, *C*. As shown in Figure 23-6, *D*, the areas between the original areola and the new inscription then are deepithelialized in preparation for application of a full-thickness skin graft to reconstruct the areola.

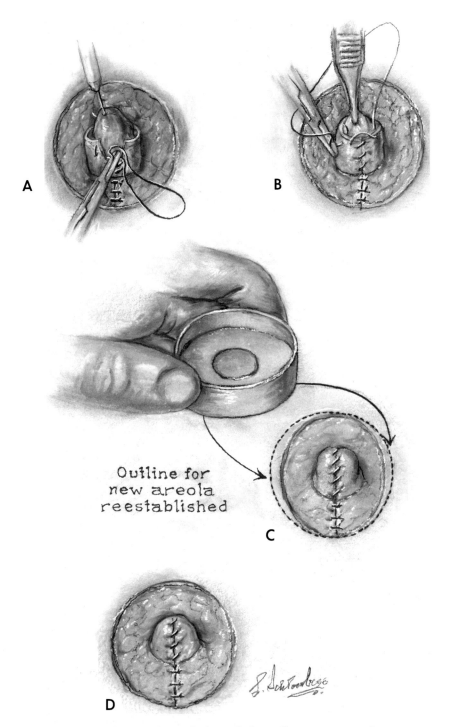

Outline for
new areola
reestablished

Fig 23-6.   Completion of skate flap reconstruction.

Areolar Reconstruction 1: Free Skin Grafting
Harvesting of the Upper Inner Thigh Skin Graft for Areolar Reconstruction (Figure 23-7)

As shown in Figure 23-7, *A*, the patient is placed in a frog-leg position and the pubic hairline is demarcated. The skin is cleansed, draped, and anesthetized locally for an upper inner thigh graft harvest. While an assistant stretches the skin taut, the surgeon inscribes a circular graft with a cookie cutter. The center of this areolar graft outline is marked with an *x* for a subsequent incision to serve as the opening for the reconstructed nipple. An ellipse is outlined around the circle to facilitate closure, and the circle is scored with a scalpel. Once the recipient site is prepared, the entire ellipse is harvested by sharp dissection as a full-thickness skin graft. The portions of skin beyond the inscribed circle are discarded, and the circular graft is defatted. When the graft has been harvested, the elliptical upper inner thigh wound is closed primarily with a running subcuticular suture or with interrupted skin sutures.

Then, as shown in Figure 23-7, *B*, the graft is positioned on the de-epithelialized areolar bed. Approximately eight interrupted sutures are placed around the periphery of the areola to attach it to the breast mound skin. The sutures are left long enough to be tied over a stent. The space beneath the graft is irrigated with saline solution to flush all blood clots. Finally a running fine chromic suture is placed around the areola periphery to secure the graft in position on the breast mound. The x mark demarcating the center of the graft is incised, and the nipple is brought out through the hole which has been created.

As shown in Figure 23-7, *C*, the surgical site is dressed with a tie-over bolster dressing of lubricated gauze covered with cotton soaked in saline solution.

Areolar Reconstruction II: Areolar Sharing
Graft Harvesting and Areolar Reconstruction (Figure 23-8)

The harvesting procedure is shown on the patient's left side. While the areola is flattened and stretched, a circle centered about the nipple is inscribed on the areola using a cookie cutter. The marked circle is incised circumferentially to the plane between the areola and the underlying gland. A second incision then is made circumferentially around the perimeter of the areola. A third incision connects the two circular incisions. The band of areolar tissue lying between the two circular incisions is harvested in the plane between the areola and the underlying gland. This strip of areolar tissue, usually 1 cm or more in width is defatted and placed in a moist sponge for areolar reconstruction on the reconstructed breast mound. Repair of the areolar defect resulting from this tissue harvesting is incorporated into the planned reduction mammoplasty or mastopexy.

Nipple reconstruction on the reconstructed breast can be performed by any of the techniques illustrated in this chapter. Following the nipple reconstruction, a cookie cutter is used to inscribe a circle around the reconstructed nipple, as shown on the patient's right side in this figure. The inside of the circle is deepithelialized, and the graft harvested from the opposite areola is

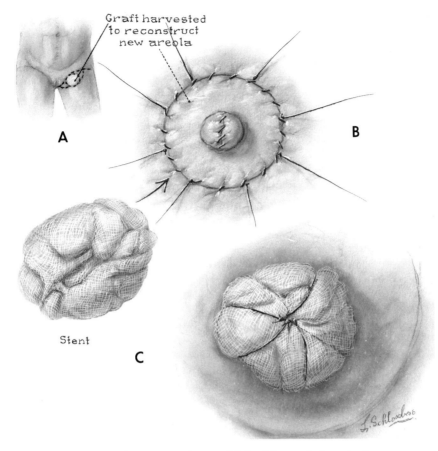

Fig 23-7. Harvesting of an upper inner thigh skin graft for areolar reconstruction.

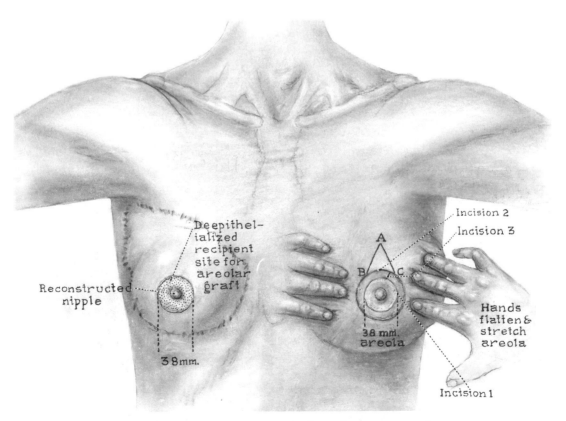

Fig 23-8. Graft harvesting and areolar reconstruction.

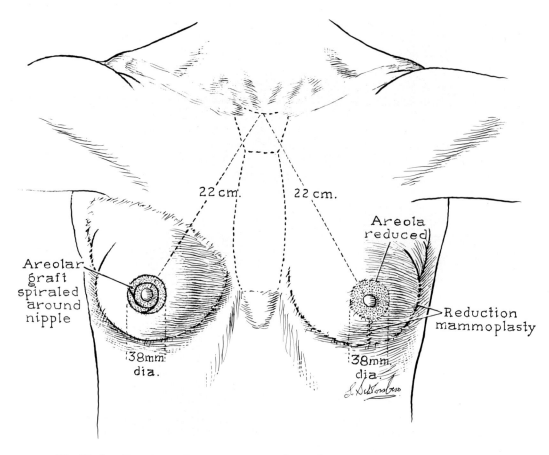

Fig 23-9. Postoperative appearance of areolar reconstruction with areolar sharing (and concurrent reduction mammoplasty).

spiraled over the deepithelialized area. The graft is sutured in place with eight interrupted sutures spaced evenly about the perimeter. The sutures are left long enough to tie over a stent for immobilization. A fine, running chromic suture then is placed around the perimeter to secure the graft in position. A stent of nonadherent gauze and moist cotton balls is placed over the reconstructed complex and held in place by the long sutures tied over it.

Postoperative Appearance of Areolar Reconstruction with Areolar Sharing (and Concurrent Reduction Mammoplasty) (Figure 23-9)

As shown here, areolae of equal diameter can be created by this procedure. A symmetrical appearance is achieved with appropriately positioned areolae of the same color and texture.

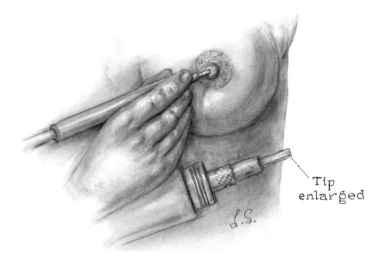

Fig 23-10. Nipple areolar tattooing.

Nipple-Areolar Tattooing (Figure 23-10)

A multineedle tattoo device is used to introduce the pigment into the nipple and into the areola. Tattoo equipment includes a color chart with guidelines for mixing the white and the colored pigments to achieve a good match with the opposite nipple and areola. For most patients a color slightly darker than the one desired should be chosen because the pigment tends to lighten over time. After a satisfactory color is selected, the pigment is mixed and the area prepared and draped in a sterile manner. A small amount of pigment is placed on the area to be tattooed, and the tattoo needle is moved in a crosshatching pattern across the area until sufficient pigment is introduced to attain the desired color. The pigment is extended and feathered slightly beyond the periphery of the reconstructed areola to camouflage the scar. The nipple, which may be mobile and therefore more difficult to tattoo than the areola, is frequently colored a darker shade to make it stand out. After tattooing is completed, the area is dressed with an antibiotic ointment and a sterile dressing is applied.

Postoperative Care

Following nipple-areolar reconstruction the dressing is left on the reconstructed nipple-areolar complex for 5 to 7 days. The donor site dressing can be removed after 2 days. The patient may resume normal activities within 1 to 2 days. When tattooing alone has been done, the dressing can be removed in 1 to 2 days and antibiotic ointment is applied daily until the tattooed skin is fully healed.

24

Treatment of a Radiation Ulcer

Introduction

Radiation-induced chest wall ulceration occurred most often in the past when radiation therapy was a common adjuvant treatment following radical resection for breast carcinoma. Such a regimen of radiation therapy is rarely used today. However, when it is administered, the improved delivery techniques are rarely associated with skin complications. Nevertheless, chest wall wounds sometimes develop following radiation therapy, and they can be difficult to manage.

Patients with chest wall radiation ulcers are often debilitated or are suffering from multiple medical problems. The surgeon must decide the most appropriate means of wound closure.

There are three major steps in the successful treatment of radiation ulcers of the chest wall: (1) adequate debridement of the involved skin and underlying soft tissue; (2) assessment of the bony thorax and resection if necessary with reconstruction that ensures normal pulmonary dynamics; and (3) closure of the wound with a vascularized muscle or myocutaneous flap.

Necrotic tissue must be excised completely from the ulcer, and the wound must be thoroughly cleaned. In severely contaminated wounds, serial debridement may be required. A portion of the chest wall may need to be resected because radiation damage can also involve the bony thorax and the underlying pulmonary parenchyma. Extensive resection of the rib cage may result in a significant physiologic deficit. The patient's preoperative pulmonary status and the amount of tissue resected during wound debridement must be considered, and synthetic material or a bone graft may be needed to provide chest wall support before wound coverage.

The preferred technique for covering radiation ulcers is to transpose muscle flaps with their blood supply. When local muscle flaps are not available, free tissue grafts can be transferred; however, the microvascular anastomosis should be performed in an area remote from the irradiated field if possible. On occasion the only option available is to transfer tissue in which the intrinsic vessels have been previously irradiated. In this setting the risk of vascular thrombosis is increased.

On the anterior surface of the body, muscle flaps can be harvested at several sites to close radiation ulcers of the chest wall. The size and location of the radiation ulcer, the availability of tissue, and the site of prior surgical procedures in the chest area determine which flap is most appropriate to use.

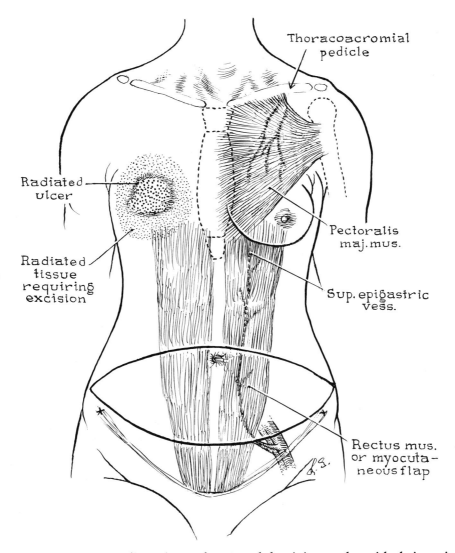

Fig 24-1. **A, Pectoralis major and rectus abdominis muscles with their major vascular supplies.**
Continued.

The pectoralis major muscle and the rectus abdominis muscles with their major vascular supplies are illustrated in Figure 24-1, *A*. The rectus abdominis can yield a vertical or a transverse flap. Because of its abundant vascular supply the pectoralis major muscle is an excellent flap for reconstruction defects caused by radiation damage. The thoracoacromial vessels (as shown here) are most often used for transposition. Other vessels, including the highest thoracic vessels, also supply the pectoralis major muscle; however, these vessels generally are not used for flap transposition. When surrounding chest and shoulder girdle muscles are present, no important loss of function results from transposition of the pectoralis major. However, when this flap is used, the ribs are visible, and this results in a significant cosmetic defect. If the lateral margin of the muscle is left intact between the chest wall and the humerus, the contour of the anterior axillary fold will be preserved and the cosmetic deformity will be diminished. The surgeon can gain access to the debrided ulcer site without repositioning the patient by using a flap based on the contralateral pectoralis major muscle or on the

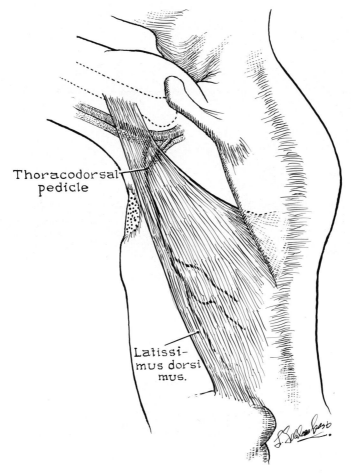

Thoracodorsal pedicle

Latissimus dorsi mus.

Fig 24-1. B, Latissimus dorsi muscle with its major vascular supply.

contralateral rectus abdominis muscle. The disadvantage of the pectoralis major flap and the vertical rectus abdominis flap relates to their size. These flaps cover only a small area of the chest (less than 10 cm). The transverse rectus abdominis muscle (TRAM) flap is large enough to cover most wounds. However, it is composed primarily of skin and subcutaneous fat and therefore is not as efficient as muscle in suppressing bacterial colonization. The TRAM flap also adds substantial bulk in obese individuals.

On the posterior surface of the body, the latissimus dorsi muscle, shown with its blood supply in Figure 24-1, B, yields a flap that frequently is used for coverage of an ipsilateral radiation ulcer.

The ipsilateral latissimus dorsi has none of the disadvantages attributed to the TRAM flap. The ipsilateral latissimus dorsi flap is used most often for closing large radiation ulcers on the anterior chest wall because it provides a large muscle mass, has a reliable vascular pedicle, and is easily rotated onto the thorax. Repositioning the patient to elevate, transpose, and inset the flap is the primary disadvantage of the ipsilateral latissimus dorsi. The omentum may be used as a flap for closure of a radiation ulcer; however, it is rarely used today because of the risk of intraabdominal infection or other complications.

The pectoralis major muscle flap used for closure of a radiation ulcer is discussed in detail in this chapter. The latissimus dorsi flap and the TRAM flap are briefly illustrated. (For full descriptions of the latissimus dorsi flap and TRAM flap procedures, see Chapters 20 and 21.)

Indications

Radiation ulcers that do not heal after 4 to 6 weeks of local wound care should be debrided and closed. Additional indications for closure include pain, foul odor, and the patient's inability to care for the wound.

Contraindications

Superficial ulcerations may develop during radiation therapy or soon after. The ulcerations often heal primarily with local wound care, and the surgeon should allow adequate time for healing. Terminally ill or severely debilitated individuals, who are unable to tolerate general anesthesia and a major surgical procedure, are not candidates for reconstruction.

Complications

The most common complication following closure of a radiation ulcer defect is necrosis of part or all of the tissue flap used to cover the defect. When a small portion of a flap is lost, the wound will usually close spontaneously. More extensive flap loss may require reoperation and coverage with additional flaps. It is preferable to use multiple flaps to gain complete closure of a large ulcer rather than to attempt coverage with a single, large flap. Although radiation wounds are heavily contaminated with bacteria, infection is rare, unless debridement is inadequate or unless a portion of the flap undergoes necrosis. Infection is less likely with a well-vascularized flap than it is with a poorly vascularized one.

Preoperative Preparation

Before surgical closure of the radiation ulcer the operative note describing the previous mastectomy and the protocol for the radiation treatment should be reviewed. If the pectoralis major muscle, the rectus abdominis muscle, or the latissimus dorsi muscle were included in the field of radiation, they might become atrophied or fibrotic and therefore unsuitable for transposition. Furthermore, interruption of the neural or vascular supply during mastectomy may have resulted in atrophy of a given muscle. Aerobic and anerobic wound cultures are obtained. If the patient's nutritional status is abnormal, total parenteral nutrition may be required to restore a positive nitrogen balance. Iron supplementation or even blood transfusion is indicated if the patient is anemic.

OPERATIVE PROCEDURE

Pectoralis Major Flap Coverage of a Radiation Ulcer

Pectoralis Major Flap Incision (Figure 24-2)

The patient is placed in the supine position. The skin is prepared and draped as a sterile field, and general anesthesia is induced. If necessary the radiation ulcer is debrided further before flap transposition. As illustrated a diagonally oriented skin incision is made *(dashed line)* extending from the acromion to the xiphoid process. This incision provides optimal exposure for skin and subcutaneous tissue detachment from the pectoralis major and for muscle elevation on a thoracoacromial pedicle. This incision will cause some distortion of the overlying breast, but this is of little consequence considering the cosmetic defect for which the muscle flap is used.

Path of Division of the Pectoralis Major Flap (Figure 24-3)

After the skin incision is made, the pectoralis major muscle is isolated circumferentially with its attached vascular pedicle. The skin and subcutaneous tissues are dissected off the muscle fascia to the midline of the sternum medially, to the clavicle superiorly, to the border of the pectoralis major laterally, and to the shoulder superiorly and laterally. The fascia at the lateral border of the pectoralis major then is incised. In this figure the arrows denote the path of the incision as the pectoralis major flap is developed. Because the pectoralis major muscle is so well vascularized, dissection should be done cautiously with meticulous hemostasis. As the muscle is elevated, the pectoral fascia should be preserved because it provides substantive tissue for suture placement when the flap is attached to the chest wall. Detachment of the muscle's origin begins at the lateral and inferior border of the pectoralis major. The muscle is raised medially and is detached from the ribs and the sternum. As the perforating vessels from the internal mammary artery are encountered near the sternum, they are ligated and divided. Mobilization progresses superiorly where the muscle is detached from the clavicle and proceeds from the most medial attachments laterally. During this portion of the procedure care must be taken not to injure the thoracoacromial pedicle supplying the muscle flap.

When the muscle is elevated almost completely, the thoracoacromial pedicle is visible on its underside. When the vascular pedicle is carefully isolated, the muscle fibers can be detached from the clavicle without injuring the vessels or the medial and lateral pectoral nerves. The muscle then is divided lateral to the thoracoacromial pedicle, with care taken first to identify and to protect the axillary and cephalic veins (not shown) that lie near the muscle's insertion on the humerus. In most instances the lateral portion of the pectoralis major and its insertion are not needed for closure of radiation ulcers, and a strip of muscle about 3 cm wide can be left attached to the chest wall. This strip of muscle will preserve the anterior axillary fold as the lateral border of the muscle is divided.

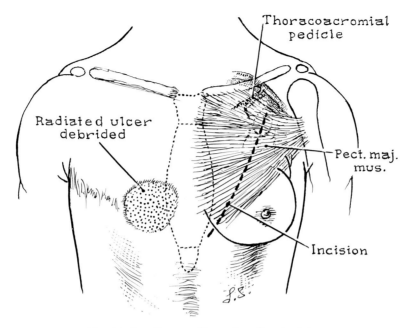

Fig 24-2.   Pectoralis major flap incision.

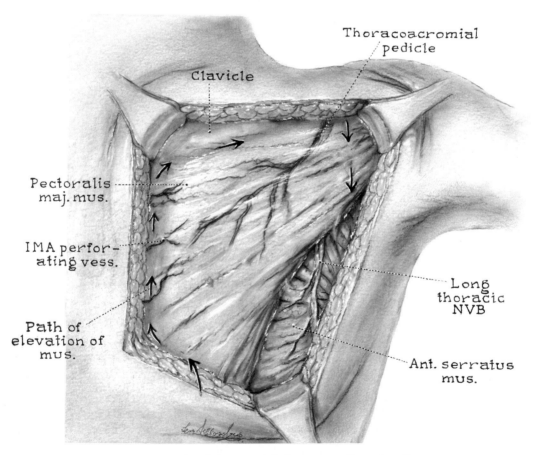

Fig 24-3.   Path of division of the pectoralis major flap.

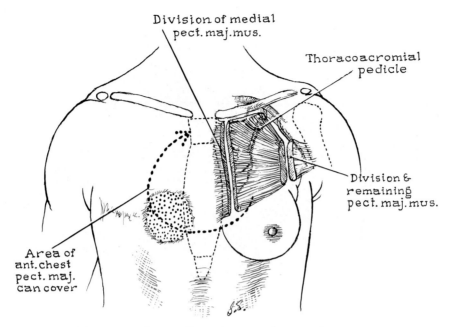

Fig 24-4. Pectoralis major muscle arc of rotation.

Pectoralis Major Muscle Arc of Rotation (Figure 24-4)

The points of division in the pectoralis major muscle are shown. Within the arc of rotation *(dashed line)* the pectoralis major muscle can cover defects over the upper sternum and for approximately 5 cm beyond the border of the sternum. It can also be rotated to reach the ipsilateral shoulder, axilla, and neck.

Fully Mobilized Pectoralis Major Flap (Figure 24-5)

When the muscle is fully mobilized, it is attached only by its vascular pedicle. The elevated muscle can be rotated out of the field of dissection. The edge of the lateral remnant of the pectoralis major and its tendon can be sutured to the chest wall to preserve the anterior axillary fold.

Pectoralis Major Flap Transposition to the Radiation Ulcer Site (Figure 24-6)

With the pectoralis major muscle ready for transposition the skin and subcutaneous tissues are dissected from the sternum to create a tunnel between the donor and the recipient sites. The elevated muscle then is rotated medially, passed through the subcutaneous tissue tunnel between the skin and sternum, and transposed into the debrided radiation ulcer wound. The flap is manipulated gently to completely cover the chest wall defect. After the transposed muscle has been satisfactorily positioned, the pectoralis major muscle is inset by attaching it to the chest wall with a layer of interrupted absorbable sutures. After the flap is secured, the portion of the muscle in the subcutaneous tunnel is inspected carefully to ensure that it is not compressed or kinked. If necessary the tunnel may be enlarged or the skin bridge may be divided to adequately accommodate the muscle and the postoperative edema that may develop. A constant vacuum drain (not shown) then is placed beneath the flap and brought to the skin through a separate stab wound.

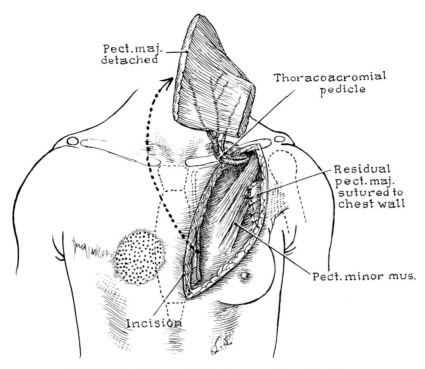

Fig 24-5.   Fully mobilized pectoralis major flap.

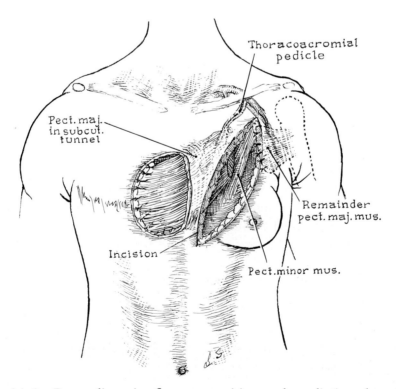

Fig 24-6.   Pectoralis major flap transposition to the radiation ulcer site.

Pectoralis Major Flap Skin Grafting (Figure 24-7)

The inset muscle is covered with a skin graft from an appropriate donor site. The preferable donor site is on the anterior surface so that the patient will not have to be repositioned during surgery and will not have to lie on the donor site during the postoperative period. The skin graft can be meshed 1 to 1½ and then sutured or stapled in place. The graft donor site is dressed with a nonadherent gauze and is covered by a sterile dressing. Finally the graft is immobilized with a bulky dressing.

Before closure of the pectoralis major donor site a constant vacuum drain (not shown) is inserted to minimize seroma formation. The drain is brought to the skin through a stab wound in the axilla. The muscle donor site is closed with a layer of absorbable subcutaneous sutures followed by skin staples. Finally the donor site is covered with a dressing of nonadherent gauze and tape.

Rectus Abdominis Flaps for Closure of Radiation Ulcers

Figures 24-8 and 24-9 depict the rectus abdominis flaps used for closure of a radiation ulcer. The reader is referred to Chapter 21 for a detailed description of the TRAM flap procedure.

Vertical Rectus Abdominis Flap (Figure 24-8)

The vertical rectus abdominis flap, which can be transposed with or without a skin island, is elevated through a vertically oriented incision extending the full length of the abdominal wall. When a rectus abdominis muscle flap is based on the superior epigastric vessels, its large arc of rotation allows it to be transposed into an area ranging from the jugular notch to about 5 cm from the apex of the contralateral axilla. Although ease of dissection and greater reliability make the pectoralis major muscle preferable for filling most chest wall defects, the pectoralis major muscle and the latissimus dorsi muscle cannot always be rotated to reach the area of the lower sternum or the central chest. To cover ulcers in these midline regions the rectus abdominis flap is usually the best option.

After muscle elevation and division the rectus abdominis usually can be transposed through a subcutaneous tunnel created between the abdominal wound and the chest wall. If the tunnel is too tight to accommodate easy passage of the muscle, a separate incision may be needed to connect the two wounds. Once the vertical rectus abdominis flap has been rotated into the chest and positioned to fill the debrided radiation ulcer, it is inset with a layer of interrupted absorbable sutures that anchor the muscle to the chest wall. The donor wound is drained and closed and the inset muscle flap is covered with a skin graft as described for the pectoralis major muscle flap procedure.

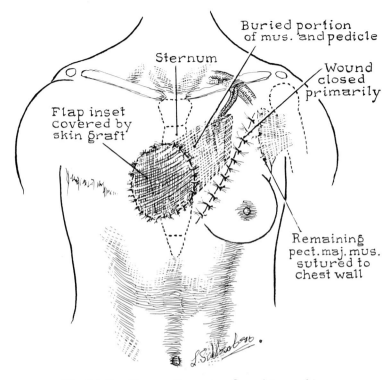

Fig 24-7. Pectoralis major flap skin grafting.

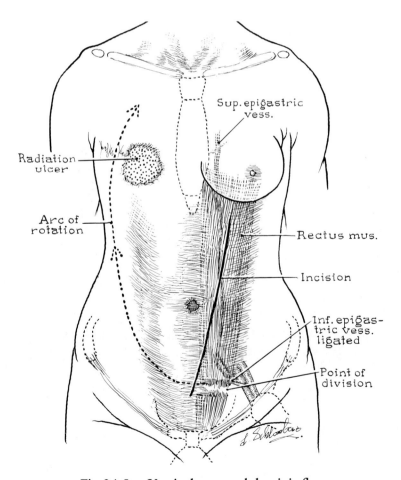

Fig 24-8. Vertical rectus abdominis flap.

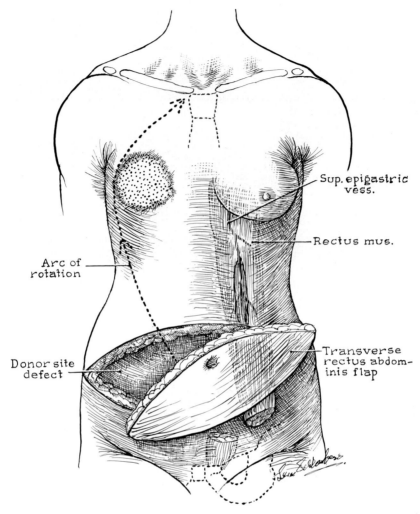

Fig 24-9. Transverse rectus abdominis muscle flap arc of rotation.

Transverse Rectus Abdominis Muscle Flap Arc of Rotation
(Figure 24-9)

A TRAM flap can be rotated to cover essentially any part of the anterior chest wall. When a standard TRAM flap is used to close a radiation ulcer, the flap should be based on the muscle contralateral to the chest wound. Because the TRAM flap includes a large skin island and a significant volume of subcutaneous tissue, it provides much more bulk and can cover a far greater area than the pectoralis major muscle flap or the vertical rectus abdominis muscle flap.

Development, elevation, and transposition of a TRAM flap based on the superior epigastric pedicle, as well as the abdominal closure, are the same for closure of a chest wall ulcer as for breast reconstruction (see Figures 21-6 through 21-19 for details). The large bulk of a TRAM flap permits breast reconstruction simultaneously with coverage of a radiation ulcer.

Latissimus Dorsi Flap for Closure of a Radiation Ulcer

(Figures 24-10 to 24-14 depict the latissimus dorsi flap used for closure of a radiation ulcer. Chapter 20 has a detailed description of the procedure.)

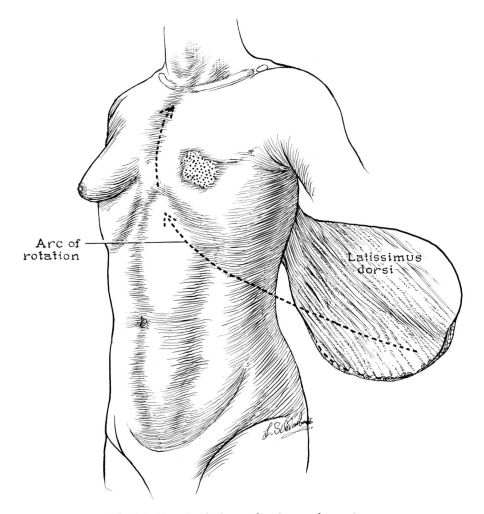

Fig 24-10. Latissimus dorsi arc of rotation.

Latissimus Dorsi Arc of Rotation (Figure 24-10)

The radiation ulcer is debrided while the patient is in the supine position. If no additional debridement is necessary and flap closure can be performed immediately, the patient is moved to a lateral position for elevation of the latissimus dorsi muscle. Specific details of patient positioning and flap elevation are given in the descriptions that accompany Figures 20-9 through 20-18. The guidelines for muscle elevation and rotation still apply when the latissimus is transposed without a skin island.

As shown in Figure 24-10 the latissimus dorsi flap can be rotated to cover almost all of the ipsilateral chest to the midline of the sternum. The flap is unreliable for coverage of the lower one third of the sternal region. In addition to coverage of the chest wall defect, the flap can be used to close ipsilateral axillary, shoulder, and neck wounds.

A latissimus dorsi flap almost always survives if the thoracodorsal vessels are intact and if the axillary area has not been heavily irradiated. During dissection of the latissimus dorsi care must be taken to identify the serratus anterior muscle to prevent its being inadvertently elevated with the latissimus dorsi. The thoracodorsal vessels and the long thoracic nerve lie close to the anterior border of the latissimus and must be protected during dissection.

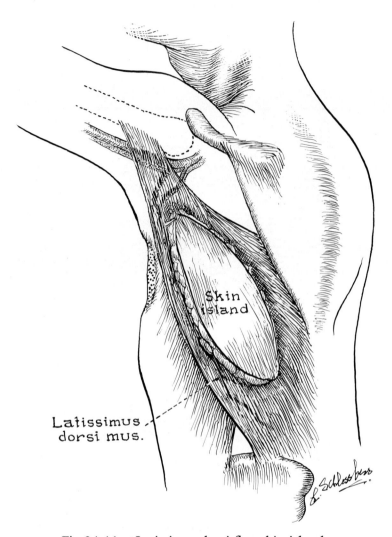

Fig 24-11.   Latissimus dorsi flap skin island.

The latissimus is completely detached from the teres major muscle before flap transposition to avoid formation of a bulge in the axilla.

Even when the donor site is drained, seroma formation is likely. Aside from this the donor site usually heals with minimal deformity, and there is little if any loss of function.

Latissimus Dorsi Flap Skin Island (Figure 24-11)

The location of the latissimus dorsi and its associated skin island most often used for wound coverage are shown. The maximum safe width of a latissimus skin island is 8 cm. Although a much larger skin island can be transposed, a skin graft would be required to close the donor site. We do not advocate skin grafts at this site for several reasons. This area of the back is highly mobile, and skin grafts heal poorly. Also a deep contour depression at the donor site may result following the creation of a large flap. The scar resulting from muscle transposition with a skin island is frequently painful. Rather than transfer a large skin island, the latissimus should be used only as a muscle flap, and it should be covered with a skin graft after it is inset on the chest, as described for the pectoralis major muscle flap coverage.

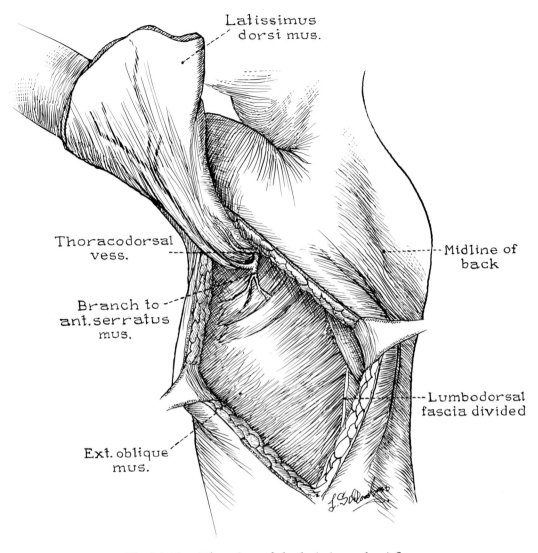

Fig 24-12. Elevation of the latissimus dorsi flap.

Elevation of the Latissimus Dorsi Flap (Figure 24-12)

The latissimus dorsi flap and its thoracodorsal vascular pedicle are shown. The vascular collateral branch to the serratus anterior is significant because if the thoracodorsal pedicle has been ligated or damaged by irradiation of the axilla, the flap can still be safely transposed on this serratus anterior branch. However, if the collateral branch is not needed, it is ligated and divided to increase the arc of rotation of the flap.

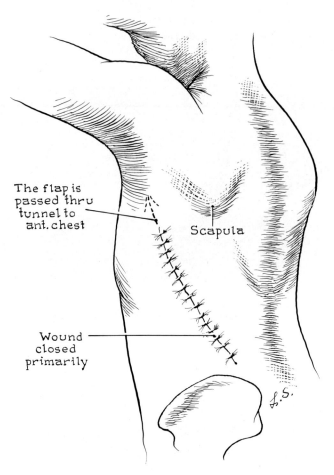

The flap is
passed thru
tunnel to
ant. chest

Scapula

Wound
closed
primarily

£.S.

Fig 24-13. Closure of the latissimus donor site.

Closure of the Latissimus Donor Site (Figure 24-13)

The latissimus dorsi flap is passed through a subcutaneous tunnel created between the back and the chest. When the flap is safely transposed to the chest wall, two 10-mm constant vacuum drains (not shown here) are inserted in the back wound and brought out near the axilla to reduce the risk of seroma formation. The donor site then is closed with a layer of interrupted sutures and followed by a layer of running subcuticular sutures.

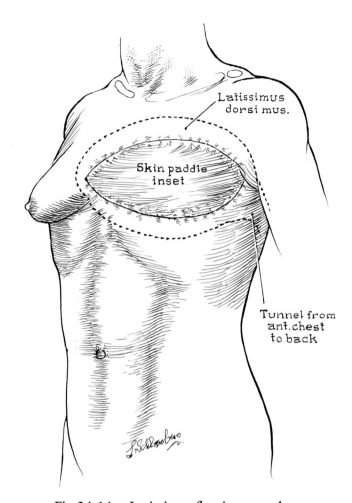

Fig 24-14.   Latissimus flap inset on chest.

Latissimus Flap Inset on the Chest (Figure 24-14)

When the flap has been transposed to the chest and the donor site is closed, the patient is again moved into a supine position. The latissimus muscle and skin then are manipulated to fill the debrided chest wall wound. The muscle is inspected in the subcutaneous tunnel to ensure that it is not kinked or compressed. If necessary the tunnel can be enlarged. The muscle is sutured to the chest wall with absorbable sutures. The skin island can be inset with absorbable subcuticular sutures or skin staples. Although staples should never be used for final insetting of a breast reconstructed with a flap, this is the most expeditious way of closing the skin in a radiation ulcer. In this context, cosmetic factors are less important than length of operative time.

Postoperative Care

Because patients with radiation ulcers may be very ill, sound postoperative care is critical. The patient's urinary output and pulmonary function should be monitored carefully. In addition, flap circulation must be observed closely to discover and promptly address any evidence of a hematoma or compromised circulation. The bulky dressing overlying the skin graft is left in place for 5 to 7 days, unless earlier removal is required to assess flap viability.

VI

COSMETIC PROCEDURES

The primary purpose of the operative procedures described in this section is to enhance or improve the appearance of the breasts. Although the operations described are typically performed bilaterally, they also are applicable for unilateral breast modification. Improved cosmetic results following breast reconstruction have resulted in increased patient expectations. Breast augmentation, reduction, or mastopexy contralateral to the mastectomy is now frequently performed to achieve symmetry and to improve the appearance of the breasts following reconstruction.

The recent controversy surrounding breast implants has resulted in a substantial decrease in bilateral augmentation mammoplasty for cosmetic purposes alone, although implants continue to be used widely for reconstruction following mastectomy. (The controversy surrounding breast implant safety is discussed in Chapter 26, "Augmentation Mammoplasty".) The final chapter in this section is devoted to a discussion of the operative treatment of gynecomastia, the most common breast disorder in males.

25

Reduction Mammoplasty

Introduction

The cause of breast hypertrophy (macromastia) is unknown; however, its development is associated with obesity and with a family history of large breasts. End organ hypersensitivity to estrogen may contribute to macromastia in thin women. Symptoms vary among individuals and are not solely dependent on the size of the breasts. Young women with markedly enlarged breasts generally have more psychological than physical discomfort and may not present with the typical symptoms of breast hypertrophy. In contrast older women are less tolerant of large breasts because they do not have the physical reserves to carry the extra weight. Generally they complain of shoulder grooving caused by the weight on brassiere straps, numbness in the ulnar nerve distribution, back and neck pain, constant fatigue, and stooped posture. When breast volume exceeds 800 g per breast, (moderate hypertrophy) the patient frequently complains of back and neck pain, intertrigo, fatigue, and general discomfort from the excess weight. When breast volume exceeds 1000 g per breast (marked hypertrophy), the patient will suffer additionally from signs of ulnar nerve compression including numbness and paresthesias. Poor posture develops among some large-breasted women, particularly teenagers, who stoop their shoulders to camouflage breast size.

Objective assessment of the nipple-areolar complex in women with macromastia usually reveals decreased sensation when compared with women with more normal-sized breasts. To assess the degree of macromastia the two most accurate objective measurements are the distance from the suprasternal notch to the nipple and the distance from the nipple to the inframammary crease. The normal distance from the suprasternal notch to the nipple ranges from 18 to 22 cm and depends on the height and age of the individual. The normal distance from the inframammary crease to the nipple ranges from 5 to 7 cm and does not differ greatly with age or height. In women with macromastia the distance from the suprasternal notch to the nipple is typically 24 cm or more and may even exceed 40 cm. The distance from the inframammary crease to the nipple is at least 10 to 15 cm. This distance is an important consideration in determining which of the two currently performed reduction mammoplasty procedures will be used for a particular individual. The inferior pedicle technique involves preservation of

295

the nipple-areolar complex on a pedicle of breast tissue with resection of excess breast tissue from multiple areas of the breast. This approach is most appropriate for reduction of mild to moderate hypertrophy, when less than 1000 g of tissue per breast is to be resected and the nipple-areolar complex is to be elevated no more than 8 cm. Healthful, young, premenopausal women who desire to maintain nipple-areolar sensation, erectile function, and the ability to lactate are candidates for this procedure. This technique offers great versatility for achieving ideal breast size and contour for the patient, and it is often the procedure of choice when a wide breast needs to be narrowed since several areas of the breast are resected. However, the inferior pedicle technique is a more complex procedure than the free nipple graft technique and should be used only in carefully selected patients.

The free nipple graft technique is used most often in postmenopausal women and in those who have large breasts that are being reduced by 1000 to 2000 g per breast. For these patients the nipple-areolar complex may need to be moved 10 cm or more. Survival of the nipple-areolar complex is better ensured by the free graft technique than it is by the inferior pedicle technique. The free nipple graft technique generally is less complicated than the inferior pedicle method. The pedicle does not have to be folded to reposition and inset the nipple-areolar complex, and tissue is resected primarily from the medial and lateral portions of the breast. The free nipple graft technique is more appropriate for older women, who typically are concerned less about loss of sensation and lactation, or for younger patients, who strongly desire a procedure that is highly likely to be successful. The free nipple graft is the technique of choice for women who are at high risk for complications, either because of tobacco smoking or significant medical problems such as diabetes mellitus or collagen vascular disease. Finally, the free nipple graft technique is preferred for obese women because their breasts have a large proportion of fat, which increases the likelihood of fat necrosis.

Breast reduction can be done in any age group, including teenagers, when the patient is physchologically prepared for the operative procedure. The benefits of early reduction in women as young as 13 or 14 years usually outweigh the disadvantages because an operation can greatly enhance the quality of life during the teenage and young adult years.

Nursing may be possible following inferior pedicle reduction mammoplasty; however, it is not possible following free nipple grafting. Therefore if breast-feeding is an important consideration, the operation should be postponed until childbearing is completed.

Indications

Reduction mammoplasty is a cosmetic and a reconstructive procedure that is indicated for symptomatic women with macromastia. There is no method of managing this disease other than surgery. Although weight loss potentially is beneficial, it will rarely reduce large breasts sufficiently to alleviate either symptoms or deformity, even when weight loss is substantial.

Unilateral reduction mammoplasty often is indicated following mastectomy when the reconstructed breast will not match a large contralateral breast. To achieve symmetry the remaining breast is reduced in a second stage procedure that is performed after the reconstructed breast has attained its final shape.

Contraindications

Reduction mammoplasty is contraindicated in women who have pulmonary, cardiac, or other systemic medical problems that would preclude safe general anesthetic administration and extensive surgery. Tobacco smoking significantly increases the risk of complications caused by impaired circulation, particularly skin, fat, and nipple-areolar necrosis. Collagen vascular disease, diabetes mellitus, and the administration of immunosuppressant drugs or corticosteroids substantially increase the likelihood of complications and are considered relative contraindications. The free nipple graft technique is associated with a lower complication rate compared to the inferior pedicle technique. Patients who are known to form keloids are poor candidates. Reduction mammoplasty also is not appropriate for women with significant psychologic instability.

Complications

Complications of reduction mammoplasty include bleeding, infection, fat and skin necrosis, malposition, necrosis or distortion of the nipple-areolar complex, hypertrophic scarring, asymmetry, standing cones, and altered breast sensation.

Hematomas develop in less than 5% of women who undergo reduction mammoplasty. Risk factors for hematoma formation include the ingestion of aspirin or other platelet-altering drugs, hypertension, and inappropriate or overly vigorous activity during the first week after surgery. The symptomatic patient, with pain and unilateral enlargement of the breast, should be promptly returned to the operating room for evacuation of the hematoma under general anesthesia. The risks of fat, nipple-areolar, or skin necrosis increase substantially if hematoma evacuation is delayed. The presence of a drain cannot prevent hematoma development, although it minimizes the risk of seroma, which contributes to postoperative discomfort and swelling.

Infection develops in fewer than 5% of patients having reduction mammoplasty. Infection usually responds to antibiotics and local wound care. Hematoma formation is associated with an increased risk of infection.

Tissue necrosis is a frequent complication of reduction mammoplasty, particularly in patients who require resection of over 1000 g of tissue per breast. Fat necrosis usually is caused by tissue devascularization during dissection or excessive tension at closure. Symptoms of fat necrosis include a low-grade temperature, pain, erythema, induration, and general malaise. Small areas of fat necrosis are inconsequential, but large areas of necrosis may result in loss of the overlying skin.

Fat necrosis may resemble delayed wound healing that is associated with tissue separation and purulent drainage. Although the differentiation of fat necrosis from infection may be difficult, bacterial cultures are negative and the body temperature elevation is usually slight with fat necrosis alone. Because it may be impossible to rule out an infection, patients with suspected fat necrosis are usually treated with antibiotics. Large areas of fat necrosis may require debridement; however, it should be done conservatively because the extent of fat necrosis is not always clear and the unwary surgeon may remove viable tissue. Fat necrosis usually results in minor contour deformities and scars, but these cosmetic problems can usually be subsequently corrected.

Nipple-areolar necrosis following inferior pedicle transposition usually results from improper patient selection, incorrect construction of the pedicle, kinking and folding of the pedicle, or excessive tension during closure. The risk of nipple-areolar necrosis is substantial with a pedicle that is more than 15 cm in length because the pedicle cannot be folded adequately to position the nipple at the desired site above the inframammary crease. The breast flaps and pedicle must be contoured correctly to eliminate excessive tension at the time of closure. If the nipple-areolar complex appears nonviable at any time during the operation, the inferior pedicle procedure should be abandoned and a free nipple graft should be constructed.

Distortion of the nipple-areolar complex is primarily caused by preparing the site for the newly positioned complex before wound closure. Distortion may also result from an improperly designed inferior pedicle that cannot be folded to produce a nipple-areolar complex that is sufficiently mobile and can be inset without tension.

The risk of scar hypertrophy increases with the presence of either excessive tension at closure, fat necrosis, or with infection. The development of scar hypertrophy may be decreased postoperatively by injecting triamcinolone or by applying silicone gel when excess scar tissue appears to form.

Obvious asymmetry following reduction mammoplasty can result from either incorrect preoperative marking of the patient or resection of unequal amounts of tissue from the breasts. This can usually be prevented by the gradual resection of tissue and by careful breast recontouring with multiple trial closures and with minor adjustments until symmetry is established. Since resected tissue cannot be replaced, excision should proceed gradually until the same amount of tissue remains in each breast. The patient should be examined a final time while she is in a semisitting position after the wounds are closed. The size, shape, and position of both breasts can be compared, and the wounds can be reopened if further modifications are needed.

Standing cones rarely resolve without surgical correction, but they can be avoided by designing the length of the superior and inferior arms of the transverse excisions to within 1 or 2 cm of each other. Standing cones also can be prevented by proper closure, which begins by suturing from the medial and lateral ends of the incision and by evenly distributing any excess tissue along the inframammary crease.

Following the free nipple graft procedure patients will lose all sensation in the nipple-areolar complex. Patients initially may lose some breast skin sensation. Approximately 50% of patients partially lose nipple-areolar and breast sensation, at least temporarily, with inferior pedicle reduction. The loss of sensation correlates with the magnitude of the resection. Breast tissue should be left attached to the chest wall at the lateral aspect of the inferior pedicle and overlying the lateral portion of the pectoralis major muscle to include the fourth intercostal nerve in the inferior pedicle. Leaving this tissue maximizes the likelihood of preserving nipple-areolar sensation. If sensation is lost, it usually returns in all patients after 1 to 2 years.

Additional complications of the free nipple graft technique include over-reduction and nipple graft failure. These problems are avoided by careful planning and meticulous operative techinque. Various precautionary steps to prevent these complications are described in the text.

A properly performed free nipple graft survives in more than 95% of cases. Factors related to graft failure are inadequate defatting, accumulation of blood and serum between the graft and the deepithelialized tissue beneath it, and inadequate immobilization of the graft after surgery. If the graft is properly thinned, if the space beneath it is irrigated to remove blood clots, and if the graft is immobilized fully with a proper stent, the likelihood of graft survival is excellent. An additional problem of the free nipple technique is the tendency for the graft to lose pigment. In dark-skinned individuals a lightened nipple-areolar complex produces an obvious cosmetic deformity. Although a depigmented graft often will darken during the first postoperative year, tattooing may be needed to produce a more appropriate color.

Preoperative Preparation

Candidates for reduction mammoplasty must be carefully selected to include only women who are psychologically well adjusted and who have realistic goals and expectations. Reduction mammoplasty produces scars and some contour irregularities. Individuals who are perfectionists and who have major concern about minimal deformity are likely to be unhappy with reduction mammoplasty no matter how successful the surgery.

Preoperatively the surgeon and patient must thoroughly discuss the desired breast size. They also must discuss the likely postoperative appearance of the breasts, which will usually be somewhat square at the base from the gradual stretching of tissues as the wounds heal. Patients should also be informed about the location of scars and about the potential loss of sensation in the nipple-areolar complex.

At least 50% of women have some degree of breast asymmetry preoperatively. Patients should understand that perfect symmetry in a bilateral breast procedure rarely is achieved. Breasts that appear symmetrical before the operation may have a 50- to 100-g difference after reduction, but this minor asymmetry is hardly noticeable and most women consider the appearance satisfactory. A mammogram should be obtained in patients over the age of 35 if they have not had one within the past year.

Usually reduction mammoplasty does not require blood replacement. However, patients should be informed that blood might be needed, and if they wish to pursue autologous blood donation, this should be done at least 2 weeks before surgery.

Patients should abstain from cigarette smoking for at least 2 weeks preoperatively. Any medications that contain aspirin should be discontinued for the same time period. The procedure is performed under general anesthesia, and perioperative antibiotics are routinely administered.

OPERATIVE PROCEDURE

Reduction Mammoplasty 1: Inferior Pedicle Technique

Preoperative Marking and Positioning (Figure 25-1)

The patient is marked for reduction mammoplasty while she is in an upright (sitting) position. The midline of the sternum, both clavicles, and both inframammary creases are marked. The breast meridian is marked by drawing a line from the midpoint of the clavicle through the nipple to the midpoint of the inframammary crease. The new nipple location is placed between 18 and 22 cm from the suprasternal notch along the breast meridian. The height of the individual and the desired breast size are considered in determining the precise location of the nipple. Marking the transposed inframammary crease on the anterior breast skin is an important reference line for determining the location of the nipple. The point at which the transposed crease crosses the breast meridian should lie approximately 2 cm above the location of the new nipple. It is preferable to place the nipple slightly lower because it easily can be raised later. Also, the nipple location should be marked slightly lower than its anticipated final position when extremely large breasts are being reduced because the natural elasticity of the skin pulls the nipple-areolar complex superiorly after extensive tissue is resected.

Two 7-cm-long lines labeled *AB* and *AC* then are drawn obliquely from the new nipple location to constitute the vertical arms of an equilateral triangle. The angle between the vertical arms can be widened to produce a breast that will be more conical; however, a wider angle results in greater tension at wound closure, with an increased risk of ischemic complications. The midpoint of the actual inframammary crease is marked as point *D* (as seen in Figure 25-1, *B*).

The extent of excision of the medial tissue next is estimated by pinching points *C* and *D* together, which defines a wedge of excess tissue. The medial apex of the wedge is the point *F* near the sternum. A line is drawn from point *C* to the medial point *F* to indicate the superior margin of the medial wedge to be excised. The inferior margin of the medial excision is determined by a line drawn from *D* to *F*. The distances of the superior *(CF)* and inferior *(DF)* excision margins are measured. If the two measurements are within 1 to 2 cm of each other, no standing cones should develop at closure. If the difference between these two measurements is greater than 2 cm, point *D* should be moved medially or laterally or the line indicating the superior arm of the excision should be curved to increase its length, until both lines measure within 2 cm of each other.

The lateral excision then is similarly estimated by pinching the tissue points *B* and *D* and by marking the lateral apex *(E)* for the lateral wedge of tissue to be excised. A line drawn from point *B* to point *E* forms the superior margin of the excision, and a line drawn from the midpoint of the inframammary crease *D* to point *E* marks the inferior margin. The measurements for the two lateral markings *(BE* and *DE)* should be within 2 cm of each other in length. If necessary the shorter of the two markings is curved to gain the needed length. The entire superior incision has a W configuration, from point *E*, laterally, through *B* to *A* to *C* to *F*, medially. The inferior

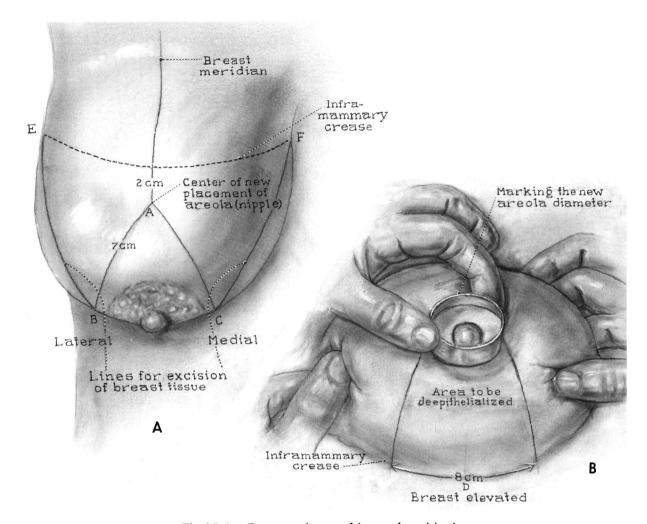

Fig 25-1. Preoperative marking and positioning.

incision is a curved line from point *E* along the inframammary crease through point *D* to point *F*. The opposite breast then can be outlined in the same manner. If one breast is substantially larger than the other, the larger breast should be supported while it is being marked or the weight of the tissue will stretch the skin and displace the measurements inferiorly.

All measurements are checked for symmetry of the breast and the nipple-areolar complex position. The patient is placed on the operating table in a supine position with her arms abducted approximately 90 degrees. General anesthesia is induced. The patient then is repositioned in a semisitting position. If the reduction will involve resection of a large amount of tissue (over 1000 g per breast), the procedure may take as long as 4 hours and a bladder drainage catheter should be inserted.

After sterile skin preparation and draping are completed, the new size for the areola, which typically will be 38 to 40 mm in diameter, is marked. This marking should be done with the areola under slight tension to eliminate wrinkles. The areola should not be marked in a constricted position because a perfect circle will not be created, and it should not be marked in a stretched position because the result will be an areola that is smaller than the diameter chosen at the time of insetting. A 38- or 40-mm cookie cutter is centered around the nipple and pressed into the areola to outline a circle, as shown in Figure 25-1, *B*. The impression made by the cookie cutter then is marked with a marking pen or brilliant green dye.

The midpoint of the inframammary crease *D* is the midpoint of the base of the inferior pedicle. The base line should be between 8 and 12 cm long. A narrow pedicle is easier to fold and inset; however, a wider pedicle tends to protect the blood supply and sensation to the nipple-areolar complex. The longer the distance from the inframammary crease to the nipple, the wider the base of the pedicle should be. The base of the pedicle can be shifted laterally or medially around the midpoint of the inframammary crease if necessary to obtain a better cosmetic result. After the base of the inferior pedicle is marked, the breast is elevated superiorly and vertical lines that gradually taper to the periphery of the new areolar marking are drawn from each end of the base line.

The superior portion of the pedicle must be carefully planned. A 5-mm margin is left around the new areolar perimeter as the vertical lines are drawn to ensure that the pedicle will not be incised too narrowly and that sufficient tissue will be present for grasping and manipulating the areola during closure. However, if the pedicle is made excessively wide in the area of the areola, insetting will be difficult.

After the markings are made, the key points that are crucial for ensuring symmetry are scored, including the new nipple location *(A)*, the inferior extent of the 7-cm lines that form the oblique arms of the triangle below the new nipple location (*B* and *C*), and the midpoint of the inframammary crease *(D)*. It is important that the markings be definitively established. If they are poorly defined, they may be obliterated as the procedure progresses.

Deepithelialization of the Inferior Pedicle (Figure 25-2)

After the marking is completed, the inferior pedicle is deepithelialized between the base line and the lower margin of the site of the new areola. The excess tissue around the existing areola also is removed. The pedicle is deepithelialized in this manner so that a raw surface overlies the tissue that will be buried when the incisions of the reduced breast are closed.

Development of the Inferior Pedicle (Figure 25-3)

After the tissue is deepithelialized, the surrounding vertical margins are beveled away from the deepithelialized segment on the medial side, and the incision is extended down to the pectoralis major fascia. On the lateral side the incision also is beveled; however it stops superficial to the pectoralis fascia so that breast tissue is left attached to the pectoralis major muscle. Preservation of this deep tissue increases the likelihood that the fourth intercostal nerve, which provides sensation to the nipple and areola, will be left intact. Facelift retractors can be used to facilitate proper beveling and dissection of the developing pedicle free from the surrounding tissue. When the incisions are completed, the developing pedicle is mobilized from the adjacent tissue superiorly by deepening the incision to the pectoralis major muscle. The inferior incision also is beveled, and a tissue margin of 5 mm is retained around the areola to facilitate its subsequent handling.

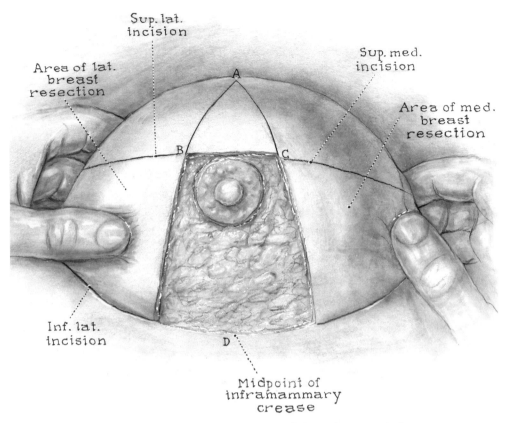

Fig 25-2. Deepithelialization of the inferior pedicle.

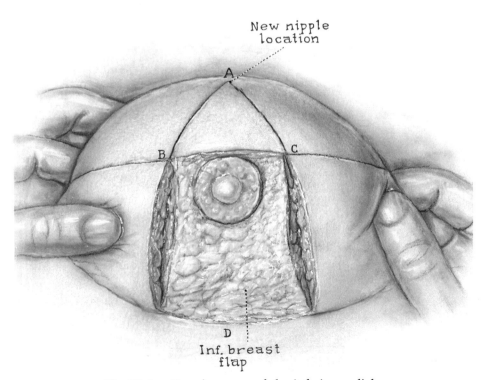

Fig 25-3. Development of the inferior pedicle.

As this dissection progresses, the pedicle is periodically palpated to ensure that it is sufficiently wide. The pedicle always can be trimmed to debulk excess tissue; however, if it is made too thin initially, adequate circulation may not be provided to the nipple-areolar complex. If signs of vascular compromise develop during this procedure, the nipple-areolar complex is harvested and reattached as a free nipple graft, as described in Figures 25-17 to 25-19.

Completed Mobilization of the Inferior Pedicle (Figure 25-4)

When the inferior pedicle is mobilized fully (as shown in the frontal view), the pectoralis major fascia will be exposed medially and superiorly. Laterally the breast tissue overlies the pectoralis major fascia in continuity with the inferior pedicle. A properly constructed inferior pedicle, as shown in the medial view, is wedge shaped and tapers from its base toward the nipple-areolar complex.

Excision of Excess Breast Tissue (Figure 25-5)

A substantial amount of breast tissue usually is left attached to the lateral edge of the pectoralis major muscle to increase the likelihood of preservation of the innervation to the nipple-areolar complex. Deliberate preservation of the excess tissue in this area (shown here) also prevents overresection, with the resulting depression and noticeable deformity at the lateral edge of the breast. Once the breast tissue within both ellipses has been resected, the wound is irrigated with saline solution and half-strength povidone-iodine and complete hemostasis is achieved.

Three areas of tissue, including a medial wedge, a triangular area subtended by points A, B, and C, and a lateral wedge now are resected. The medial wedge can be resected first by making an incision along the previously marked line CF. A second incision is made from the medial edge of the inferior pedicle to point F. The incisions are deepened to the pectoralis major fascia, beveling them away from the tissue that will remain in the breast. This wedge of tissue then is sharply dissected off the underlying pectoralis major fascia and is removed.

The triangular area of tissue subtendinal by points A, B, and C is incised. The incisions are deepened directly to the pectoralis major fascia, without beveling. This triangle of tissue then is sharply dissected off the underlying pectoralis major fascia and is removed. Finally the lateral wedge of tissue is resected by making an incision along the previously marked line BE. A second incision is made from the lateral edge of the inferior pedicle to point E. The incisions are deepened to the pectoralis major fascia (or to the serratus anterior muscle laterally), beveling them away from the tissue that will remain in the breast. The tissue then is sharply dissected by beginning medially and proceeding through the breast tissue so that some residual breast tissue remains lying over the pectoralis major fascia in the region of the fourth intercostal nerve. All of the breast tissue resected then should be weighed and recorded to document the absolute amount of breast tissue resected and to compare the amounts of tissue resected in the medial and lateral wedges for symmetry.

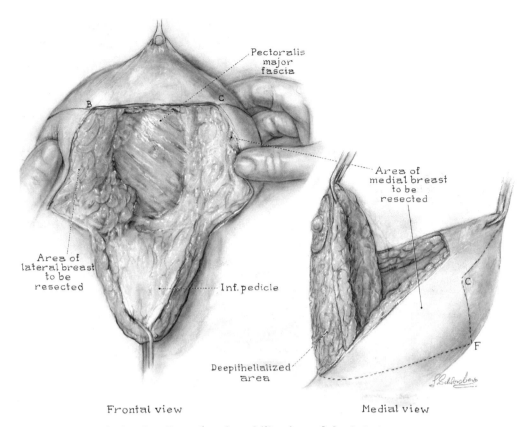

Frontal view

Medial view

Fig 25-4. Completed mobilization of the interior pedicle.

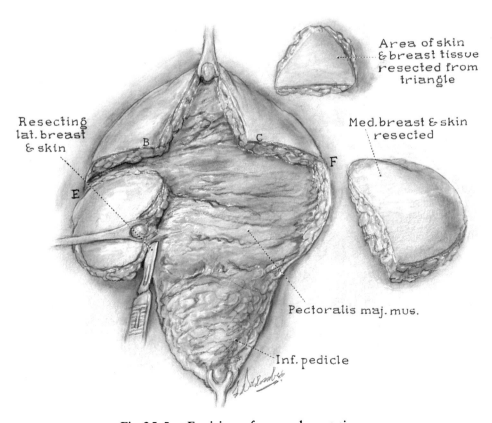

Fig 25-5. Excision of excess breast tissue.

Contouring of the Residual Breast (Figure 25-6)

After the lateral, medial, and triangular resections are completed, the breast tissue in the superior breast flap is undermined at the level of the pectoralis major fascia to just below the clavicle superiorly, a few centimeters lateral to the midline of the sternum medially, and to the border of the pectoralis major muscle laterally. Elevation of the breast provides the mobility needed to drape the remaining tissue and skin around the inferior pedicle without undue tension at closure.

With this tissue elevated, points *B* and *C* are brought toward point *D* to determine the amount of tension on the flaps and to assess the size and shape of the breast mound. A trial draping is performed. Based on the appearance, usually it is necessary to resect additional tissue from the middle portion of the superior flap to create a space of sufficient size for insetting the inferior pedicle.

Final contouring is performed cautiously because overreduction cannot be corrected. It is preferable to make several trial closures and resect small amounts of tissue from obvious areas of excess than to attempt a single complete resection and create a deformity that can be corrected only by insertion of an implant.

When a bilateral reduction mammoplasty is performed, one breast is first reduced, contoured, and initially closed. Once a satisfactory breast mound is produced with regard to size, shape, and tension, the other breast is reduced, until a symmetrical appearance is achieved. If the breast sizes differ, the larger one is reduced first and the smaller breast then is reduced if necessary to match it. The breast symmetry is evaluated while the patient is in a semisitting position and before the nipple-areolar complex is brought out and the final contouring and closure are completed. Any further adjustments needed to achieve symmetry are made while the patient remains in a semisitting position.

Initial Suturing of Points B, C, and D (Figure 25-7)

After contouring is completed, points *B* and *C* are sutured to point *D*. The inferior pedicle is placed beneath the triangle. It is folded or oriented so that the nipple is beneath point *A* when points *B* and *C* are sutured to point *D*. If this placement makes the suturing of points *B* and *C* to point *D* difficult, the inferior pedicle can be temporarily displaced laterally and inferiorly, until the suture is securely tied and then is manipulated back into its proper location. It is not necessary to suture the inferior pedicle to the chest wall to maintain its position. Such suturing could be detrimental because it might restrict the surgeon's ability to mobilize the nipple-areolar complex for final insetting.

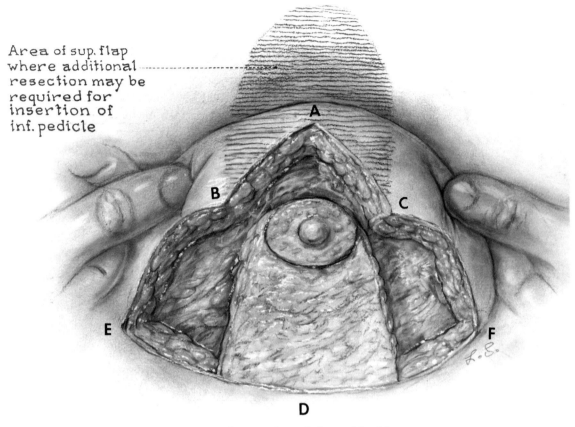

Area of sup. flap where additional resection may be required for insertion of inf. pedicle

Fig 25-6. Contouring of the residual breast.

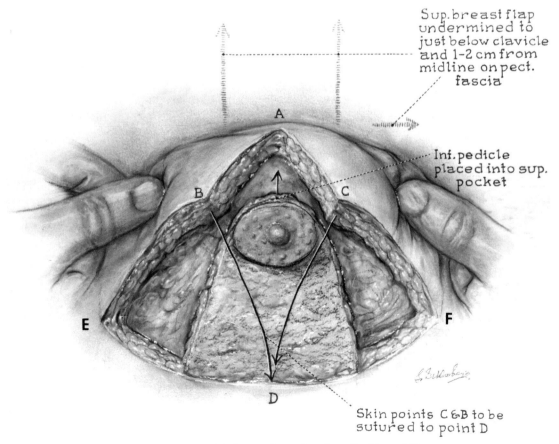

Sup. breast flap undermined to just below clavicle and 1-2 cm from midline on pect. fascia

Inf. pedicle placed into sup. pocket

Skin points C & B to be sutured to point D

Fig 25-7. Initial suturing of points B, C, and D.

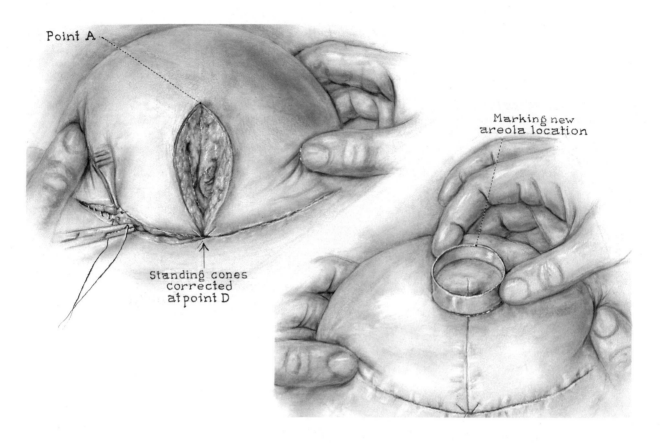

Point A

Standing cones
corrected
at point D

Marking new
areola location

Wound Closure and Marking the Location of the New Nipple-Areolar Complex (Figure 25-8)

A constant vacuum drain, 7 to 10 mm in diameter, is inserted and brought out laterally through a stab wound in a minimally noticeable part of the axilla (not shown). After the symmetry of both breasts is evaluated and any needed adjustments are made, the breast incisions are closed in layers with absorbable sutures. To prevent the formation of standing cones the closure is started at the medial and lateral ends of the horizontal incision and the closure is advanced toward point D with skin staples. Any discrepancy in the lengths of the incisions can be corrected, and if necessary any skin excess can be excised at the midpoint of the inframammary crease. The skin staples are subsequently removed as interrupted sutures are placed between them at the level of the deep dermis. Closure is completed with a running subcuticular suture. Once the horizontal incisions are completely closed, the nipple and the inferior pedicle are positioned as closely as possible to the new nipple location. The vertical incision then is closed in the same manner as the horizontal incision. At this point the nipple-areolar complex is completely buried beneath the closed incisions.

As shown in Figure 25-8, B, the final site for the new nipple-areolar location can be marked with a 38- to 40-mm cookie cutter. The inferior edge of this cutting apparatus is positioned 4.5 to 5 cm above the new inframammary crease. Although this measurement is an initially short nipple-

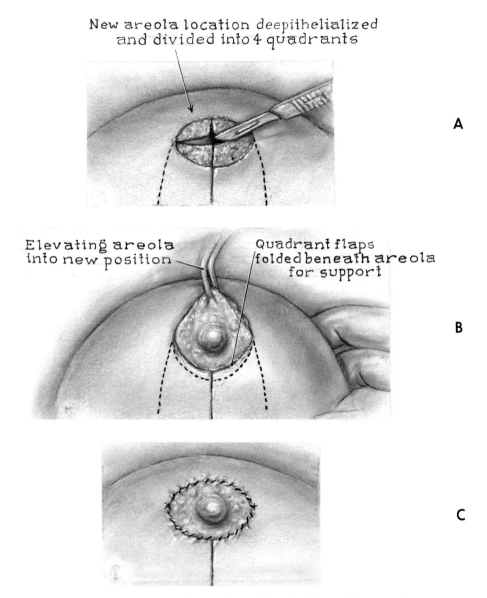

New areola location deepithelialized and divided into 4 quadrants

A

Elevating areola into new position   Quadrant flaps folded beneath areola for support

B

C

Fig 25-9.   Elevation and insetting of the nipple-areolar complex.

to-inframammary crease distance, the distance will increase over time and the nipple ultimately will be properly positioned. If the inferior edge of the cookie cutter is placed higher than 5 cm above the inframammary crease, the nipple will eventually appear too high as the breast tissues soften, stretch, and remodel.

Elevation and Insetting of the Nipple-Areolar Complex
(Figure 25-9)

After the new nipple-areolar location is marked, the circle is deepithelialized and divided into four quadrants, as shown in Figure 25-9, *A*. These four small skin flaps can be folded under if additional tissue is needed to support the nipple-areolar complex. The skin flaps are discarded if the de-epithelialized quadrants are not needed, or if they produce too much bulk. The nipple-areolar complex then is elevated into position through the incisions that divide the newly marked areolar location, as shown in Figure 25-9, *B*. Usually it is necessary to core out some of the underlying fat and breast tissue from the superior breast flap around the new site of the nipple-areolar complex to reduce tension on the inferior pedicle as the areola is pulled into its new location. However, tissue should not be resected from the inferior pedicle.

Once the nipple-areolar complex is in position, the circulation is evaluated. If venous congestion is present, the pedicle is probably kinked or is under excessive tension. The vertical and horizontal incisions should be reopened to allow inspection of the pedicle. Kinking can be corrected through gentle manipulation of the pedicle; however, excessive tension at points *B*, *C*, and *D* requires resection of additional breast tissue from the superior breast flaps to relieve the venous congestion. Any excision of tissue from the inferior pedicle must be performed judiciously to avoid producing a pedicle that is too thin to provide reliable circulation for the nipple-areolar complex. If arterial inflow is inadequate, the nipple and areola should be harvested as a full-thickness graft and should be replaced as a free nipple graft. When one breast requires further resection with bilateral reduction to remove excess bulk, the other breast likely will need additional revision as well if symmetry is to be maintained.

When the circulation to the nipple-areolar complex is satisfactory, the complex is inset with several interrupted absorbable sutures evenly positioned around the areolar perimeter. Additional sutures are placed at equal distances around the areola to distribute the tension evenly. The closure is completed with a fine, running subcuticular chromic suture, as shown in Figure 25-9, *C*.

The incisions and the nipple-areolar complex are covered with a nonadherent, lubricated gauze dressing and light gauze packs. The dressing should not constrict the breast in any way.

Reduction Mammoplasty 2: Tissue Excision with Free Nipple Grafting
Preoperative Marking and Patient Positioning (Figure 25-10)

The patient should be marked preoperatively in a sitting or standing position. The preliminary new nipple location is marked between 18 and 22 cm from the suprasternal notch on the breast meridian. An additional guideline for the location of the new nipple-areolar complex is the level of the midpoint of the transposed inframammary crease on the anterior surface of the breast. That point should be 2 cm above the new nipple location. However, the final nipple location is determined in relation to its distance from the inframammary crease and can be adjusted at the end of the operation. A distance of 22 cm from the suprasternal notch at the breast meridian reliably produces an acceptable nipple location in the average individual. After the nipple location is marked, two oblique lines (*AB* and *AC*) are drawn inferiorly from the nipple location. These lines are drawn obliquely and inferiorly from point *A* and are 7 cm in length. The lines connecting points *A*, *B*, and *C* form an equilateral triangle. This triangle can be distributed evenly around the breast meridian or can be shifted either medially or laterally to allow adjustment in the transverse incision lines *CF* and *BE* (to be described). Generally, however, the triangle is centered with 3.5 cm on each side of the breast meridian along an imaginary line drawn between

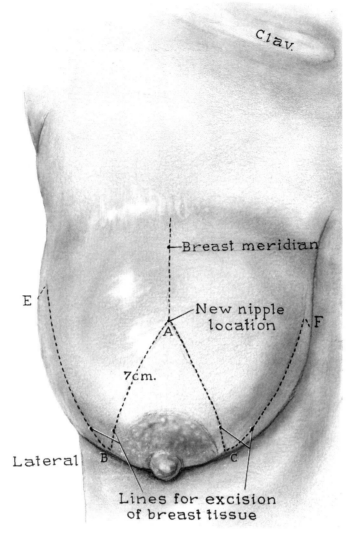

Fig 25-10. Preoperative marking and patient positioning.

B and C. The midpoint of the inframammary crease is marked D (not shown here). After the 7-cm oblique lines are drawn, the medial and lateral breast excision lines are drawn. In this figure the superior incisions are labeled CF and BE. CF typically is drawn first, and can be estimated by pinching point C to point D to define a wedge of tissue. The apical point (F) of the wedge is marked medially. The distance from C to F is measured and compared with the distance from D to F. If CF is less than DF, then CF is curved to increase its length; if CF is greater than DF, then CF is drawn as a straight line; and if these two distances are within 1 to 2 cm of each other, no further adjustment is necessary. If CF is more than 2 cm longer than DF, the midpoint of the inframammary crease should be shifted to make CF and DF within 2 cm of each other. BE is similarly drawn, and BE and DE then are modified as necessary to ensure that their lengths are within 2 cm of each other. Point F can be shifted inferiorly or the respective lines can be curved to gain length. After marking, the patient is placed on the operating table in a supine position with her arms abducted. General anesthesia is induced. The skin is prepared and draped, then the patient is placed in a semisitting position. If an operation in excess of 4 hours is anticipated, a bladder drainage catheter should be inserted.

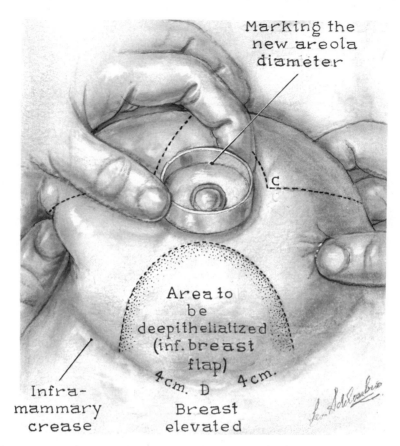

Fig 25-11. Marking of the nipple-areolar complex and inferior breast flap.

Marking of the Nipple-Areolar Complex and Inferior Breast Flap
(Figure 25-11)

The nipple-areolar complex is marked with a 38-mm cookie cutter with the patient in a semisitting position. This marking should be done with the areola slightly under tension to eliminate wrinkles. The areola should not be marked in a constricted position, or a circle will not be created; also it should not be marked in a stretched position or the areola will be smaller than the chosen diameter at the time of grafting. The cookie cutter is centered on the areola and the nipple and is pressed into the areola to produce a circular impression. The impression then is marked with either brilliant green or a marking pen. After the nipple-areolar complex is marked, the inferior breast flap is outlined by measuring and marking 4 cm lines along the inframammary crease from its midpoint (point *D*) medially and laterally. An arc is drawn superiorly to just below the areola to form an inverted ∪. This arc subtends the inferior breast flap that is to be deepithelialized and mobilized to provide central bulk for the breast.

After the markings are made, the key points that will be crucial for obtaining symmetry are scored, including the new nipple location *(A)*, the inferior extent of the 7-cm lines that form the oblique arms of the triangle below the new nipple location (*B* and *C*), and the midpoint of the inframammary crease *(D)*. Because these markings may be obliterated as the procedure progresses and then cannot be reliably relocated, they need to be clearly defined.

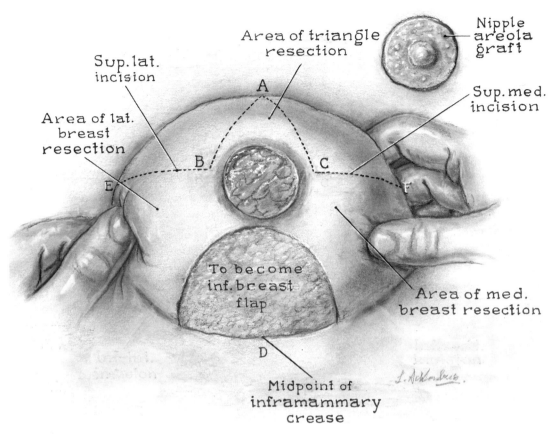

Fig 25-12. Harvesting of the nipple-areolar graft and deepithelialization of the inferior breast flap.

Harvesting of the Nipple-Areolar Graft and Deepithelialization of the Inferior Breast Flap (Figure 25-12)

The nipple-areolar graft is harvested as a full-thickness graft by incising the previously inscribed circle about the nipple. The graft is harvested in the relatively avascular plane between the areola and the superficial fascia. At the level of the nipple the ductal tissue is divided so that the nipple is approximately 5 mm in vertical thickness. If the nipple is thicker than 5 mm, it should be thinned by excision of ductal tissue from its deep surface, until the maximum thickness is 5 mm. Excess fatty tissue should be excised from the deep surface of the areolar graft. The graft then should be stored in a cool, moist sponge and marked left or right. The inferior breast flap is deepithelialized after incising along the outlined inverted U and the 8-cm inframammary crease line. If possible some dermis is left to reepithelialize the area if the incision separates.

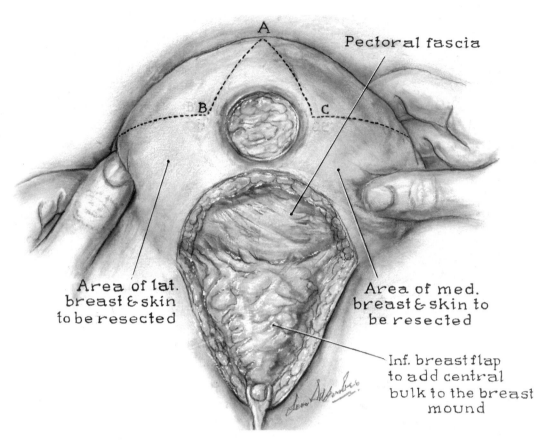

Fig 25-13. Mobilization of the inferior breast flap.

Mobilization of the Inferior Breast Flap (Figure 25-13)

The inferior flap is mobilized by making incisions along the periphery of the deepithelialized inverted ∪. These incisions then are deepened toward the chest wall, and they bevel away from the flap. Facelift retractors should be used to separate the flap from the adjacent breast tissue. The development of an inferior flap with an excessively narrow base can be avoided by consciously dissecting medially, laterally, and superiorly away from the flap with the electrocautery or the scalpel. Initially the flap will be excessively bulky; however, it can be subsequently recontoured.

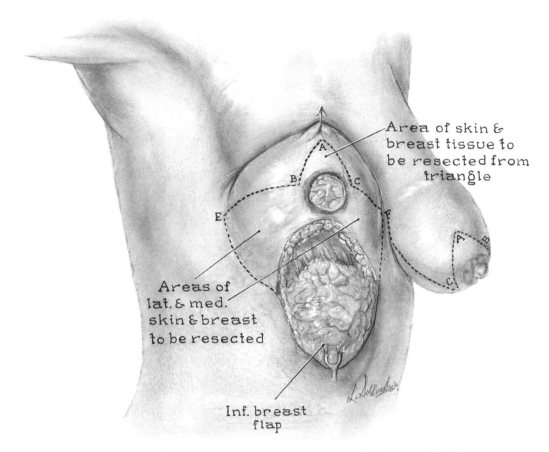

Fig 25-14. Mobilized inferior breast flap and incisions for medial, lateral, and triangular areas of breast resection.

Mobilized Inferior Breast Flap and Incisions for the Medial, Lateral, and Triangular Areas of Breast Resection (Figure 25-14)

The inferior breast flap easily can be retracted downward after it has been separated from the surrounding breast tissue. At this point the inferior breast flap should be well vascularized with sufficient bulk to provide the essential mass to the central breast following tissue resection and wound closure.

Essentially all the breast tissue and skin shown with the dotted lines (depicted on the patient's right breast) are excised en bloc. After the marked skin incision is made, it is extended to the pectoralis major fascia and beveled away from the tissue to remain in the breast. The tissue then is sharply dissected off the underlying pectoralis major fascia and is excised.

All of the resected breast tissue then should be weighed and recorded to quantitate the amount of tissue removed and to compare it with the amount of tissue resected on the opposite side.

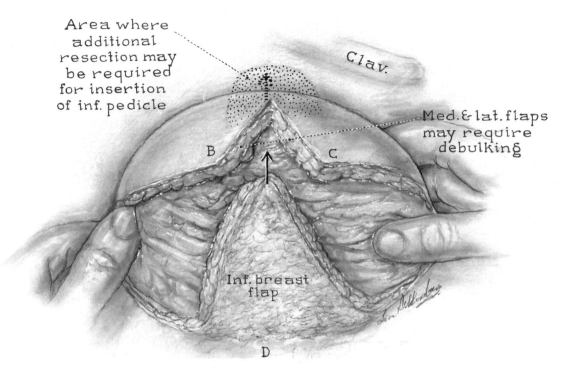

Area where
additional
resection may
be required
for insertion
of inf. pedicle

Clav.

Med.& lat. flaps
may require
debulking

B

C

Inf. breast
flap

D

Fig 25-15. Contouring of the residual breast.

Contouring of the Residual Breast (Figure 25-15)

The remaining superior breast flap then is elevated at the level of the pectoralis fascia to just inferior to the clavicle superiorly, 1 to 2 cm lateral to the sternum medially, and 1 to 2 cm to the border of the pectoralis major laterally. With this tissue elevated a trial draping is performed by bringing points *B* and *C* toward point *D* (the midpoint of the inframammary crease) to determine the amount of tension on the flaps and to assess the size and shape of the breast mound. Usually it is necessary to resect additional tissue from the middle portion of the superior flap to create a space of sufficient size for insetting the inferior flap.

Wound Closure (Figure 25-16)

After contouring is completed, wound closure begins by suturing points *B* and *C* to point *D*. The inferior breast flap is positioned beneath the center of the breast mound. A constant vacuum drain, 7 to 10 mm in diameter, is inserted and brought out laterally through a stab wound in a minimally noticeable part of the axilla (not shown).

After the symmetry of both breasts is evaluated and after any needed adjustments are made, the incisions are closed in layers with absorbable sutures, as shown in Figure 25-16, *B*. To prevent the formation of standing cones, the closure is started at the medial and lateral ends of the horizontal incision and the tissues are advanced toward the midpoint *D* with skin staples. Any discrepancy in the lengths of the incisions can be corrected, and if necessary any excess skin can be excised at the midpoint of the inframammary crease. The skin staples subsequently are removed as interrupted sutures are placed between them at the level of the deep dermis. Closure is completed with a running subcuticular suture. Once the horizontal incisions are completely closed, the vertical incision is closed in the same manner.

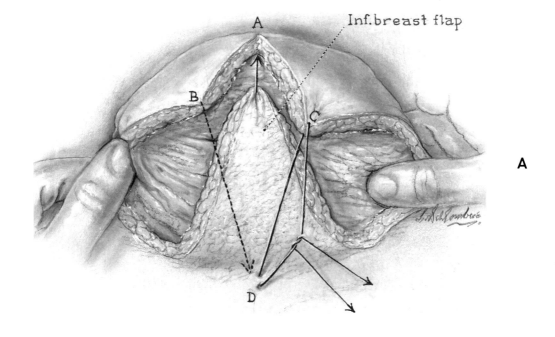

A

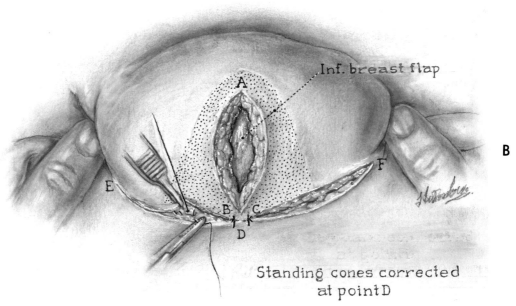

B

Standing cones corrected
at point D

Fig 25-16. Wound closure.

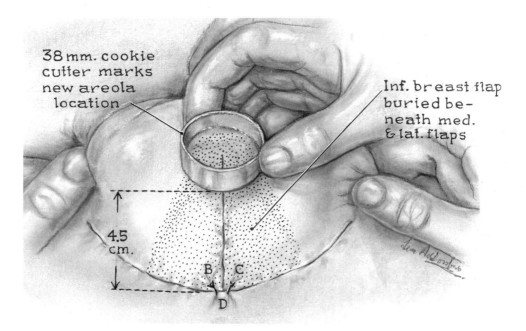

Fig 25-17. Marking the final location of the nipple-areolar.

Marking the Final Location of the Nipple-Areolar (Figure 25-17)

The actual location of the nipple-areolar complex is finalized after wound closure. The final location of the nipple-areolar complex to be marked with a 38-mm cookie cutter is chosen by centering the cookie cutter around the predetermined position for the nipple at point *A*. With the cookie cutter centered on point *A*, the distance from the inferior margin of the cookie cutter to point *D* should be measured. If this is in excess of 4.5 cm, the cookie cutter should be lowered slightly and then pressed into the breast tissue to leave a temporary mark. This mark then should be viewed to be certain that the nipple-areolar complex will not be too high. It is better to err on the low side in locating the nipple-areolar complex because the remodeling and stretching of tissues will result in a superior migration of the nipple-areolar complex. The ultimate placement of the nipple-areolar complex should be near the summit of the breast mound or slightly below that. However, it is more important that the nipple-areolar complex not be more than 5 cm from point *D* in the inframammary crease. After the location of the nipple is decided, the cookie cutter should be pressed against the breast tissue to leave a circular mark, which then is marked with a pen or brilliant green.

318

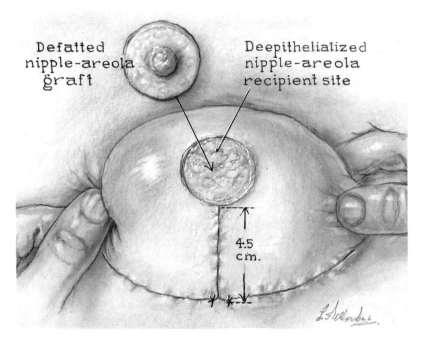

Fig 25-18. Deepithelialization of the recipient site for the nipple-areolar complex.

Deepithelialization of the Recipient Site for the Nipple-Areolar Complex (Figure 25-18)

Once the final site for the nipple-areolar complex is determined, the circle inscribed with the cookie cutter is deepithelialized, and as much dermis as possible is left. Hemostasis is obtained, and the wound is irrigated with saline solution. Complete hemostasis is necessary to ensure satisfactory attachment of the nipple-areolar complex to the underlying dermal bed. Blood clots or persistent bleeding will prevent graft survival. The nipple-areolar graft is inspected and defatted further if necessary. Then it is placed in position on the deepithelialized circle.

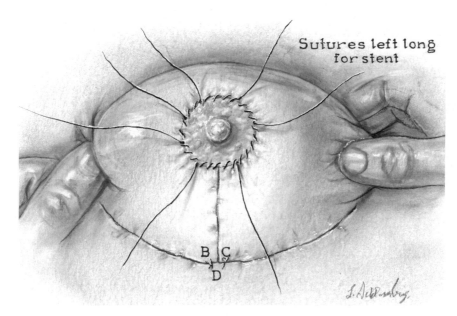

Fig 25-19. Suturing the nipple-areolar complex to the breast mound.

Suturing the Nipple-Areolar Complex to the Breast Mound (Figure 25-19)

The nipple-areolar complex should be sutured with a least eight non-absorbable sutures that are distributed evenly around the perimeter of the areola (as shown here). The sutures should be left long enough to permit them to be tied over a stent. A fine, running chromic suture then is placed around the periphery to complete the closure. Before this closure is finished, the undersurface of the graft is irrigated with saline solution to flush any residual blood clots. After the closure is complete, the graft is immobilized with a stent consisting of nonadherent gauze and moist cotton balls. The eight long sutures are tied over the stent to immobilize the graft.

Postoperative Care

Postoperative care consists of the application of antibiotic ointment to the incisions. An elastic sports brassiere is worn or a bulky dressing is applied. The dressing is removed in 2 to 3 days; however, the stent is left in place for 7 to 10 days. After the stent is removed, the patient can shower and resume moderate activities. The drains are removed when the drainage is less than 30 ml for a 24-hour period. Patients are typically discharged on the first day after surgery unless they are elderly or have had extensive resections that may result in significant blood loss and require more prolonged hospitalization.

26

Augmentation Mammoplasty

Introduction

Augmentation mammoplasty is a cosmetic procedure designed to enhance the size and contour of the breast. It involves placement of an implant beneath the breast either in a subglandular or a subpectoral position. In the past, silicone gel-filled implants and saline-filled implants have been used widely for augmentation mammoplasty. Ill-defined autoimmune symptoms developing in patients with silicone gel-filled implants have been reported; however, objective evidence that links these implants causally with rheumatologic disorders does not exist. Nevertheless, because of the controversy concerning complications associated with these prostheses, only saline-filled implants are available at present for augmentation mammoplasty.

Subglandular implants are preferable to subpectoral implants because they produce a more natural-appearing breast while also correcting minor or moderate ptosis. It is important to use implants with a textured surface, rather than a smooth surface, because the latter are associated with an increased incidence of capsular contractures.

However, an important advantage of the subpectoral position is that the implant is only partially in contact with the breast parenchyma and can be displaced away from the breast more easily. Therefore mammographic images of breast tissue are clearer when the implant is in the subpectoral position as compared with the subglandular location. There are two limitations to the use of subpectoral implants. Subpectoral augmentation alone will not correct ptotic changes, and subpectoral implants often produce unsatisfactory results in athletic women because their increased muscularity distorts the implant and the breast contour.

Periareolar, inframammary, or transaxillary incisions (shown in Figure 26-1) may be used for augmentation mammoplasty. A periareolar incision is best suited for augmentation when the areola is large (over 35 mm in diameter) and when the inframammary crease is poorly defined. The submammary or subpectoral spaces can be reached through a periareolar incision by incising directly through the breast parenchyma or by tunneling subcutaneously to the inferior margin of the breast. Subcutaneous tunneling avoids injury to the breast parenchyma, but gaining access to the pocket site may be difficult. An incision directly through the parenchyma gives excellent

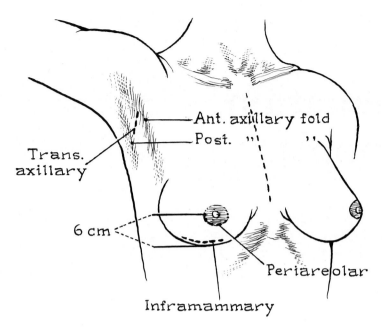

Fig 26-1. Incisions used for augmentation mammoplasty.

exposure to the entire pocket. However, division of ductal tissue may result in contamination of the implant pocket with *Staphylococcus epidermidis*, which is abundant in ductal secretions. Low-grade infections from this organism have been associated with the development of capsular contractures. A rare complication of the periareolar incision and subsequent approach through the breast parenchyma is lactation through the incision. The incidence of denervation of the nipple-areolar complex following a periareolar incision is the same for the transglandular and the subcutaneous tunnel approaches.

The inframammary approach, which does not involve division of breast tissue, is appropriate for either subglandular or subpectoral augmentation. The incision should be placed in or just above and parallel to the inframammary crease, 6 or 7 cm below the nipple, which will allow the nipple to be centered over the implant. If the existing inframammary crease needs to be lowered so that it will be at least 6 cm from the nipple, the incision should be planned to hide the scar. A 4- to 5-cm incision is adequate for the insertion of an implant. An inframammary incision should begin at or just lateral to a vertical line drawn inferiorly from the center of the nipple. The main disadvantages of the inframammary approach are that access to the upper quadrants of the breast pocket is limited and occasionally a noticeable scar is produced. Implant extrusion also is more frequent with this approach when compared with the transaxillary or periareolar approach.

The transaxillary approach should be used only for subpectoral augmentation. This incision leaves no scar on the breast, but the exposure of the pocket is poor. Some of the dissection must be performed blindly, and it is difficult to obtain hemostasis. Hematoma formation in the subpectoral space is rare, however. Creation of a symmetrical pocket and insertion and positioning of the implant also are more difficult through this incision. If a capsular contracture later requires open release, a second incision will be necessary. The intercostobrachial nerve is at risk of being injured during the dissection, and therefore it must be identified and protected.

Regardless of which incision is chosen for augmentation, precise positioning is important particularly for textured implants, which tend to adhere to the surrounding soft tissues. Occasionally, two implants are placed one on top of the other to gain projection. In such cases the smaller implant is placed beneath the larger one so that the curvature of the larger implant will mask the edges of the one beneath it. If only one breast is being augmented, the pocket should be configured and an implant size should be chosen to match the contralateral breast.

When a single surgeon is performing a bilateral augmentation, the implant pocket in one breast should be dissected and a sizing implant should be inserted to determine which size implant will provide satisfactory projection and cleavage without excessive tension on the skin. The adequacy of the pocket's size and configuration is assessed, and any irregularities are corrected. The other pocket then can be more precisely dissected and, with a sizing implant placed in the second pocket, the appearance of the breasts can be compared for symmetry. Any final modifications of the pockets can be made before the permanent implants are inserted. Before wound closure the symmetry of the breasts should be evaluated again from different perspectives by viewing the contour, size, position, and skin flow of the breasts while the patient is in both a semisitting and a supine position.

When two surgeons are operating and creating bilateral pockets at the same time, a careful evaluation for symmetry with the patient in a semisitting position is especially important.

Indications

The ideal candidate for augmentation is a patient with small breasts who desires a change in body image. Also women whose breasts have undergone substantial involution after pregnancy and lactation are good candidates for augmentation mammoplasty. Such individuals have usually had larger breasts and wish to maintain that size permanently.

Augmentation mammoplasty also is indicated to correct congenital breast asymmetry or to establish symmetry following breast reconstruction. Augmentation alone is the preferred treatment for correction of minor ptosis and for correction of moderate ptosis in patients who do not require skin excision and nipple elevation. The correction of breast ptosis is discussed in Chapter 27.

Contraindications

Women with a strong family history of breast cancer should probably be advised against augmentation because all currently available implants are radiopaque and may interfere with the mammographic detection of breast cancer. The procedure is also contraindicated in women who have psychiatric illness or other medical problems that make elective surgery unwise. Finally, augmentation mammoplasty alone is contraindicated for the correction of major ptosis, which always requires skin excision and nipple elevation, as well as insertion of an implant.

Complications

Bleeding is the most common early complication of augmentation mammoplasty, and approximately 5% of patients require reexploration for evacuation of a hematoma. Hematomas are more common when the implant is placed in the subglandular position. Factors predisposing to bleeding include aspirin ingestion, hypertension, postoperative emesis, and overexertion during the postoperative period. Evacuation of a hematoma should always be performed expeditiously under general anesthesia because delay may result in necrosis of the skin, the fat, or the nipple-areolar complex. Hematoma formation increases the incidence of infection and the subsequent development of capsular contracture.

Infections following augmentation can involve the superficial wound or the periprosthetic pocket. Superficial wound infections when treated by incision and drainage, local wound care, and antibiotics often resolve without removal of the prosthesis. Acute infections of the periprosthetic space, which may occur 5 to 10 days postoperatively, are usually caused by *Staphylococcus aureus*. Delayed infections, which may become evident weeks or even months after augmentation, are manifest by persistent pain, induration, and swelling. Acute and delayed infections are treated by implant removal, irrigation of the pocket with povidone-iodine solution, insertion of a vacuum drain, and parenteral antibiotics. The implant can be reinserted when the infection has resolved and when the tissues are soft and supple. The risk of infection may be decreased by irrigation of the pocket with an antibiotic solution before insertion of the implant.

The most common late complication of augmentation mammoplasty is capsular contracture, which can range from mild to severe. Factors associated with the development of capsular contracture include low-grade infections with *Staphylococcus epidermidis* and hematoma formation. Most capsular contractures occur within the first year of implant placement. Capsular contracture can be minimized by subpectoral placement, irrigation of the implant pocket with antimicrobial solutions at the time of implant insertion, and the use of textured, rather than smooth, implants.

Currently the treatment of established contractures requires reoperation. A contracture associated with a smooth implant in a subglandular position is treated by removing the implant, by performing capsulectomy, and by placing a textured implant in a subglandular or a subpectoral position. When a contracture develops with a smooth implant in a subpectoral position, the treatment is capsulectomy and replacement with a textured implant in the subpectoral location or placement of a subglandular textured implant. For contracture associated with a textured implant in a subglandular position the treatment is implant removal and replacement in a subpectoral location. Finally, when a contracture develops with a textured implant in a subpectoral position the implant is moved to a subglandular postion.

A long-term complication of smooth, gel-filled implants is periprosthetic capsular calcification, which occurs in about 20% of patients who have had implants in place for at least 10 years. Treatment is capsulectomy. The frequency of calcification in the presence of saline-filled implants is unknown.

Postoperative asymmetry may result from preexisting abnormalities or from malpositioned implants. Any preoperative asymmetry should be documented, and treatment options should be discussed with the patient. Asymmetry caused by uneven implant positioning or dissimilar inframammary creases results from technical errors and can be prevented by proper planning, precise dissection of the pockets, and careful comparison of both breasts when the sizing implants are in place. If an inframammary crease is too high, it can be easily corrected by enlarging the pocket inferiorly. A low inframammary crease is difficult to elevate, and proper correction may require removal of the implant and a repeat augmentation several months later. Inferior excision of the capsule with suturing of the skin to the chest wall also is used to correct this problem, although the results of this approach are often unsatisfactory. Asymmetry caused by migration of a prosthesis, usually inferiorly or laterally, almost always involves a smooth implant. Implant migration is corrected by capsulectomy and by repeat augmentation with a textured implant, which will better retain its position.

Subtle chest wall deformities and abnormally shaped breasts (such as those which are tubular, constricted, or markedly ptotic) may be more pronounced following augmentation. The considered correction of abnormalities should be discussed with the patient. Ptosis can be corrected with mastopexy and augmentation, but the added scarring associated with mastopexy is often unacceptable to the patient.

Most patients who undergo augmentation are willing to accept the resulting scars, but improper placement of incisions, depigmentation, and hypertrophy of scars can produce unsatisfactory results. Placement of the inframammary incision above or below the true inframammary crease can produce a noticeable scar. Periareolar incisions should be located at the periphery of the areolae. If the incision is placed inside the areola perimeter, the resulting scar will be depigmented. Although scar hypertrophy and keloid formation are uncommon following augmentation, patients who heal abnormally should be informed of these complications.

The risk of implant leakage or spontaneous rupture increases with time, but the overall risk appears to be only about 5% over the lifetime of an implant recipient. Rupture also can occur with trauma. Implant rupture is usually obvious from the change in size and shape of the breast. A ruptured gel-filled implant releases free silicone that must be removed promptly to prevent migration and formation of multiple granulomas. Implants can be replaced after the silicone has been extracted.

Inflatable implants may deflate because of valve failure or because of fold flaw failure. The latter occurs when a fold develops in the implant and its edges rub together until friction causes a rupture of the membrane. Saline-filled inflatable implants are associated with a noticeable deformity in the appearance of the skin overlying the upper quadrants of the breast. This *skin rippling* is related to the fluid dynamics of the saline and is most pronounced when the patient is in an upright position.

The onset of lactation following augmentation is rare and poorly understood. In most cases the lactation subsides spontaneously, but some patients require hormonal treatment.

Approximately 15% of patients have permanent alteration of sensation in the breast or the nipple following augmentation mammoplasty. Temporary alterations in sensation are common, and normal sensation usually returns in 2 or 3 months.

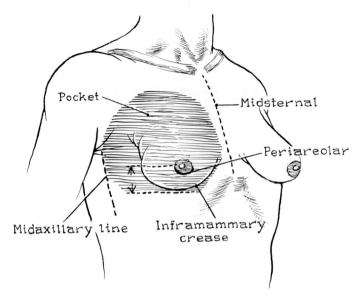

Fig 26-2. Preoperative marking.

Preoperative Preparation

A detailed medical history, particularly of any bleeding or rheumatologic disorders, is obtained, and current medication use is reviewed. Prior mammograms and biopsy reports are reviewed. A history of breast cancer in the family is questioned. The patient should be examined in the sitting and the supine positions. The presence and degree of ptosis and breast asymmetry, as well as the location of any scars, are recorded. The diameter of the areolae and the distance between the nipples and the suprasternal notch are measured. The flow of the breast is observed when the patient lies down because this natural mobility should be preserved after augmentation. The general shape of the patient's body and thoracic cage, as well as the proportions of her torso, are evaluated to help determine the ideal breast size and position. The appearance of a woman with a wide chest and breasts that seem too narrow can be improved when wider implants are used. The patient with a narrow chest will look better if the implants have a narrow base. While the appearance of obese women can be improved with augmentation, the operation may not produce ideal results because of abdominal fullness. Patients should be given a realistic assessment of the end result. The breasts are examined thoroughly to make certain that no masses are present.

Augmentation can be performed under local or general anesthesia. Local anesthesia, with subcutaneous and submammary infiltration or with an intercostal nerve block, usually requires supplementation with intravenous sedation. Prophylactic intravenous antibiotics are administered preoperatively.

Preoperative Marking (Figure 26-2)

Preoperative marking, except for the location of the incision, is essentially the same for all augmentation mammoplasty procedures. The midline of the sternum, the inframammary crease, and the proposed implant pocket are outlined with a marking pen or with brilliant green dye. The inframammary crease is marked while the patient is in an upright (sitting) position.

Most implants are 12 to 14 cm in diameter. If the original inframammary crease is less than 6 to 7 cm below the midpoint of the nipple, the crease should be lowered to center the nipple over the implant. If the nipple is not centered, the implant will appear too high. When the inframammary crease needs to be lowered, planning for its ideal location should initially be conservative; otherwise the implant pocket may be created too low, which will make the nipple appear too high. As the procedure progresses, the crease gradually can be lowered another centimeter or so until the best position is found. Usually the inframammary crease will be 7 cm below the nipple, but the exact measurement is less important than centering the nipple on the augmented breast mound. The implant pocket is marked while the patient is in a supine or semisitting position with her arms abducted. The pocket should extend superiorly to just beneath the clavicle, medially to within 1 or 2 cm lateral to the midline of the sternum, laterally to the midaxillary line, and inferiorly to the inframammary crease (or to a distance 7 cm below the nipple if this distance is greater). If a periareolar or transaxillary incision is to be used for implant placement, it is also marked.

The patient then is placed on the operating table in the supine position with both arms abducted. General anesthesia is induced, the skin is prepared with an appropriate antiseptic solution from the clavicle to the umbilicus, and sterile drapes are placed.

OPERATIVE PROCEDURE

Augmentation Mammoplasty 1: Subglandular Augmentation Through a Periareolar Incision

Creation of a Subglandular Pocket (Figure 26-3)

The periareolar incision extends from the 3 o'clock to the 9 o'clock positions at the junction of the pigmented areola and the nonpigmented breast skin. Either the transglandular approach or the subcutaneous approach can be used to gain access to the subglandular space. In the subcutaneous approach, as shown in Figure 26-3, *A*, a tunnel from the periareolar incision to the chest wall near the level of the inframammary crease is created by sharp dissection between the subcutaneous tissue and the breast tissue. When the inferior border of the breast tissue is reached, the breast parenchyma is elevated until the pectoralis fascia is encountered. Alternatively, in the transglandular approach, as shown in Figure 26-3, *B*, the dissection extends slightly inferior to the initial skin incision and then directly through the glandular tissue with sharp dissection to the pectoralis fascia.

With either approach, once the pectoralis fascia is reached, a pocket is created between the pectoralis major fascia and the breast parenchyma. Most of this subglandular pocket can be developed using blunt dissection with a finger to separate the tissue planes; however, some sharp dissection usually is required medially and inferiorly. Superiorly the pocket extends to just beneath the clavicle. Medially the dissection extends to 1 or 2 cm lateral to the sternal midline because dissection too close to the midline can result in tenting of the skin over the sternum (synmastia), which is difficult to correct. The distance from the nipple to the inframammary crease determines the

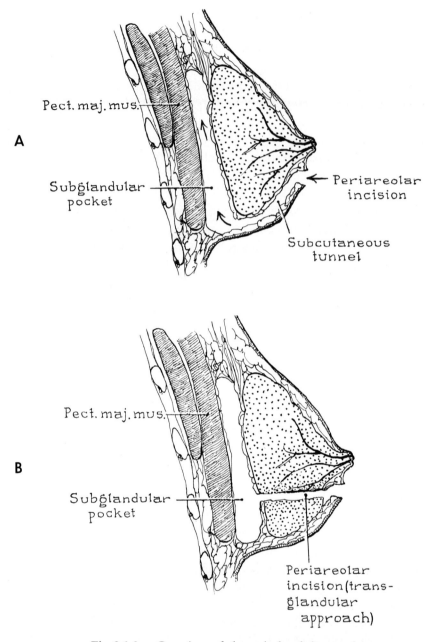

Pect. maj. mus.

A

Subglandular
pocket

Periareolar
incision

Subcutaneous
tunnel

Pect. maj. mus.

B

Subglandular
pocket

Periareolar
incision (trans-
glandular
approach)

Fig 26-3. Creation of the subglandular pocket.

lower extent of the dissection. If the nipple-to-crease distance is 6 to 7 cm or greater, the dissection stops at the original crease to preserve a normal fold and center the nipple on the augmented breast mound. When the nipple-to-crease distance is less than 6 cm, a new crease is established 6 or 7 cm below the nipple. Laterally the pocket extends to the midaxillary line. The final lateral dissection must be done cautiously to minimize the risk of injury to the sensory nerves that supply the nipple and breast.

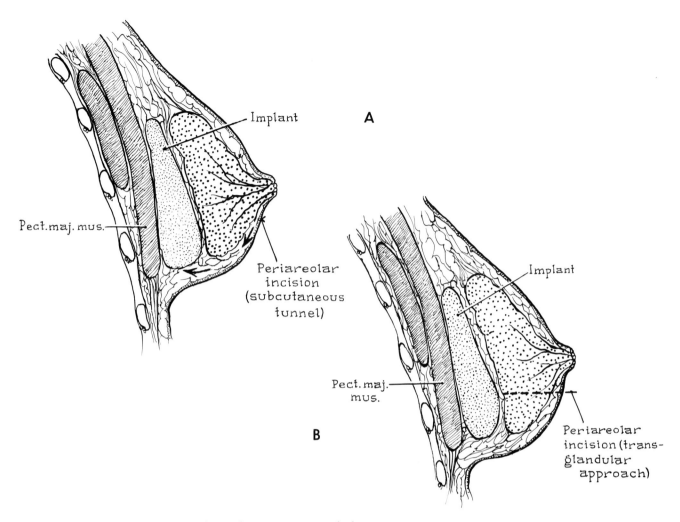

Fig 26-4. Implant placement; wound closure.

Implant Placement; Wound Closure (Figure 26-4)

When both pockets are symmetrically configured, the sizing implants are removed and the wounds are irrigated with saline solution and are assessed for any residual bleeding. The pockets then are irrigated with half-strength povidone-iodine solution. Before implant placement a constant vacuum drain is inserted into the pocket to prevent the accumulation of serum and blood around the implant. The drain is brought out through a separate stab wound in a minimally visible area of the axilla. The deflated implant is inserted through the subcutaneous tunnel, as shown in Figure 26-4, *A*, or through the transglandular tunnel, as shown in Figure 26-4, *B*, inflated with saline solution, and positioned in the pocket. Before the wound is closed, symmetry of the contour, size, and position of the breasts is evaluated carefully, while the patient is placed in an upright position and then in a supine position. If necessary final adjustments are made in the pockets or in the placement of the implants. The superficial fascia just beneath the dermis is closed with a layer of absorbable sutures, and the skin is closed with a layer of intracuticular running sutures. The skin closure can be reinforced with adhesive paper strips. Nonadherent gauze is placed over the incision and is covered by a layer of gauze sponges with a central hole for the nipple. The dressing is secured with tape.

Augmentation Mammoplasty 2: Subpectoral Augmentation through a Periareolar Incision

Location of the Subpectoral Pocket (Figure 26-5)

The superomedial aspect of the implant pocket that is to be developed through the marked periareolar incision will underlie the pectoralis major muscle. Inferolaterally and beyond the lateral border of the pectoralis muscle the implant will overlie the serratus anterior muscle in a subcutaneous location. The margins for development of the subpectoral pocket and the subglandular pocket are essentially the same. The pocket extends medially to 1 to 2 cm lateral to the sternum, superiorly to the infraclavicular region, laterally almost to the midaxillary line, and inferiorly to the inframammary crease.

The patient then is placed on the operating table in the supine position with both arms abducted. General anesthesia is induced, the skin is prepared with an appropriate antiseptic solution from the clavicle to the umbilicus, and sterile drapes are placed.

Exposure of the Lateral Border of the Pectoralis Major Muscle (Figure 26-6)

After the periareolar incision is made, a subcutaneous tunnel from the skin to the inferior border of the breast parenchyma is created by sharp dissection, which separates the subcutaneous tissue from the breast. The glandular tissue then is elevated until the pectoralis major muscle is exposed, and its lateral border identified by direct vision. Alternatively a transglandular dissection by sharp division of the breast parenchyma from the skin to the pectoralis fascia can be used. When the fascia is exposed, the dissection is extended inferiorly and laterally until the lateral border of the pectoralis major muscle is identified.

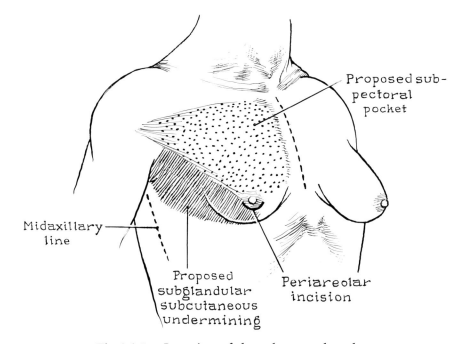

Fig 26-5.   Location of the subpectoral pocket.

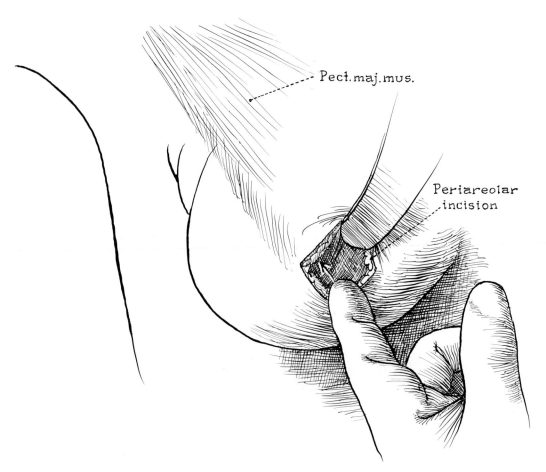

Fig 26-6.   Exposure of the lateral border of the pectoralis major muscle.

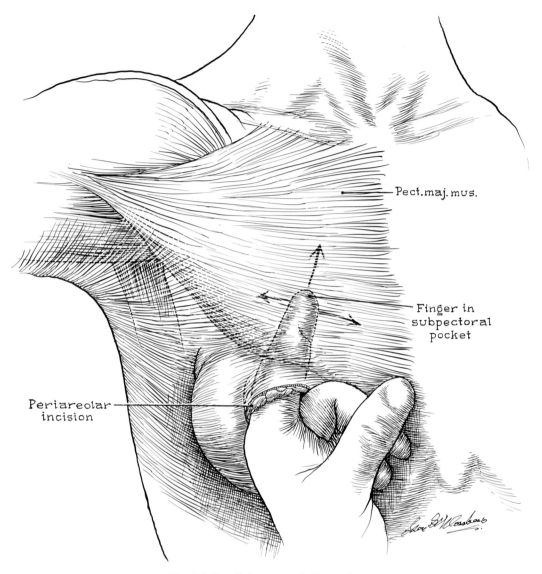

Fig 26-7. Subpectoral dissection.

Subpectoral Dissection (Figure 26-7)

Once the lateral edge of the pectoralis major muscle has been identified, the pectoralis fascia that overlies the muscle along its lateral border is incised. Then a finger is inserted beneath the muscle. A subpectoral pocket for the implant, which corresponds to the limits of the preoperative markings, is created by blunt dissection. During dissection laterally, care must be taken to avoid injury to the intercostal neurovascular bundles—particularly the fourth intercostal bundle, which is the major sensory nerve of the nipple-areolar complex. Use of only blunt dissection for creation of the pocket will minimize the risk of nerve injury.

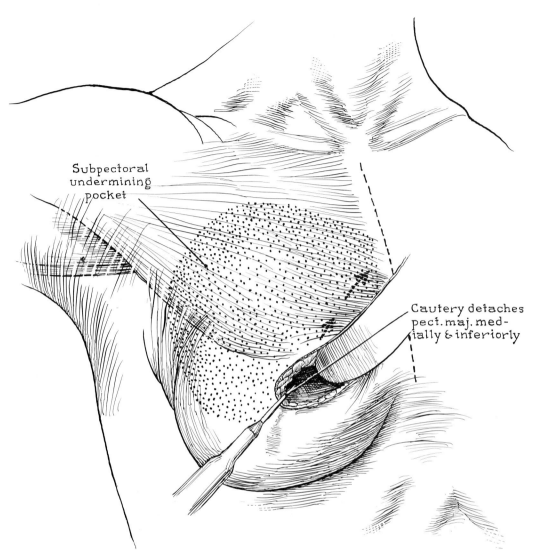

Subpectoral
undermining
pocket

Cautery detaches
pect. maj. med-
ially & inferiorly

Fig 26-8. Inferomedial detachment of the pectoralis major muscle.

Inferiomedial Detachment of the Pectoralis Major Muscle (Figure 26-8)

After the preliminary pocket is dissected, a sizing implant is inserted to assess the size and configuration of the pocket. Frequently the implant appears tight and constricted medially and inferiorly, and the sternal and costal attachments of the pectoralis major muscle must be divided. To enlarge the pocket the pectoralis major muscle fibers are detached inferiorly and medially from their costal and sternal origins by use of the electrocautery. Only the muscle fibers are divided. Fibers are detached until the constricted and tight appearance of the inferior and medial area of the pocket is relieved and a sizing implant fits appropriately in position. As perforating branches from the internal mammary artery are identified, they are carefully secured either with ligation or electrocoagulation and then divided. The fat and subcutaneous tissue medial to the origin of the pectoralis major are left attached to the sternum to prevent synmastia.

Completion of the Pocket (Figure 26-9)

Because the creation of a complete submusculofascial pocket would require mobilization of the serratus anterior muscle, a totally submuscular pocket is not routinely used for augmentation mammoplasty. Instead, most of the implant will be positioned beneath the pectoralis major muscle, and some of it will lie in a subglandular subcutaneous pocket that is lateral and inferior to the pectoralis major.

When the subcutaneous portion of the implant pocket is created, most of the dissection is done bluntly to minimize the risk of neurovascular injury. However, in the lateral portion of the pocket beneath the subcutaneous tissue, sharp dissection is needed to complete the pocket. The scissors are held to position the blades parallel to the intercostal nerves, which run from lateral to medial. The blades are spread vertically and the tissue is divided gently until the pocket is gradually enlarged to the midaxillary line. The subglandular and submuscular components of the completed pocket are illustrated in Figure 26-9, *A*. Figure 26-9, *B,* shows a sagittal view of the completed pocket to demonstrate its relationship to the pectoralis major and pectoralis minor muscles. After the pocket dissection is completed, a sizing implant is inserted and the adequacy and configuration of the pocket are assessed and modified as required to obtain a symmetrical appearance.

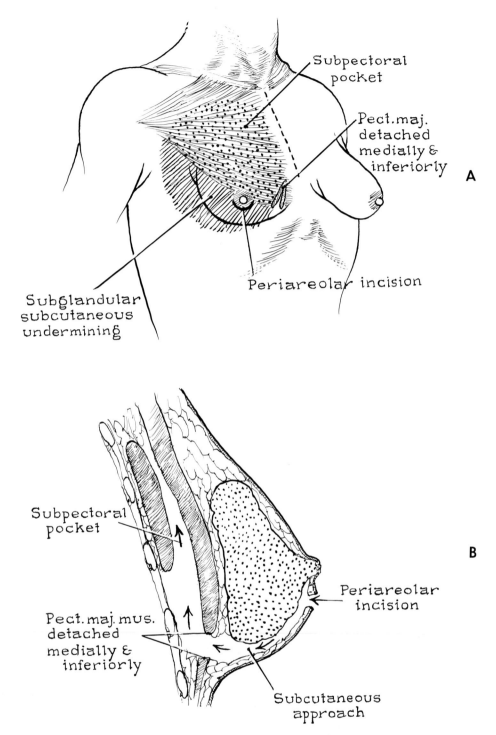

Subpectoral pocket

Pect.maj. detached medially & inferiorly

A

Periareolar incision

Subglandular subcutaneous undermining

Subpectoral pocket

B

Periareolar incision

Pect.maj.mus. detached medially & inferiorly

Subcutaneous approach

Fig 26-9. Completion of the pocket.

Sagittal Section of the Chest Wall with Subpectoral Implant
(Figure 26-10)

Figure 26-10, *A*, illustrates the subpectoral placement of an implant inserted through a periareolar incision by the subcutaneous approach, and Figure 26-10, *B*, illustrates the transglandular approach.

After the sizing implant is removed, the pocket is irrigated with saline solution followed by half-strength povidone-iodine solution, and complete hemostasis is achieved. The patient is placed in a semisitting position, and breast symmetry is assessed again. A constant vacuum drain is placed in the implant pocket and is brought out through a separate stab wound in a minimally visible area of the axilla. An appropriately sized permanent implant is inserted, inflated, and properly positioned. After symmetry is evaluated again, the superficial fascia is closed with a layer of absorbable sutures. A running intracuticular suture is used to close the skin incision. The skin closure can be reinforced with adhesive paper strips. The incision is dressed with nonadherent gauze, and gauze sponges with a hole for the nipple are placed over the breast. The dressing is secured with tape.

Augmentation Mammoplasty 3: Subglandular Augmentation Through an Inframammary Incision
Skin Marking; Creation of a Subglandular Pocket (Figure 26-11)

The primary landmarks, the location of the incision, and the borders of the subglandular implant pocket are shown. After marking, the patient is placed on the operating table in the supine position with both arms abducted. General anesthesia is induced, the skin is prepared from the clavicle to the umbilicus with an appropriate antiseptic solution, and sterile drapes are placed. The skin incision is made at or just lateral to a vertical line drawn inferiorly from the center of the nipple. The incision continues laterally and curves to match the inframammary crease for about 5 or 6 cm. If necessary the incision is placed below the existing inframammary crease (as shown here) so that the distance between the nipple and the new inframammary crease will be 6 to 7 cm.

The skin incision is deepened inferior to the glandular tissue and is extended to the chest wall to expose the serratus anterior and pectoralis major muscles. The lateral margin of the pectoralis major is identified. Then sharp and blunt dissection are used to create an adequate subglandular pocket, with care taken to avoid subpectoral dissection. The superior extent of the pocket lies just below the clavicle, with the lateral margin anterior to the midaxillary line. The medial dissection ends 1 or 2 cm lateral to the midline of the sternum. Inferiorly, the pocket extends to the inframammary crease or to 6 cm below the nipple if the inframammary crease needs to be lowered.

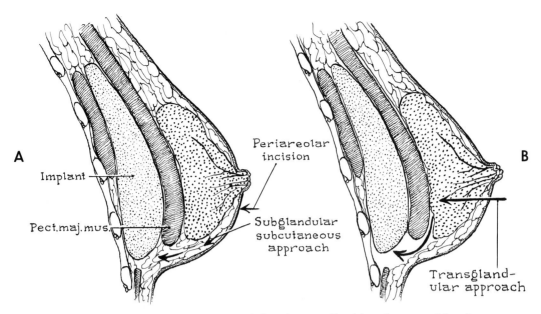

Fig 26-10.   Sagittal section of the chest wall with subpectoral implant.

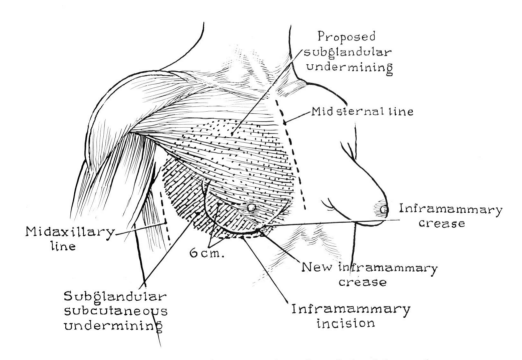

Fig 26-11.   Skin marking; creation of a subglandular pocket.

Sagittal Section of Chest Wall with Subglandular Implant
(Figure 26-12)

After the subglandular pocket is created and the sizing implant is inserted, final adjustments in the pocket size and configuration are made to achieve symmetry. An appropriate sized implant is then selected. The pocket is irrigated with saline solution followed by half-strength povidone-iodine solution, and complete hemostasis is achieved. Before implant placement a constant vaccum drain is inserted into the pocket and brought out through a stab wound in the axilla. The implant is inserted, inflated, and carefully positioned to ensure that the implant's inferior edge will lie at the postoperative inframammary crease and that the nipple will be centered on the augmented breast mound.

Once the implant is positioned properly, the patient is placed in a semi-sitting position and the breasts are again evaluated for symmetry. The superficial fascia is closed with interrupted absorbable sutures followed by a running subcuticular closure of the skin with adhesive paper strip reinforcement. A dressing consisting of nonadherent gauze is placed over the incision and secured with tape.

Augmentation Mammoplasty 4: Subpectoral Augmentation Through an Inframammary Incision
Marking; Incision Placement (Figure 26-13)

The operative landmarks and relationships of the subpectoral and subglandular subcutaneous portions of the pocket for subpectoral augmentation are shown. The guidelines for incision placement and for extent of the chest wall dissection for the implant pocket were described in Figure 26-2. After marking, the patient is placed on the operating table in the supine position with both arms abducted. General anesthesia is induced, the skin is prepared from the clavicles to the umbilicus with an appropriate antiseptic solution, and sterile drapes are placed.

The initial inframammary crease incision is made and is deepened to the chest wall. Blunt subglandular dissection proceeds superiorly and medially until the lateral border of the pectoralis major muscle is identified. The pectoralis fascia is sharply incised to expose the subpectoral space.

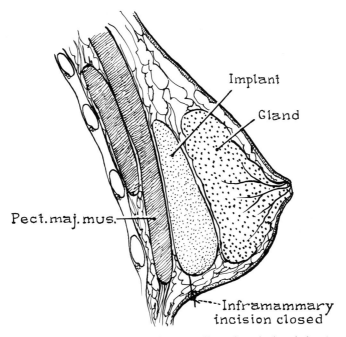

Fig 26-12. Sagittal section of chest wall with subglandular implant.

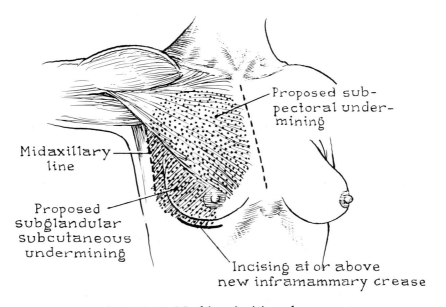

Fig 26-13. Marking; incision placement.

Creation of a Subpectoral Pocket (Figure 26-14)

With the subpectoral space exposed, most of the implant pocket is easily created by blunt dissection beneath the pectoralis major muscle. The pocket is extended superiorly to just below the clavicle, medially to approximately 2 cm lateral to the midline of the sternum, and inferiorly to the planned level of the inframammary crease.

In the area between the midaxillary line and the lateral border of the pectoralis major muscle, sharp dissection may be necessary to create the subcutaneous portion of the subglandular pocket. Scissors are used with the blades lying parallel to the intercostal nerves, which run from lateral to medial. The blades are spread vertically, and the remaining tissue is divided gently until the pocket is gradually enlarged to the midaxillary line. This technique will decrease the risk of damage to the intercostal nerves, which are vulnerable in the area between the lateral border of the pectoralis major and the midaxillary line.

Division of the Pectoralis Major Muscle (Figure 26-15)

After dissection of the preliminary pocket is performed, a sizing implant is inserted to assess the size and configuration of the pocket. Frequently the implant appears tight and constricted medially and inferiorly, and the sternal and costal attachments of the pectoralis major muscle must be divided. Using the electrocautery the pectoralis major muscle fibers are detached inferiorly and medially from their costal and sternal origins to release the pocket. Only the muscle fibers are divided. Fibers are detached until the constricted and tight inferior and medial area of the pocket is relieved with a sizing implant in position. As perforating branches from the internal mammary artery are identified, they are carefully secured, either by ligation and division or by electrocoagulation. The fat and subcutaneous tissue beyond the origin of the pectoralis major are left attached to the sternum to prevent synmastia.

As previously described for subpectoral augmentation through a peri-areolar incision in Figure 26-9, the lateral portion of the pocket is developed subcutaneously to the midaxillary line. Total submusculofascial coverage of an implant for augmentation mammoplasty is unnecessary.

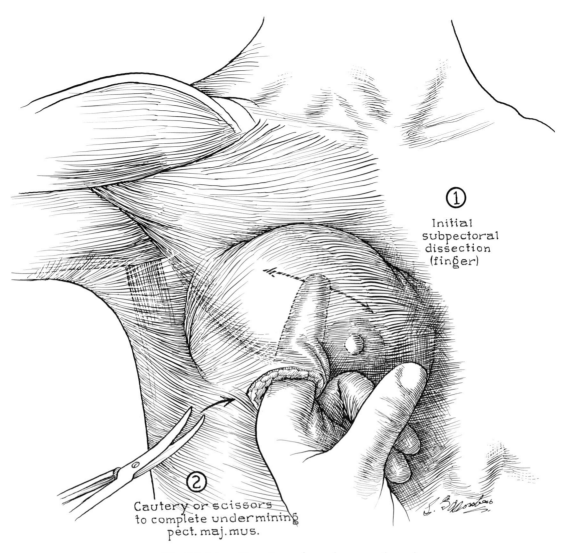

① Initial subpectoral dissection (finger)

② Cautery or scissors to complete undermining pect. maj. mus.

Fig 26-14.   Creation of a subpectoral pocket.

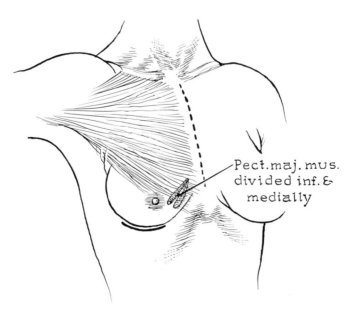

Pect. maj. mus. divided inf. & medially

Fig 26-15.   Division of the pectoralis major muscle.

341

Sagittal Section of Chest Wall with Subpectoral Implant
(Figure 26-16)

A sizing implant should be inserted to assess the pocket size and configuration. With the pocket dissected and the sizing implant in position, symmetry is assessed again and any final modifications are made before insertion of the permanent implant. After an appropriately sized permanent implant is selected, the sizer is removed, the pocket is irrigated with saline solution and half-strength povidone-iodine solution, and hemostasis is achieved. Before implant insertion a constant vacuum drain is inserted and brought out through a stab wound in the axilla.

The implant is inserted, inflated, and positioned to lie smoothly in the pocket. Its inferior edge is at the level of the postoperative inframammary crease, and the nipple is centered on the breast mound. The symmetry of the breasts is again evaluated, while the patient is in a semisitting position. The inframammary crease wound is closed in layers by approximation of the superficial fascia with interrupted absorbable sutures followed by a running subcuticular closure of the skin that is reinforced with adhesive paper strips. A sterile dressing of nonadherent gauze is secured over the closed incision.

Augmentation Mammoplasty 5: Subpectoral Augmentation Through a Transaxillary Incision

Skin Marking; Location of the Implant Pocket (Figure 26-17)

The operative landmarks and the outline of the pocket, which are marked before the beginning of the procedure, are shown. Proper marking of the inframammary crease placed 6 to 7 cm below the nipple is particularly critical with the transaxillary approach because changing the position of the inframammary crease through the transaxillary incision is impossible if the crease is made too low. The margins for the area of dissection for the implant pocket are the same as described in Figure 26-2. The intercostobrachial nerve lies in close proximity to the transaxillary incision. After marking, the patient is placed on the operating table in the supine position with both arms abducted. General anesthesia is induced, the skin is prepared with an appropriate antiseptic solution from the clavicle to the umbilicus, and sterile drapes are placed.

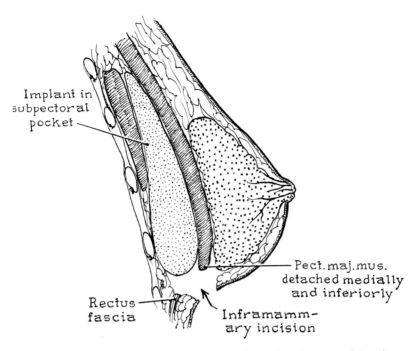

Implant in subpectoral pocket

Pect. maj. mus. detached medially and inferiorly

Rectus fascia

Inframamm-ary incision

Fig 26-16.   Sagittal section of chest wall with subpectoral implant.

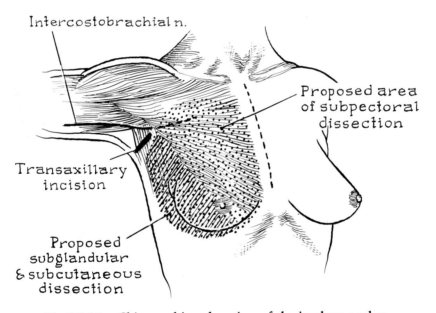

Intercostobrachial n.

Proposed area of subpectoral dissection

Transaxillary incision

Proposed subglandular & subcutaneous dissection

Fig 26-17.   Skin marking; location of the implant pocket.

Creation of the Subpectoral Pocket (Figure 26-18)

A 5-cm transverse incision is made starting just behind the anterioax-illary fold and extending obliquely across the hair-bearing portion of the axilla. The incision is high enough in the axilla so that the scar will be well concealed. Once the initial skin incision has been made, the lateral border of the pectoralis major muscle is identified by palpation. The incision then is deepened through the subcutaneous tissue to expose the intercostobrachial nerve. Inadvertent injury to the intercostobrachial nerve is avoided by the use of blunt dissection until the nerve is visualized in the operative field. Sharp and blunt dissection then is used to expose the lateral border of the pectoralis major muscle. The pectoralis fascia is sharply incised to allow insertion of a finger or blunt instrument in the subpectoral space. The implant pocket constructed through a transaxillary incision is created blindly. The majority of the subpectoral pocket can be developed by finger dissection.

Completed Dissection of the Pocket (Figure 26-19)

A urethral sound or a comparable blunt instrument then is used to dissect the inferior and the medial portions of the subpectoral pocket by detaching the costal and sternal origins of the pectoralis major. The progress of the dissection should be evaluated frequently by assessing the position of the urethral sound in relation to the proposed pocket margins that are marked preoperatively. A sizing implant also can be inserted intermittently during the pocket dissection and can be moved to delineate the pocket margins and to identify any irregularities.

Through a transaxillary approach difficulties may be encountered with dissection in establishing the correct position of the inframammary crease. When the inferior portion of the subpectoral pocket is created, the dissection must not extend below the desired level of the inframammary crease because a separate incision then would be necessary to subsequently raise the crease. After the muscle is detached medially, the lateral subcutaneous portion of the pocket is created bluntly with the urethral sound. The use of blunt dissection alone minimizes the risk of damage to the intercostal nerves during the creation of the lateral portion of the implant pocket.

After the dissection has been completed, the pocket is irrigated with saline solution. If any bleeding occurs, pressure is applied to the chest for 5 minutes. When significant bleeding persists (a rare occurrence), an infra-mammary incision may be required for adequate exposure to obtain he-mostasis. Once complete hemostasis is obtained, the pocket is irrigated with half-strength povidone-iodine solution. A sizing implant then is inserted and manipulated to determine the configuration of the pocket, to detect any irregularities, and to select the properly sized implant. Symmetry is checked when the patient is in a semisitting position. Minor changes in pocket con-figuration or correction of pocket irregularities are completed by using the urethral sound. The sizing implant is then removed, and the wound is irri-gated again with half-strength povidone-iodine solution. The permanent im-plant is inserted, inflated, and properly positioned. In contrast to the other approaches to implant insertion that have been described here, drains are not routinely used with insertion of a transaxillary implant.

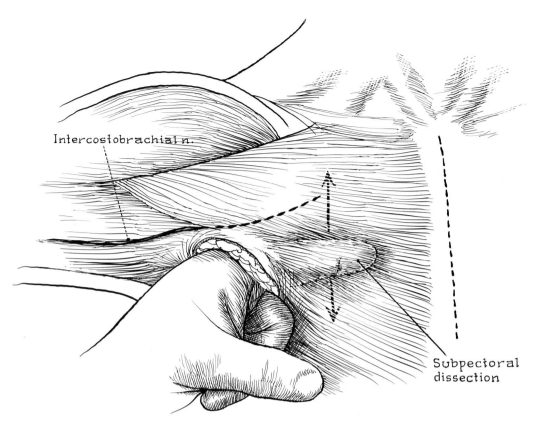

Fig 26-18.   Creation of the subpectoral pocket.

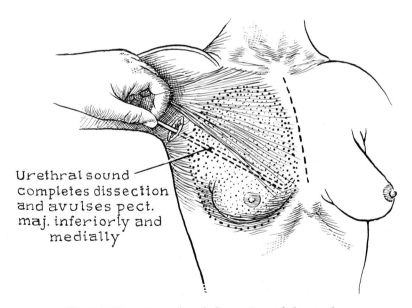

Fig 26-19.   Completed dissection of the pocket.

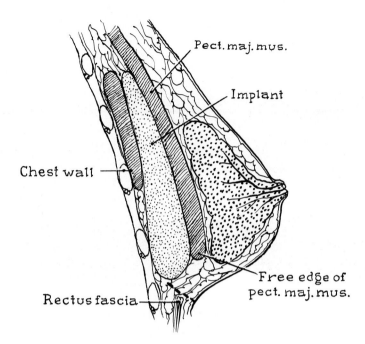

Fig 26-20. Sagittal section of chest wall with subpectoral implant.

Sagittal Section of Chest Wall with Subpectoral Implant
(Figure 26-20)

After the implant is inserted and positioned, the inferior margin of the implant should lie at the inframammary crease (indicated by the dashed line in the figure) and the nipple should be centered on the implant. After both implants are positioned, symmetry and configuration of the breasts are checked again while the patient is in a semisitting position. The axillary incision then is closed with running subcuticular absorbable sutures. The incision is reinforced with adhesive paper strips, and a sterile gauze dressing is taped over it.

Postoperative Care

The patient can be discharged from the outpatient recovery center when she is alert and is tolerating liquids. Oral analgesics are prescribed for pain. The patient is instructed to remain in bed overnight and to contact the surgeon if severe unilateral pain or swelling develops. She is instructed in drain care if drains were placed. The patient returns to the office in 3 to 5 days for evaluation and drain removal. She should wear a properly fitting and lightly supportive sports brassiere for 6 weeks. She is reexamined periodically during the first month for postoperative complications. All patients should be followed at least annually thereafter, and a mammogram should be obtained at intervals as indicated.

27

Management of Ptosis

Introduction

Breast ptosis is defined as inferior displacement of the nipple-areolar complex in relation to the clavicle and suprasternal notch. The condition is part of the aging process and results from glandular atrophy, loss of skin elasticity, and weakness of the ligamentous supportive structures of the breast. Ptosis is enhanced by pregnancy within its associated glandular hypertrophy and subsequent atrophy. The overall effect of these changes is unesthetic drooping or sagging of the breasts.

In the youthful breast the nipple is usually at the level of the fourth rib, as shown in Figure 27-1, *A*. The junction between the youthful breast and chest wall is indistinct, and the inframammary crease is not well defined. All the breast lies above the point where the inferior portion of the breast joins the chest wall. The lower defining point of the breast mound is usually at the sixth rib, and most of the breast mass overlies the pectoralis major muscle.

Women who are over age 30 or who have had at least one pregnancy and subsequent glandular atrophy are considered to have mature breasts. In the mature breast the nipple-areolar complex is usually at the level of the fifth rib and a well-defined inframammary crease typically lies at the level of the seventh rib (Figure 27-1, *B*). In general the breast's inferior aspect has a convex contour, and the breast mound above the nipple has a gentle slope. Most of the breast mass still overlies the pectoralis major muscle.

Breast ptosis is classified by the relationship of the nipple to the breast parenchyma with respect to the inframammary crease. The inframammary crease remains constant, usually at the level of the seventh rib, but the locations of the nipple-areolar complex and the breast parenchyma change as ptosis progresses. In addition, some degree of drooping exists in all grades of ptosis. Drooping makes the breast appear lower than normal and makes the upper portion of the breast look flattened.

The initial ptotic changes are classified as minor ptosis (grade 1), as shown in Figure 27-2, *A*. The nipple is located at the level of the inframammary crease. Although a significant portion of the breast lies below the inframammary crease, the nipple-areolar complex still is superior to a portion of the breast mass. As changes progress to moderate, or grade 2 ptosis, the nipple-areolar complex and a large portion of the breast parenchyma have

347

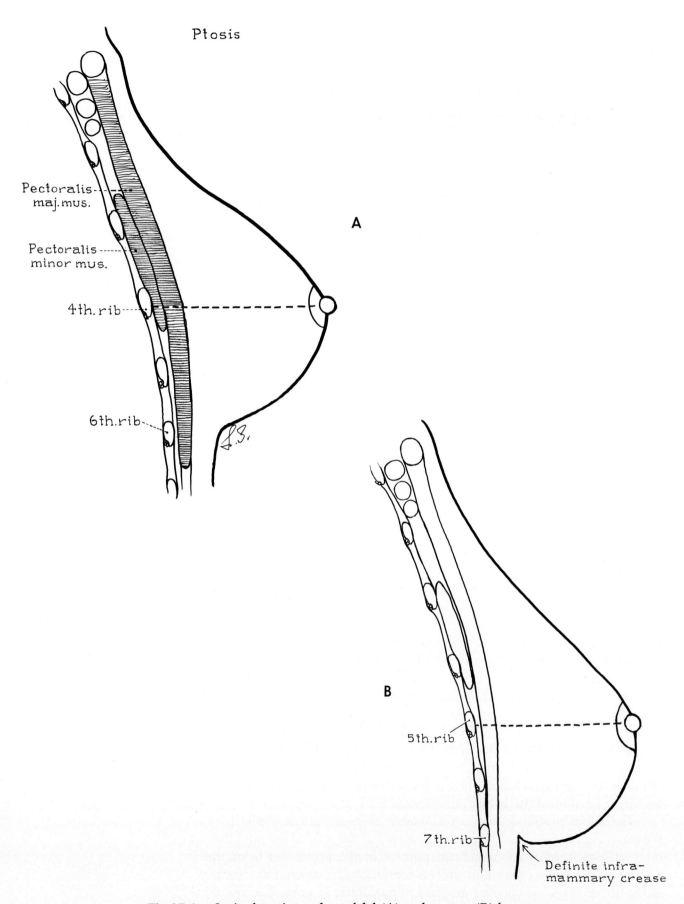

Ptosis

Pectoralis
maj. mus.

Pectoralis
minor mus.

4th. rib

6th. rib

A

B

5th. rib

7th. rib

Definite infra-
mammary crease

Fig 27-1. Sagittal sections of youthful (A) and mature (B) breasts.

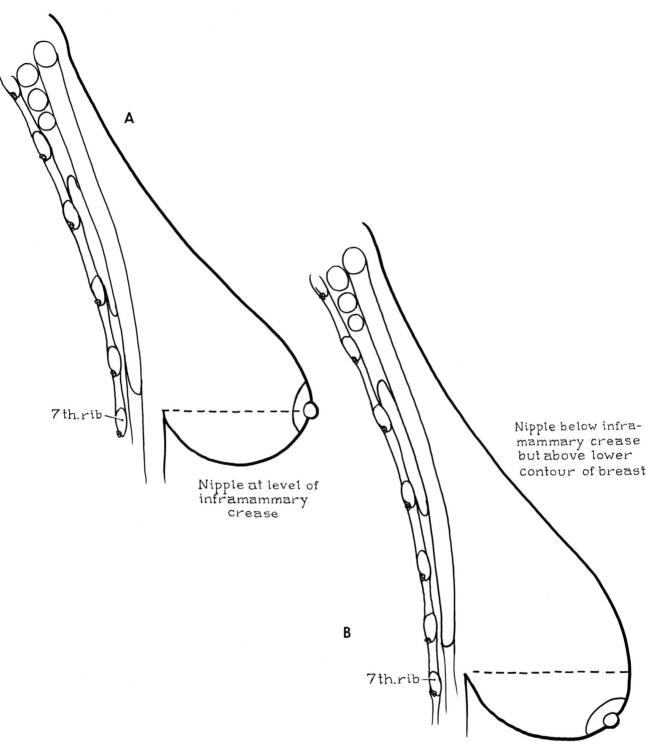

A

7th. rib

Nipple at level of
inframammary
crease

Nipple below infra-
mammary crease
but above lower
contour of breast

B

7th. rib

Fig 27-2.   Sagittal sections of breasts with A, minor ptosis and B, moderate
ptosis.

Continued.

moved below the inframammary crease and a small amount of breast tissue
still lies inferior to the nipple, as shown in Figure 27-2, *B*. There is a moderate
excess of skin in proportion to glandular tissue. In major ptosis (Grade 3)
the nipple-areolar complex lies inferior to virtually all of the breast paren-

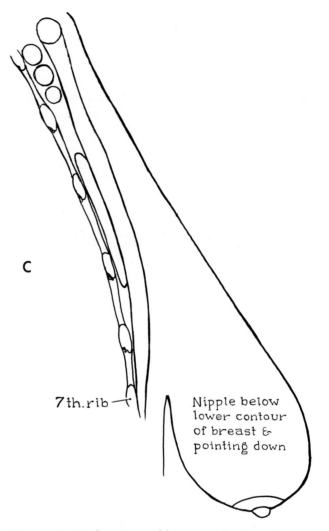

C

7th.rib ─┬

Nipple below
lower contour
of breast &
pointing down

Fig 27-2.   Sagittal section of breast with C, major ptosis.

chyma. Most of the breast and the nipple-areolar complex lie inferior to the inframammary crease (Figure 27–2, C).

Pseudoptosis and glandular ptosis are two other conditions that are characterized by an excess of skin in the portion of the breast inferior to the nipple-areolar complex. In pseudoptosis the nipple-areolar complex remains in its normal position, usually at the fourth or fifth rib, but most of the glandular tissue lies beneath the nipple-areolar complex and some lies below the inframammary crease as shown in Figure 27-3, A. Typically a well-defined inframammary crease is located at or slightly inferior to the level of the seventh rib. The breast mound possesses an abnormally full and convex contour below the nipple, but the breast has a normal slope above the nipple. In glandular ptosis the nipple-areolar complex is located in a relatively normal position at or about the fifth rib level, as shown in Figure 27-3, B. Below this complex the breast mound has a convex curvature, but only a minimal portion of the glandular tissue lies below the inframammary crease.

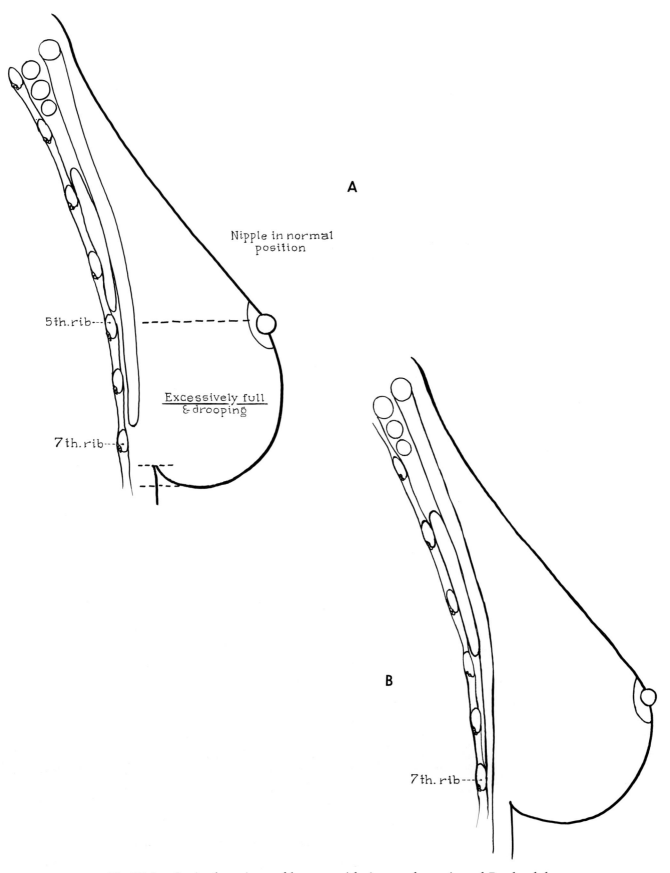

Fig 27-3.   Sagittal sections of breasts with A, pseudoptosis and B, glandular ptosis.

Minor ptosis almost always can be corrected by augmentation alone with placement of an implant in the subglandular position. Textured implants are preferred for correction of ptosis. To correct moderate ptosis, the skin envelope must be filled and the projection of the nipple-areolar complex must be enhanced. This may be done by inserting an implant, by skin excision, or by both. Use of a textured implant with a narrow base diameter and a high profile will usually increase the projection of the nipple and areola on the breast mound, while an implant with a large base diameter will tend to enlarge the overall breast diameter but produce less nipple-areolar projection. A high profile implant that is placed over a low-profile, large-base diameter implant will fill the breast envelope and enhance nipple-areolar projection. In achieving a naturally shaped breast, this combination of implants often is better than a single implant; however, combining the two implants will substantially increase the breast size. If the patient is concerned about the large breast size, the ptosis may be corrected by skin excision. The correction of major ptosis, pseudoptosis, or glandular ptosis always requires skin excision. In procedures where tissue is resected the cosmetic results can usually be enhanced by the insertion of an implant to modify the breast contour.

Indications

Mastopexy to produce a rounder and a firmer breast with improved projection and proper nipple-areolar positioning is primarily a cosmetic procedure to correct breast sagging. The procedure also may be used to correct asymmetry that results from a congenital deformity or to restore symmetry in conjunction with breast reconstruction. Following mastectomy, mastopexy is often performed on a contralateral ptotic breast as a second-stage procedure after the reconstructed breast mound has attained its final contour.

Contraindications

Mastopexy is contraindicated in patients who have pulmonary, cardiac, renal, or other systemic problems that would preclude the safe administration of general anesthesia. Correction of ptosis with an implant, which can obscure suspicious lesions on mammography, may be inappropriate for the patient with a strong family history of breast cancer. Results of mastopexy often are poor in obese women. Tobacco smoking is a contraindication to correction of major ptosis.

Complications

Patients who are to receive an implant as part of the mastopexy should be informed of the potential risks associated with implants, including contracture formation, rupture, and the impaired interpretation of mammograms.

Patients having mastopexy also should be informed that ptosis can only be corrected temporarily and that the condition usually recurs because of progressive aging, pregnancy, or weight fluctuation. Because a repeat procedure may be necessary to correct ptosis, the surgeon should carefully plan and execute the initial operation accordingly. Women who have moderate or major ptosis should be told that following correction the inferior half of the breast will appear boxy. After correction of major ptosis the breast rarely looks normal or naturally youthful, although some contour irregularities improve with time.

Mastopexy can improve the breast shape and position, but it is inevitably accompanied by scarring. Substantial risks are associated with the correction of moderate or major ptosis. Undermining of the skin can cause delayed healing and necrosis of the skin, fat, and nipple-areolar complex. Infection is uncommon, and usually responds to antibiotic therapy.

Preoperative Preparation

Mastopexy procedures usually are performed on an outpatient basis, with the patient under general anesthesia. Prophylactic perioperative antibiotics are routinely administered to patients receiving breast implants. For all mastopexy procedures the patient is marked and then placed on the operating table in a supine position with both arms abducted on arm boards. After general anesthesia is induced, both breasts are prepared and draped in a sterile field for correction of unilateral or bilateral ptosis. Later the patient is placed in a semisitting position to assess the implant's position and the breast symmetry.

OPERATIVE PROCEDURE

Correction of Minor Ptosis

Insertion of a Subglandular Implant (Figure 27-4)

The breast augmentation procedures described in Chapter 26 may be used to correct minor ptosis. The inframammary approach with subglandular postioning of the implant (as shown) usually is associated with minimal scarring and gives the most satisfactory result. An incision is made in the inframammary crease, and dissection is deepened to the chest wall until the fascia overlying the pectoralis major muscle is visualized. Blunt and sharp dissection then is used to create a subglandular pocket large enough to receive the selected implant. The pocket should extend superiorly to just below the clavicle, laterally to the midaxillary line, medially to within 1 or 2 cm lateral to the midline of the sternum, and inferiorly to the inframammary crease.

After dissection of the subglandular pocket is completed, a sizing implant is inserted and final adjustments in pocket size and configuration are made. The pocket then is irrigated with saline solution and half-strength povidone-iodine solution, and complete hemostasis is achieved. A constant vacuum drain is inserted before insertion of the implant to minimize the collection of blood and serum around the implant, which can interfere with tissue adherence to the textured surface. The drain is brought out through a stab wound in the axilla. The implant then is inserted and inflated. Textured implants usually project more and are slightly larger than the smooth implants. When a textured implant is used, it should be soaked first in saline solution or in povidone-iodine solution to facilitate insertion. After insertion the implant must lie flat in the pocket with no folding or crumpling. The incision is closed by approximation of the superficial fascia with interrupted absorbable sutures followed by a running subcuticular closure of the skin. The incision is dressed with a sterile gauze bandage. After placement of the implant the superior aspect of the breast has a full contour and the nipple-areolar complex has been elevated to lie at the level of the fifth rib.

Correction of Moderate Ptosis

Marking for Elevation of the Nipple-Areolar Complex (Figure 27-5)

Correction of moderate ptosis, with elevation of the nipple-areolar complex and reduction of the areolar size, often requires excision of a vertical ellipse of skin, as well as insertion of an implant.

The patient is marked before surgery, while she is in a sitting or standing position. The new location of the nipple-areola complex and the existing locations of the breast meridian, the inframammary crease, and the midpoint of the inframammary crease are marked. The positions of these points will change when the patient is supine.

The breast meridian is identified by drawing a line from the midpoint of the clavicle through the nipple to the midpoint of the inframammary crease. To define the new location of the nipple, a point between 18 to 22 cm from the suprasternal notch and not more than 7 cm above the inframammary crease on the breast meridian is marked. It is better to err on the

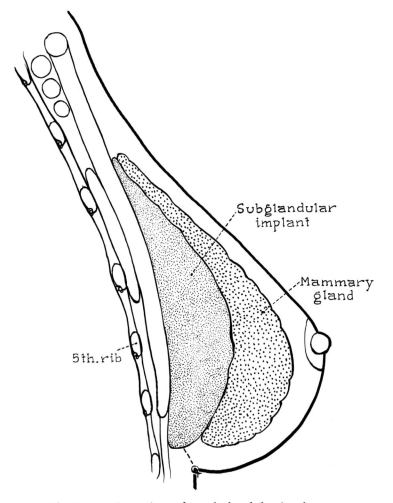

Fig 27-4.   Insertion of a subglandular implant.

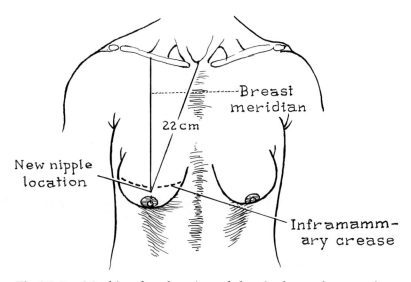

Fig 27-5.   Marking for elevation of the nipple-areolar complex.

355

low side for the new nipple-areolar position because the complex cannot be subsequently moved inferiorly without creating a noticeable scar above the areola. Conversely to raise the nipple-areolar complex further would require that the procedure to be described here be repeated, but the reoperation is straightforward and does not add unsightly scars.

Marking for Skin Excision and Insertion of the Implant (Figure 27-6)

After the patient is placed on the operating table in a supine position and general anesthesia is induced, the midline of the sternum is marked. The nipple-areolar complex then is marked while it is under minimal tension. Excessive stretching results in an areola that is smaller than desired at insetting. For the areolar circle a cookie cutter is centered about the nipple and pressed into the areola skin. The imprinted circle is outlined with brilliant green or a marking pen.

Next a vertical segment of tissue at the base of the breast and inferior to the nipple-areolar complex is pinched between the thumb and index finger to displace the nipple superiorly to its new location. This identifies the extent of the skin ellipse (labeled as the area of preliminary skin excision) to be resected in the vertical axis. The ellipse is drawn from the center of the inframammary crease and extended superiorly around the existing areola to the new location of the nipple. Sutures then are placed from one side of the proposed ellipse to the other. The sutures are tied to bring the breast tissue together over the oval area (labeled as area of preliminary skin excision). After the breast contour is evaluated, additional sutures can be placed if necessary. Based on the suture placement the final shape of the resultant vertical ellipse is marked and the sutures are removed. A conservative resection is planned initially because the ellipse can be enlarged later if necessary.

The upward transposition of the nipple and the final skin closure are facilitated by undermining of the skin and the subcutaneous tissues laterally, medially, and superiorly. The margin of the area to be undermined is marked with an inverted ∪ around the nipple-areolar complex and around the ellipse. The guidelines for pocket location described in Figure 27-4 can be used to mark the outline of the proposed subglandular pocket.

Correction of Moderate Ptosis
Incision for Placement of the Implant (Figure 27-7)

A 6-cm incision is made along the inframammary crease, and placement of the implant proceeds as described for Figure 27-4. The implant should be placed before excision of the vertical ellipse described in Figure 27-6.

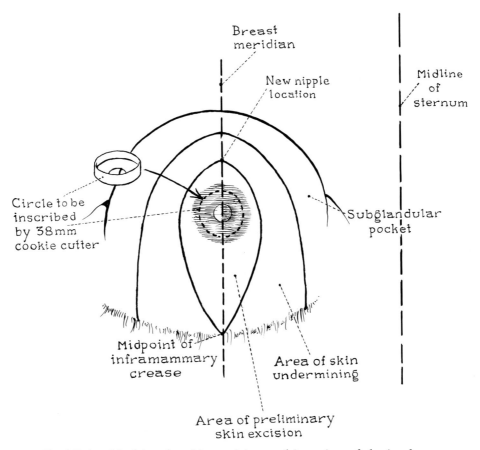

Fig 27-6.   Marking for skin excision and insertion of the implant.

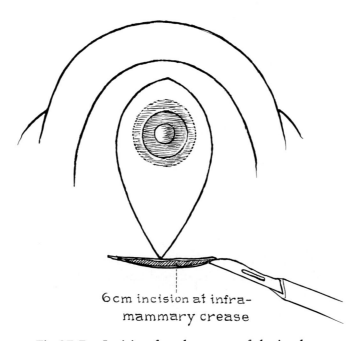

Fig 27-7.   Incision for placement of the implant.

Positioning of the Implant (Figure 27-8)

This sagittal section shows the appropriate location of an implant for correction of moderate ptosis. Because the positioned implant adheres to the surrounding tissues, it needs to be carefully placed to ensure that it is centered beneath the proposed location of the new nipple. When two implants (not shown here) are used one on top of the other to gain projection, it is best to place the smaller implant beneath the larger one so that the curvature of the larger implant will mask the contour of the smaller one beneath it.

Skin Excision from within the Ellipse (Figure 27-9)

Incisions are made in the marked imprint on the areola to separate it from the surrounding skin. The vertical ellipse of skin then is excised. The tissue medial and lateral to the excised vertical ellipse is undermined, as described in Figure 27-6. Now medial and lateral flaps exist. They are draped in sequence across the site of the excised vertical ellipse so that the surgeon can determine how much of the flap needs to be excised to provide a suitable cosmetic result. If the skin and the subcutaneous tissues appear excessively tight, they should be undermined further. When a satisfactory appearance is obtained with the patient in a semisitting position, the nipple-areolar complex is pushed superiorly beneath the skin to its new location and the final draping of the flap is completed. If the nipple-areolar complex appears tethered after it has been moved into its new location, tissue at the base of the breast near the inframammary crease is mobilized.

To perform the final draping and skin excision, a point is marked on each skin flap 7 cm inferior to the new location of the nipple. These two points will be sutured to the midpoint of the inframammary crease after the skin flaps are draped and after the excess skin is excised. The medial skin flap is pulled laterally and slightly inferiorly toward the midpoint of the inframammary crease, and the flap is anchored by suturing the 7 cm point to the midpoint of the inframammary crease (not shown here). Then a vertical line on the flap is marked for the line of skin excision, and the skin is resected. This procedure is repeated for the lateral skin flap, which is pulled medially and slightly inferiorly.

The flaps may be mobilized further as they are pulled toward the breast median by extending the incision along the inframammary crease. If skin excision alone is being performed without insertion of an implant, an inframammary incision still may be needed to eliminate standing cones as the flaps are pulled toward the center of the breast.

When bilateral mastopexies are performed, one breast at a time is corrected, contoured, and initially closed. Once satisfactory size, shape, and tension of the breast mound are established on one side, the other breast is corrected until a symmetrical appearance is obtained. The breast symmetry is assessed, and any needed adjustments are made while the patient is in a semisitting position, before the nipple-areolar complex is brought out and the final contouring and closure are performed.

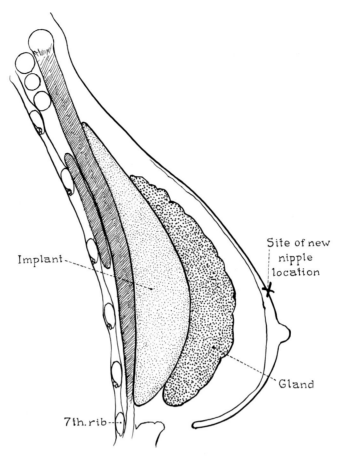

Fig 27-8. Positioning of the implant.

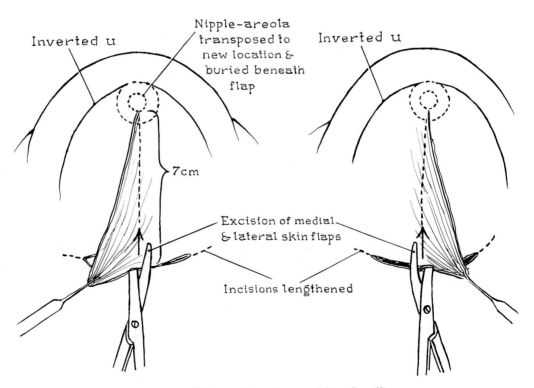

Fig 27-9. Skin excision from within the ellipse.

Wound Closure; Nipple-Areolar Marking (Figure 27-10)

The wound closure is started at the medial and the lateral ends of the inframammary incision. Skin staples are used initially to advance and to distribute evenly the edges of the skin flaps along the inframammary crease to allow excision of any excess skin at the midpoint. The skin staples then are removed, and a layer of interrupted absorbable sutures is placed between them. This is followed by a running subcuticular suture layer. A similar two-layer closure is used for the vertical incision.

With both incisions closed the nipple-areolar complex now is buried completely beneath the skin at its new location. The cookie cutter is used to mark a circle that is centered over the site of the new nipple-areolar complex. The distance between the proposed inferior areolar border and the inframammary crease is measured. When an implant has been placed, this distance should not exceed 5 cm with the nipple positioned at or slightly below the center of the implant. If no implant has been inserted, the distance from the proposed inferior border of the areolar to the inframammary crease should be approximately 4.5 cm. Placement of the nipple-areolar complex low on the breast mound at the time of surgery will result in a properly positioned complex once the wound has healed and the tissues have softened and stretched.

Insetting of the Nipple-Areolar Complex (Figure 27-11)

Before the nipple-areolar complex is inset, the symmetry of the marked circles is assessed. Then the skin inside the circle is deepithelialized, and the underlying fat and breast tissue are divided into four quadrants. The four small skin flaps can be folded under to support the nipple-areolar complex, as shown in the inset. If the skin flaps are bulky or if the additional support for the nipple-areolar complex is unnecessary, the flaps are excised and discarded.

The nipple-areolar complex then is brought into position through the incised tissue. The areola is anchored in position with four to eight interrupted sutures evenly distributed around the perimeter. If necessary, additional sutures can be placed between the original ones to align the complex correctly. The closure is completed with a running layer of fine chromic skin sutures around the perimeter of the areola.

Correction of Major Ptosis

Preoperative Marking (Figure 27-12)

Preoperative marking is done while the patient is in an upright position. The midline of the sternum, the inframammary crease (shown projected through the breast to its anteriorsurface), and the midpoint of the inframammary crease (defined as point *d*) are marked. To determine the new position of the nipple, (point *a*), the breast meridian, is marked from the midpoint of the clavicle through the nipple to the midpoint of the inframammary crease (not shown here). Then a point along the breast meridian between 18 and 22 cm from the suprasternal notch is marked. This point should place the new nipple location on the anterior breast skin approximately 2 cm below the anterior projection of the inframammary crease.

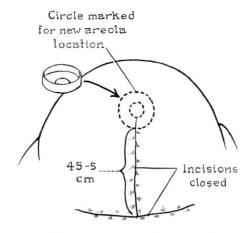

Fig 27-10.   Wound closure; nipple-areolar marking.

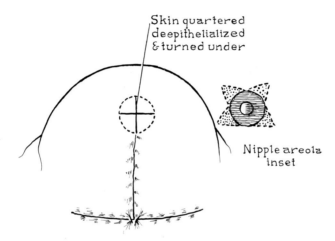

Fig 27-11.   Insetting of the nipple-areolar complex.

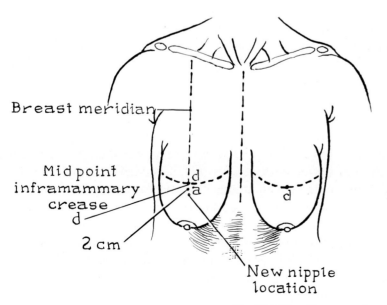

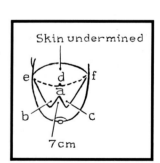

Fig 27-12.   Preoperative marking.

Oblique lines 7 cm long (labeled *ab* and *ac* on the inset drawing) then are drawn inferiorly from the site of the new nipple. These lines subsequently will establish the distance from the nipple to the inframammary crease. Points *b* and *c* later will be sutured to point *d*—the midpoint of the inframammary crease. These oblique lines are marked as two of the three sides of an equilateral triangle with its apex at the site of the new nipple. The angle between lines *ab* and *ac* will determine the tension of the final closure and influence the final breast shape. A wider angle produces a more conical breast, but it increases the skin tension at closure.

Oblique lines then are drawn superiorly, medially and laterally (labelled *cf* and *be*), from the inferior points *b* and *c* to complete the outline of the skin excision. The appropriate locations for points *e* and *f* can be judged by pinching the breast tissue above the nipple and noting where the standing cones of skin end medially and laterally. The apices of these cones are marked as the medial *f* and lateral *e* end points of the incision. Finally lines are drawn from the midpoint of the inframammary crease to points *e* and *f*.

After the area to be excised has been outlined, the superior and inferior lines are measured and compared. For example, the length of *cf* should be within 1 cm of the length of df to prevent a standing cone at closure. If *df* is too short, it should be curved until the lengths *df* and *cf* are within 1 cm of each other. If *cf* is too short, it can be curved laterally and lengthened. This process then is repeated for the lateral lines *be* and *ed*.

Areola Marking for Reduction; Scoring Key Points (Figure 27-13)

After the patient is placed in the supine position on the operating table and general anesthesia is induced, the nipple-areolar complex is marked for reduction of its diameter. A cookie cutter is centered over the nipple and pressed into the areola to make an imprint, and the imprinted circle is marked with brilliant green or a marking pen. The areola should not be under tension when the imprint is made.

The following key points are then scored with a needle or scalpel blade: the new nipple location *a*, points *b* and *c* (representing the inferior points of the 7-cm oblique lines), and point *d* (the midpoint of the inframammary crease). It is important to score these points because the ink may be erased or obliterated during the procedure and it may be impossible to reestablish the landmarks accurately once the patient is in a supine or a semisitting position.

Creation of the Implant Pocket (Figure 27-14)

An implant, which is almost always needed to correct major ptosis, is inserted before the skin excision. The implant is placed as illustrated in Figure 27-4 for correction of minor ptosis. A 6-cm transverse incision is centered around the midpoint *d* of the inframammary crease. The incision is deepened to the pectoralis major fascia, and an implant pocket is created by blunt and sharp dissection that extends superiorly to just below the clavicle, laterally to the midaxillary line, inferiorly to the inframammary crease, and medially to within 1 or 2 cm lateral to the midline of the sternum. When the pocket is completed, sizing implants are inserted to determine the appropriate size for proper projection and volume.

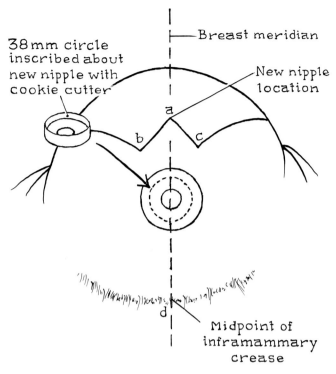

Fig 27-13.   Areolar marking for reduction; scoring key points.

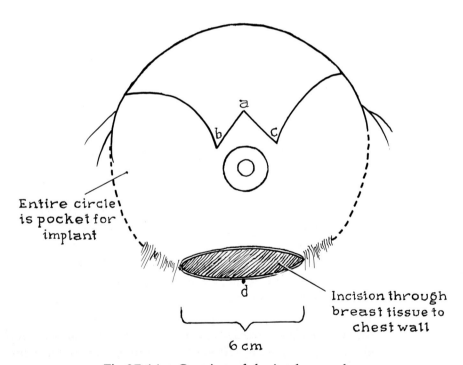

Fig 27-14.   Creation of the implant pocket.

With the sizing implant in position, points *b, c,* and *d* are sutured together to evaluate the tension of the skin flaps. This trial closure, before the excess skin has been resected and the skin flaps have been undermined, defines the amount of tension. It then can be determined if a smaller implant will be necessary to avoid excessive tension. Once the most appropriate implant is selected, the sizer is removed and hemostasis is achieved. The pocket then is irrigated with saline solution and with half-strength povidone-iodine solution. If a textured implant will be used, a 10-mm constant vacuum drain is inserted and brought out through the stab wound in a minimally visible area of the axilla. A permanent implant then is inserted, and the subcutaneous tissue flaps are reapproximated to cover it.

Resection of Excess Skin; Reduction of Areola (Figure 27-15)

The circular imprint marked on the areola is incised. The outlined incisions that indicate the limits of skin excision are scored. After these incisions have been made, the excess areola is resected and the skin within the excision boundary is removed at the junction between the dermis and the subcutaneous fat (area of skin to be excised is shown by stippling).

To facilitate nipple-areolar transposition and skin flap redraping, the skin is undermined between the subcutaneous tissue and the breast parenchyma in an area about 5 cm wide above the oblique lines *ab* and *ac* (as shown by parallel lines).

Draping of Flaps; Wound Closure (Figure 27-16)

After the skin around the excised area has been undermined, points *b* and *c* are sutured to point *d* and the breast mound is inspected. If excessive tension is present or if the tissues do not redrape smoothly, the sutures are removed and the skin is undermined further until it is adequately mobilized for uniform and tension-free draping of the flaps. After the ideal breast contour has been determined by trial closures and has been assessed with the patient in a semisitting position, the nipple-areolar complex is buried beneath the skin and the final draping is completed.

When bilateral mastopexy is performed, one breast at a time is corrected, contoured, and initially closed. Once the satisfactory size, shape, and tension of the breast mound are achieved, the other breast should be corrected until the two match. Before the nipple-areolar complex is brought out and the final contouring and closure are performed, breast symmetry is checked and adjustments are made while the patient is in a semisitting position.

Final closure begins by suturing points *b, c,* and *d* together with absorbable sutures. Closure of the transverse incision can be performed by starting at the medial *f* and lateral *e* incision end points and working toward the inframammary crease midpoint (*d*) or by starting at the midpoint of each incision (indicated by arrows on the illustration) and then by splitting the difference as the closure progresses toward the edges. This latter method should be used only if the superior and inferior arms of the excisions are equal in length. Skin staples are placed first to distribute the skin evenly along the incision. Then the staples are removed while a layer of interrupted absorbable sutures is added. Finally a layer of running subcuticular sutures is placed. As closure proceeds, the skin flaps are gently and evenly redraped as they are secured in position.

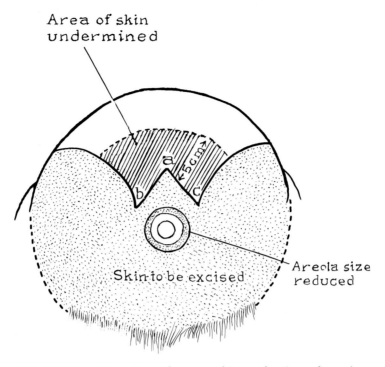

Fig 27-15. Resection of excess skin; reduction of areola.

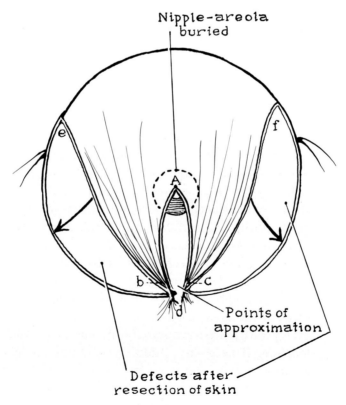

Fig 27-16. Draping of flaps; wound closure.

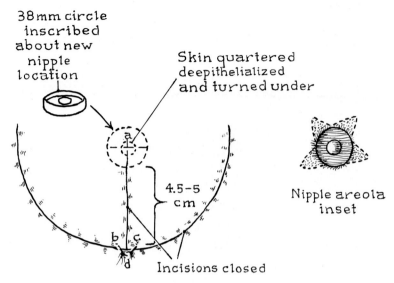

Fig 27-17. Insetting of the nipple-areolar complex.

Once the horizontal incision is closed, the mobility of the nipple-areolar complex is checked to confirm that it is sufficient to allow transposition of the complex to the new location. If the complex will appear distorted because of excessive tension, tissue at the base of the breast is mobilized. Adequately mobilized tissue is essential for the nipple-areolar complex to be inset without kinking or enfolding. The vertical incision between the new location of the nipple and the inframammary crease then is closed with two layers of absorbable sutures.

Insetting of the Nipple-Areolar Complex (Figure 27-17)

After the breast mound incisions have been closed, a cookie cutter is used to mark the new location of the nipple-areolar complex. The inferior border of the cookie cutter is placed approximately 4.5 to 5 cm above the inframammary crease, and the nipple should lie on or slightly below the center of the breast mound. When an implant has been inserted, the nipple should overlie its center. If bilateral mastopexy is being performed, the symmetry of the outlined circles is checked before the final insetting is begun. The tissue inside each circle is divided into four quadrants to form tissue flaps. The flaps are deepithelialized and are folded beneath the areola to add support if needed. If these flaps add too much bulk, they may be discarded.

The nipple-areolar complex that was buried earlier then is brought out through the divided circle and inset. Four to eight interrupted sutures are evenly distributed around the perimeter to anchor the areola in its new location. If necessary, additional sutures are placed between the original sutures to align the complex correctly. The closure is completed with a running fine chromic layer through the skin around the perimeter of the areola.

Postoperative Care

Following all mastopexy procedures a light dressing of bandages and tape is required for approximately 3 days. Occasionally a patient requires overnight hospitalization. After the bandage is removed, the patient can shower. Drains are removed when 24-hour accumulation is less than 50 ml per drain. The patient should wear a sports brassiere continuously for 3 weeks after surgery. Normal activities can be resumed in 2 or 3 weeks, but heavy lifting should be avoided for a minimum of 3 weeks.

28

Correction of Gynecomastia

Introduction

Gynecomastia accounts for more than 65% of male breast disease. Histopathologically it has a variable picture. In nonobese adolescents it is characterized by proliferation of mammary ducts and periductal tissues. In obese individuals it is the result of fat deposition. In men who have lost a large amount of weight, excess skin can mimic gynecomastia.

Physiologic pubertal gynecomastia is the transient growth of breast tissue, probably related to the normal development of the testes and a short-lived increase in plasma estrogen relative to plasma testosterone. In over 90% of young males the condition resolves within a year. When it does not resolve, a careful clinical and biochemical evaluation rarely reveals a pathologic cause, such as an estrogen-secreting tumor, a trophoblastic tumor, hyperthyroidism, or chronic liver disease. In adults, gynecomastia is associated with increasing age. The onset of breast enlargement in older adults correlates closely with the onset of testicular hypofunction and increased adiposity; the latter leads to enhanced peripheral aromatization of androgens to estrogens.

A number of conditions are associated with gynecomastia. Chronic renal failure, hypogonadism, and ingestion of alcohol or various drugs (most notably cimetidine) diminish androgen levels and can cause gynecomastia. A variety of pulmonary conditions, including tuberculosis, chronic obstructive pulmonary disease, cystic fibrosis, and hypertrophic pulmonary osteoarthropathy, have been associated with gynecomastia. Some tricyclic antidepressants, benzodiazepines, phenothiazines, and digitalis derivatives are associated with gynecomastia. Because gynecomastia without apparent endocrinopathy has been reported in several families, greater genetic predisposition may be a factor.

Medical treatment of gynecomastia has been uniformly unsuccessful. Operative treatment in the past consisted of direct excision of the breast tissue, usually through a periareolar or an inframammary incision. Unfortunately, the outcome of such procedures was often disappointing because they resulted in obvious contour deformities. With the advent of suction-assisted lipectomy (SAL), operative results have substantially improved and the procedure has become safe and efficacious.

Gynecomastia may currently be treated by direct surgical excision, surgical excision plus SAL, SAL alone, or skin excision plus nipple grafting. Generally a combination of direct excision and SAL is the most widely used approach to correcting gynecomastia.

Young, thin adolescents, who develop gynecomastia primarily because of glandular hypertrophy, are best treated by direct excision. Obese adolescents may have components of glandular hypertrophy and excess fat, so they are most effectively managed by a combination of direct excision and SAL. This combined procedure is appropriate for the majority of adults who have some glandular tissue beneath or adjacent to the areola and who also have a significant component of fat. Only obese adults may be candidates for SAL alone. For a few individuals who have lost large amounts of weight and are left with a redundant skin and some glandular excess, direct excision of breast tissue and skin with replacement of the nipples as free grafts is the treatment of choice. The various surgical techniques described here generally are applied after considering an individual's age, body morphology, and the type of deformity.

Indications

Gynecomastia does not involve functional impairment, but the cosmetic reasons for operation may be compelling. The condition can produce significant emotional problems for adult males, and the psychologic effect on young boys and teenage males may be even greater.

Contraindications

Because gynecomastia often resolves spontaneously in adolescent males, correction generally is contraindicated if the condition has been present for less than 2 years. Occasionally, however, the emotional factor of the condition may warrant earlier surgery. On medical grounds, surgery for gynecomastia is contraindicated in individuals with hemophilia or with severe cardiac or pulmonary disease that would make general anesthesia unsafe.

Complications

Early complications resulting from an operation for gynecomastia are hematomas and seromas. Strict attention to hemostasis and the insertion of constant vacuum drains reduce the risk of these complications. Nipple-areolar necrosis, skin necrosis, infection, and malpositioning of the graft may occur with skin excision and free nipple grafting.

Cosmetic complications associated with the correction of gynecomastia (excision and lipectomy procedures) are generally contour irregularities. The most frequent contour irregularities include palpable breast tissue edges on the chest wall, a depressed nipple-areolar complex, and a rippling or denting of the skin. In addition, if the skin lacks sufficient elasticity to contract, excess skin may be present when large amounts of gland and fat are removed. Hypertrophic scarring can occur following skin excision and free nipple grafting. In contrast, direct excision and SAL, through a periareolar incision, rarely produce a hypertrophic scar.

Preoperative Evaluation and Preparation

A history of childhood diseases, such as mumps (the most common cause of testicular failure in young adults), and any concurrent disease is sought, as well as a history of other medical problems, such as cirrhosis, alcoholism, or malignant disease. In all age groups a drug history and information about environmental exposure to chemicals are obtained to determine whether the patient has been exposed to endocrinologically active substances. On physical examination the presence, size, and consistency of the testicles, thyroid, and liver are noted. Breast abnormalities suggestive of malignancy should be confirmed histologically. Laboratory evaluation for gynecomastia may include liver and renal function studies. The determination of serum and urine concentrations of various sex steroids and their metabolites rarely is indicated. Correction of gynecomastia is performed on an outpatient basis with the patient under general anesthesia.

OPERATIVE PROCEDURE

Correction of Gynecomastia 1: Direct Surgical Excision

Preoperative Marking (Figure 28-1)

A periareolar incision site is marked along the lower halves of the areolae. The distinct, firm peripheral edge of the glandular tissue, which is to be directly excised, can be readily palpated. After marking, the patient is placed in the supine position, general anesthesia is induced, and the chest from neck to umbilicus is prepared and draped as a sterile field.

Periareolar Incision (Figure 28-2)

The periareolar incision is made at the junction of the pigmented areolar skin and the nonpigmented breast skin. Precise placement of the incision is important to obtain an optimal cosmetic result. After the periareolar incision is made, sharp and blunt dissection is used to free the nipple-areolar complex from the underlying glandular tissue. As the areola is mobilized, approximately 7 to 10 mm of breast tissue is left attached to its undersurface to provide padding and projection for the nipple-areolar complex. If this is not done, the areola will appear sunken postoperatively. If the nipple-areolar complex is too thick at closure, additional tissue can be readily excised from the deep surface to produce a proper contour.

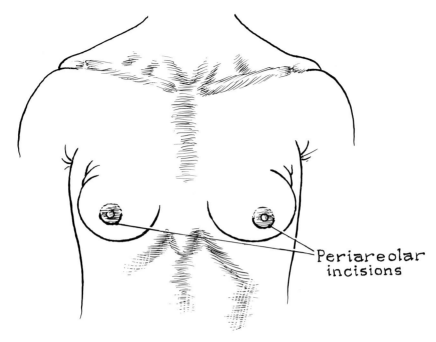

Fig 28-1.   Preoperative marking.

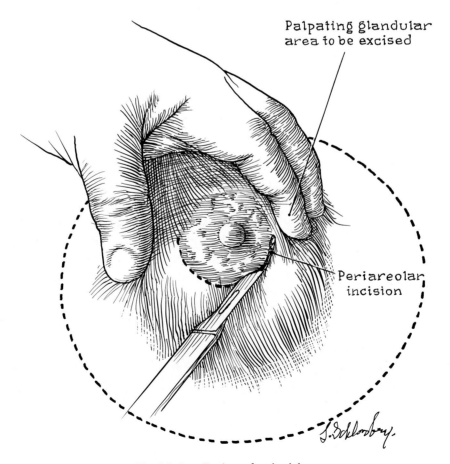

Fig 28-2.   Periareolar incision.

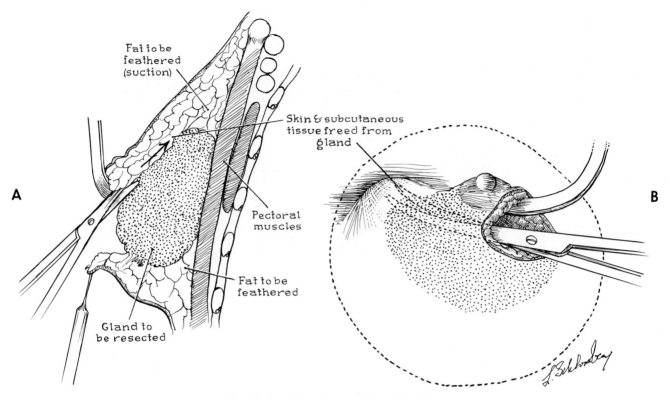

Fig 28-3. Elevation of the skin flap.

Elevation of the Skin Flap (Figure 28-3)

The breast is shown in sagittal section in Figure 28-3, *A*, and in the frontal view in figure 28-3, *B*, after the nipple-areolar complex has been elevated. The glandular tissue is shown by stippling. Detachment of the skin and subcutaneous fat from the underlying breast parenchyma is done most easily with facelift scissors, which are sharp enough to divide the glandular attachments but will not penetrate the skin. The scissors are placed in the subcutaneous space overlying the gland and then gently pushed forward, while the blades are slowly moved back and forth to divide any fibrous attachments. This is done multiple times to create several small tunnels that then are connected by division of any residual attachments. Detachment of the skin and subcutaneous tissue from the anterior surface of the gland is associated with bleeding, which necessitates hemostasis by electrocautery. Visualization for the dissection is aided by the use of a headlight or a lighted retractor.

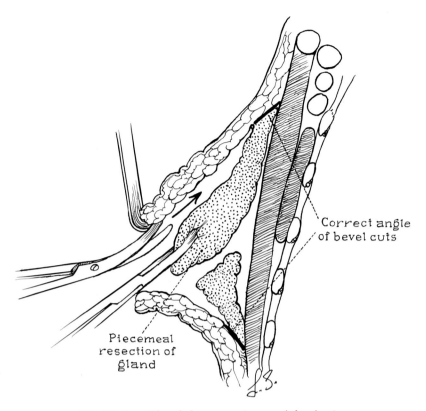

Correct angle
of bevel cuts

Piecemeal
resection of
gland

Fig 28-4. Glandular resection and feathering.

Glandular Resection and Feathering (Figure 28-4)

After the gland is freed from its overlying attachments to the subcutaneous tissue, the deep surface of the glandular tissue is separated sharply from the underlying pectoralis fascia. Occasionally the entire gland can be excised in one step. Usually, however, the parenchyma is divided (as shown here) and the dissection then is extended down to the pectoralis fascia to free the gland. The glandular tissue then is divided sharply and is removed segmentally.

After the glandular tissue is completely excised, the cavity is irrigated with saline solution, and hemostasis is obtained with electrocautery. Excision of the glandular tissue alone often leaves a palpable tissue edge. To attain a smooth contour this edge is feathered by direct excision and the tissue is beveled with scissors (indicated in the figure by the solid black lines). The excision must proceed carefully and gradually with only small pieces of tissue excised sequentially. Excess resection produces a depression that can be corrected only with further resection. This may ultimately result in an abnormally flat-appearing chest. During this part of the procedure the area of excision must be continually assessed visually and by palpation until an esthetic contour is achieved.

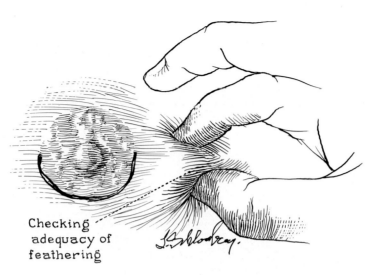

Checking adequacy of feathering

Fig 28-5. Wound closure.

Wound Closure (Figure 28-5)

After constant vacuum drains are inserted to prevent seroma development, the periareolar incision is closed with a single layer of interrupted or running subcuticular absorbable sutures. After closure the contour is checked by palpation to ensure that the chest has no uneven areas and that a smooth transition exists at the excision periphery. As tissue is moved back and forth between the thumb and index finger, irregularities that may need additional feathering can be palpated. If any irregularities are detected, the incision is reopened and additional fat is excised.

Correction of Gynecomastia 2: Direct Excision and Suction-Assisted Lipectomy

Preoperative Marking for Excision Plus Lipectomy (Figure 28-6)

Preoperative markings, consisting of an inner concentric circle that overlies the gland to be excised and an outer concentric circle that surrounds the area that will require feathering of fat, are made with the patient in an upright position.

As illustrated in Figure 28-6, *A,* the inner circle defines the distinct, firm peripheral edge of the glandular tissue as determined by palpation. The correct location of the outer circle is determined by palpating the thin underlying layer of adipose tissue. The area between the inner and outer concentric circles represents the fat surrounding the glandular tissue. Suction-assisted lipectomy is used to complete the resection within the area of the outer circle and to obtain a satisfactory contour following direct excision of the glandular tissue. The lateral extent of the concentric circles that mark the areas of planned tissue resection is illustrated in Figure 28-6, *B.*

After marking, the patient is placed in the supine position, general anesthesia is induced, and the chest from neck to umbilicus is prepared and draped as a sterile field.

374

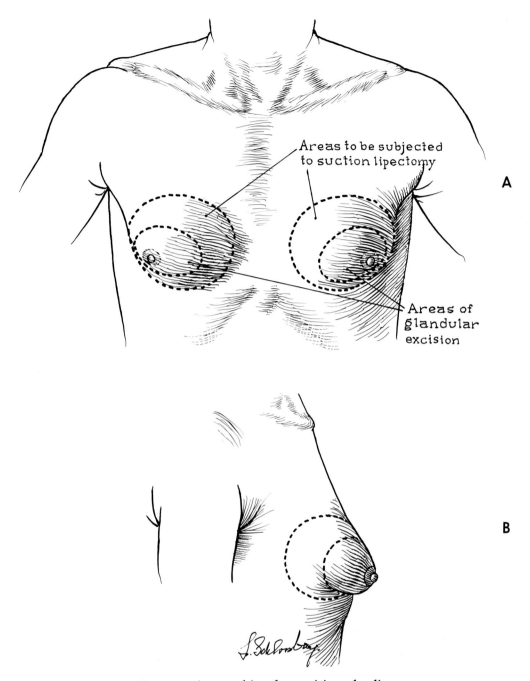

Fig 28-6. Preoperative marking for excision plus lipectomy.

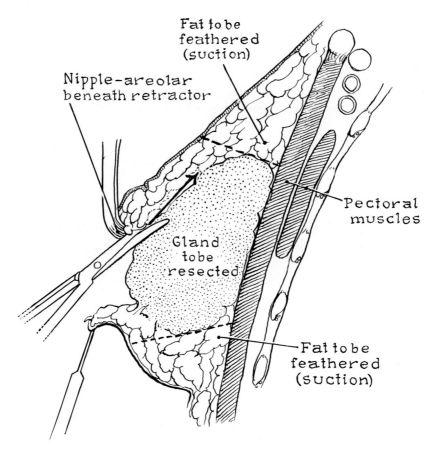

Fig 28-7. Elevation of the skin and subcutaneous tissue from the gland.

Elevation of the Skin and Subcutaneous Tissue from the Gland
(Figure 28-7)

A standard periareolar incision is made, and sharp dissection is used to free the nipple-areolar complex from the underlying glandular tissue (shown in the sagittal section). Approximately 7 to 10 mm of breast tissue is left beneath the areola to serve as padding and to prevent depression of the nipple-areolar complex postoperatively. After the areola is elevated, facelift scissors are inserted into the subcutaneous space and the blades are gently pushed back and forth to divide the attachments between the gland and the overlying skin and subcutaneous tissue.

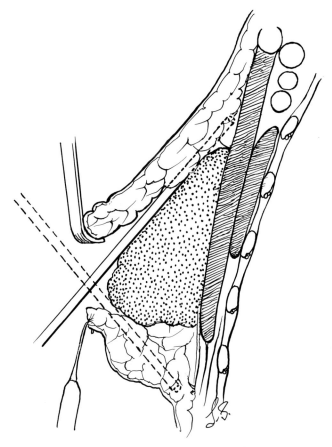

Fig 28-8. Resection of fat by suction-assisted lipectomy.

Resection of Fat by Suction-Assisted Lipectomy (Figure 28-8)

After the skin flaps are elevated, excellent exposure is obtained for advancing the lipectomy cannula in the area between the inner and outer concentric circles. The fat in this region is aspirated. Suction-assisted lipectomy produces less bleeding than sharp dissection of fatty tissue between the inner and outer concentric circles. However, caution must be taken to avoid overresection because prediction of the final contour can be extremely difficult at this stage. A lipectomy cannula, usually 4 to 6 mm in diameter, is initially used. The tissue is held between the thumb and the index finger, and the cannula is passed back and forth in multiple directions to aspirate the fat. As the resection proceeds, the smaller cannulas are used to avoid excessive resection of the fatty tissue and to feather the resection edges. After this is completed, the glandular tissue (indicated by stippling) is directly excised in a segmental manner as illustrated in Figure 28-4.

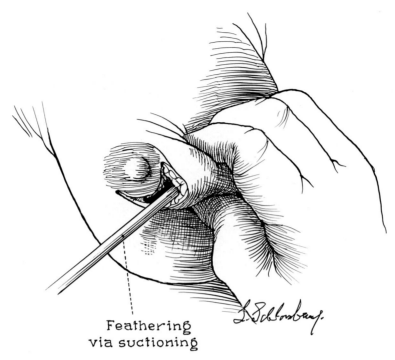

Feathering
via suctioning

Fig 28-9. Feathering the edges.

Feathering the Edges (Figure 28-9)

When the glandular resection is completed, the excision of the edges can be feathered by SAL. Any residual fat from the outer concentric circle and from the excision periphery is removed to produce a smooth contour. To refine the feathering and to avoid excessive resection, suction is performed with 2- to 4-mm cannulas.

Constant vacuum drains are inserted when the feathering has been completed. The wound is closed with a layer of interrupted or running subcuticular sutures. By palpation and visualization the contour is assessed after the incision is closed. In some patients an excess of skin may be evident. However, excision of additional skin should not be attempted at this time because most of the excess will eventually contract and adopt an acceptable contour. If necessary the skin can be excised several months later as a second-stage procedure. The incisions are dressed with nonadherent gauze and tape.

Direct Excision Combined with Suction-Assisted Lipectomy: Final Result (Figure 28-10)

The locations of the periareolar scars and the final frontal appearance of the chest achieved by the combined excision and lipectomy procedure are shown. The new breast contour, typical of a normal adult male, is more apparent in the lateral view.

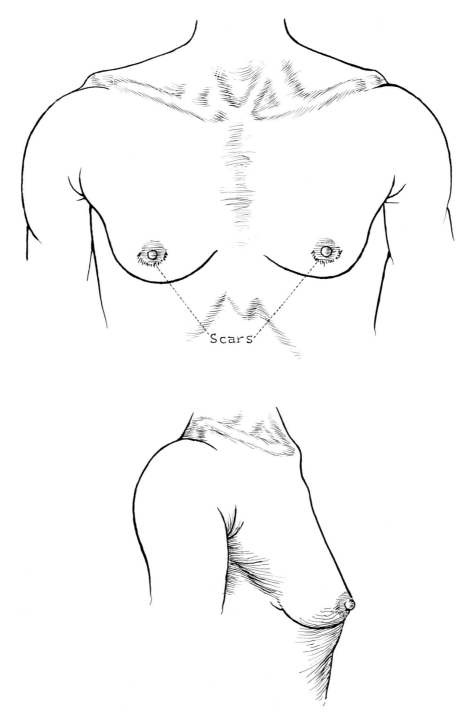

Fig 28-10.   Direct excision combined with suction-assisted lipectomy; final result.

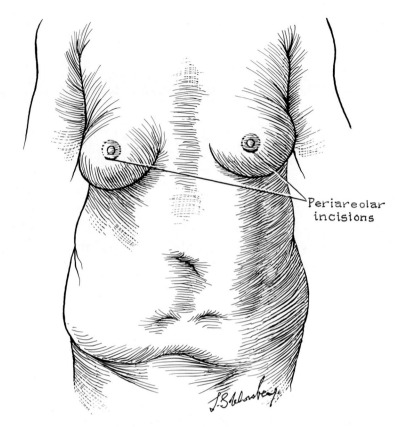

Fig 28-11. Placement of incision.

Correction of Gynecomastia 3: Suction-Assisted Lipectomy Alone
Placement of Incisions (Figure 28-11)

The patient depicted here with an obese body habitus and predominantly fatty breasts typifies the individual who would be a candidate for correction of gynecomastia by SAL alone.

This procedure is performed through a small incision, approximately 1 cm in length, along a premarked standard periareolar incision line. A 6-mm cannula is introduced, and SAL is performed by passage of the cannula in radial directions. The cannula paths are crisscrossed for gradual removal of the fat. The breast should be recontoured carefully, and the adequacy of resection should be assessed often by visualization and palpation. As the resection proceeds, progressively smaller cannulas are used to complete the lipectomy. Care should be taken to avoid rippling or denting contour irregularities. If a satisfactory contour is achieved with suction lipectomy alone, the wound can be closed with a layer of interrupted or running subcuticular absorbable sutures.

If SAL alone produces an unsatisfactory contour and some direct excision becomes necessary, the premarked periareolar incision is extended and the residual breast tissue is directly excised as illustrated in Figure 28-4.

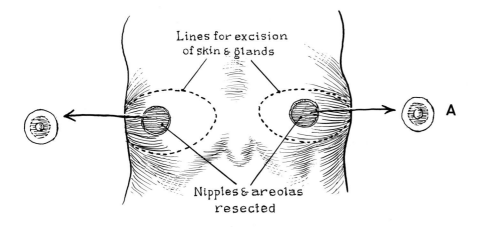

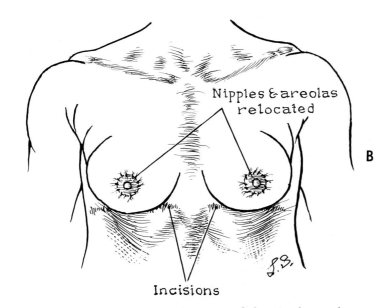

Fig 28-12. Harvesting and relocation of the nipple-areolar.

Correction of Gynecomastia 4: Skin Excision and Free Nipple Grafting

Harvesting and Relocation of the Nipple-Areolar (Figure 28-12)

The lenticular-shaped area of excess skin and gland to be excised (identified by visualization and palpation) should be marked as shown in Figure 28-12, *A*, while the patient is in a sitting or standing position. The patient then is placed in the supine position, with the arms abducted 90 degrees, and general anesthesia is induced. The chest is prepared and draped as a sterile field. A 3-cm circle that is centered around the nipple is inscribed on the areola. The 3-cm-diameter nipple-areolar complexes are incised circumferentially and are harvested as full-thickness skin grafts. The nipple-areolar complexes then are defatted to remove any underlying fat or muscle. The right and left grafts are marked to differentiate them and then are kept moist and cool until relocation.

Resection of the gland and the excess skin is begun by making the outlined incision *(dashed lines)*. The incisions are deepened to the level of the pectoralis fascia. At this level the glandular tissue and overlying skin are excised and the pectoralis fascia is left intact. After hemostasis is obtained, the wound is closed in layers with interrupted absorbable sutures in the dermis followed by a running intradermal absorbable suture. At this point the adequacy of tissue resection is assessed and any residual deformity is corrected by SAL performed through an opening in the incision. Insertion of a constant vacuum drain is optional.

As shown in Figure 28-12, *B,* the harvested nipple-areolar complexes are relocated above the closed incisions. The new nipple-areolar locations are chosen at approximately the level of the fourth or fifth rib. To determine the ideal location the border of the pectoralis major muscle is palpated when the patient is in an upright position. The nipple usually lies along the midclavicular line just above the rounded edge of the muscle's inferior margin. An equilateral triangle that connects the suprasternal notch and the new locations of the nipples is marked to ensure that symmetrical locations have been selected. After the positions of the nipple-areolar complexes are marked by drawing circles that are 3 cm in diameter, the inscribed circles are deepithelialized. The defatted grafts are inset into their new locations. Eight or twelve sutures are distributed equally around the areolar perimeter and are left long enough to be tied over a stent. The space beneath the graft is irrigated with saline solution. Then a running layer of fine chromic suture is placed around the areolar periphery to secure the nipple areolar complex in the new location. To immobilize the graft the long sutures are tied over a stent consisting of nonadherent gauze and moist cotton. All wounds then are dressed with absorbent gauze and tape.

Postoperative Care

After all of the described gynecomastia procedures that require direct excision of tissue are completed, constant vacuum drains are inserted and sterile dressings are left in place for 1 week. Physical activity, such as exercise and heavy lifting, should be restricted for 2 weeks. The patient also should be monitored for hematoma formation. After gynecomastia with SAL is corrected, significant swelling often is present for the first month postoperatively. The swelling gradually resolves within 4 to 5 months. Ecchymosis associated with SAL may last for 6 weeks.

Index